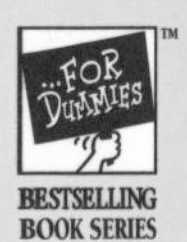


# Dieting For Dummies®, 2nd Edition

## Finding Your Healthy Weight Range

You can quickly estimate your healthy weight range with these simple formulas:

**Men** 106 pounds for 5 feet, plus 6 pounds per inch over 5 feet or minus 6 pounds per inch under 5 feet; plus and minus 10 percent.

**Women** 100 pounds for 5 feet, plus 5 pounds per inch over 5 feet or minus 5 pounds per inch under 5 feet; plus and minus 10 percent.

For example, a six-foot man would calculate his healthy weight range like this:

106 + (6 x 12) = 178

178 +/- 10% = 160 to 196 pounds

A woman who measures 5 feet and 5 inches, would calculate her healthy weight range like this:

100 plus (5 x 5) = 125

125 +/- 10% = 113 to 137 pounds

You'll be at the higher end of the range if you're large-framed or carry more muscle, and at the lower end of the range if you're small-framed with less muscle.

## The Health Risks of Being Overweight

If you're having trouble staying motivated to eat healthy and exercise, remember that you're making changes that will allow you to maintain or improve your health. You can improve the quality of your life by preventing the following weight-related health problems:

- Asthma
- Bladder control problems
- Depression
- Diabetes
- Gallbladder disease
- Gout
- Heart disease
- Hypertension (high blood pressure)
- Increased surgical risk
- Menstrual irregularities
- Osteoarthritis
- Pregnancy complications
- Respiratory problems
- Some forms of cancer
- Stroke

## Where Calories Come From

Protein, carbohydrate, and fat make up the calorie content of all foods. Although not considered a nutrient, alcohol also provides calories. Take a quick look at what various foods add up to calorie-wise:

- 1 gram of protein contains 4 calories.
- 1 gram of carbohydrate contains 4 calories.
- 1 gram of fat contains 9 calories.
- 1 gram of alcohol contains 7 calories.

The remaining nutrients — water, minerals, and vitamins — don't provide calories, nor does fiber or cholesterol.

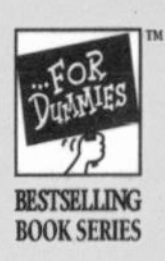


# Dieting For Dummies®, 2nd Edition

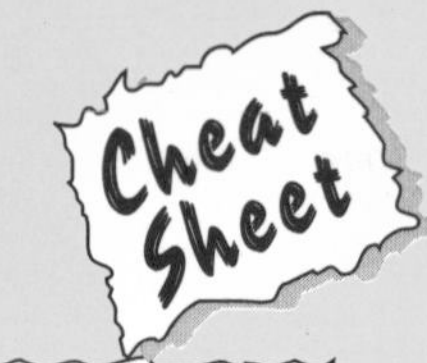


## Knowing How Many Calories You Need to Burn to Lose Weight

Because there are 3,500 calories in a pound and 7 days in a week, you must cut your daily calorie intake by 500 to lose 1 pound a week (3,500 ÷ 7 = 500).

To lose 1½ pounds, you need to cut 750 calories a day. A 2-pounds-a-week loss means eliminating 1,000 calories a day. A faster rate of weight loss is generally associated with weight regain and yo-yo dieting. Eating less is one way to cut calories, but if you add exercise, you don't have to restrict your intake so severely to lose the weight that you want to lose.

## Trimming Fat to Trim Calories

If you're looking to cut some of the fat (and therefore calories) out of your diet, follow some of these helpful hints:

- Use fats and oils sparingly.
- Eat plenty of grain products, vegetables, and fruits.
- Choose lean or extra-lean meats, fish, and poultry, and trim off any visible fat. For beef, look for the word *round* or *loin* in the name, which indicates that it's a lower-fat cut — such as sirloin, ground round, or top round.
- Use small amounts of lowfat salad dressing, whipped butter or margarine, and lowfat or fat-free mayonnaise.
- Use herbs, spices, lemon juice, and fat-free or lowfat salad dressings for seasoning.
- Consume few high-fat processed meats, such as sausage and cold cuts.
- Up your intake of beans, such as kidney, pinto, and Great Northern, and bean products. Not only are most of these foods nearly fat-free, but they're also a good source of protein and fiber.
- Choose fat-free or lowfat (1%) milk, fat-free or lowfat yogurt, and reduced-fat or lowfat cheeses.

## Ten Rules for Eating Well

Living and eating well involves more than just counting calories. Remember these ten easy guidelines:

- Eat a minimum of 3 servings of vegetables and 2 servings of fruit each day.
- Eat at least 3 servings of whole grains each day.
- Eat at least 4 servings of beans, lentils, or peas each week.
- Eat 3 meals and 2 to 3 small snacks a day.
- Eat breakfast.
- Limit soft drinks and drink plenty of water.
- Limit caffeine to two servings or less a day.
- Limit salty foods and the amount of saturated fat that you eat.




Item 4149-8.
For more information about Wiley Publishing, call 1-800-762-2974.

# Dieting FOR DUMMIES®

2ND EDITION

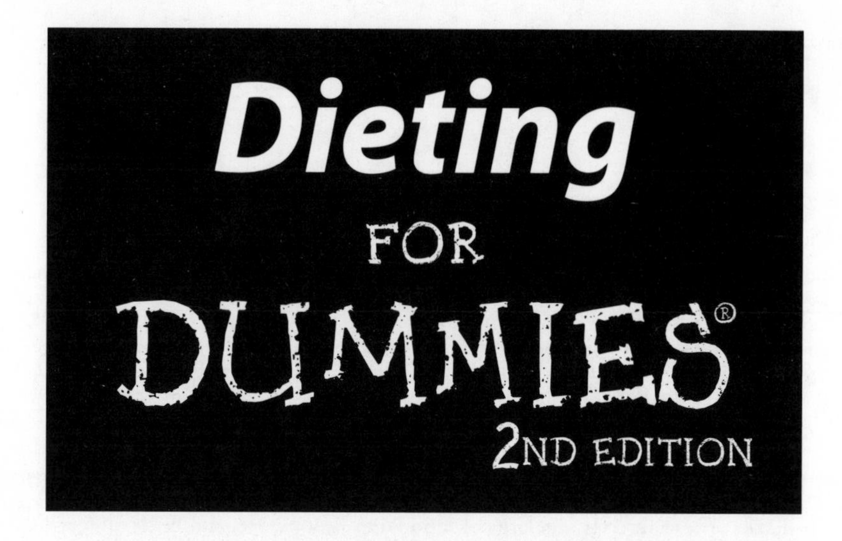


**by Jane Kirby, RD, for the American Dietetic Association**

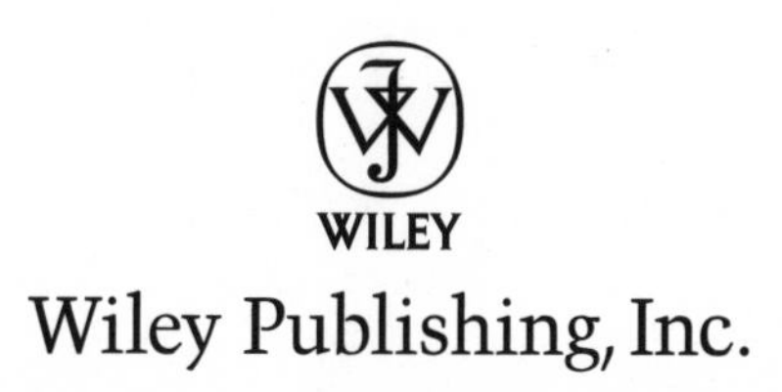


Wiley Publishing, Inc.

**Dieting For Dummies®, 2nd Edition**

Published by
**Wiley Publishing, Inc.**
111 River St.
Hoboken, NJ 07030
www.wiley.com



Library of Congress Control Number: 2003114568

ISBN: 0-7645-4149-8

Manufactured in the United States of America

10 9 8 7 6 5 4 3 2 1

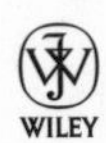

# About the Author

The American Dietetic Association is the largest group of food and health professionals in the world. As the advocate of the profession, the ADA serves the public by promoting optimal nutrition, health, and well-being.

Jane Kirby, a registered dietitian and member of the American Dietetic Association, is the food and nutrition editor of *Real Simple* magazine and owner of the Vermont Cooking School in Charlotte, Vermont. She is the former editor of *Eating Well* magazine and the food and nutrition editor for *Glamour.* She served on the dietetics staff of the Massachusetts General Hospital in Boston, where she completed graduate work in nutrition. She holds a Bachelor of Science degree from Marymount College.

Jane has written for numerous food and nutrition articles in magazines and on the Internet. She often shares her food and nutrition expertise on *The View, The Food Network,* and *The CBS Early Show* and appears regularly on *The Today Show.* Jane's work has been published in *The Journal of the American Dietetic Association* and *Nutrition Today.* She is the author of the first edition of *Dieting For Dummies, Eat More Weigh Less* (Rodale, 2000), *The 50 Best Salsas and Dips* (Broadway Books, 1998), and *Glamour's Guide to 30 Minute Meals and Effortless Entertaining* (Villard, 1987). She received the American Dietetic Association's 1994 Media Excellence Award.

Originally from the Boston area, Kirby now lives on her farm in Vermont with her son, husband, and 28 hens, one rooster, 30 sheep, one dog, and three cats.

# Dedication

To everyone who has ever wanted to weigh less.

# Author's Acknowledgments

Although the cover of *Dieting For Dummies,* 2nd Edition, bears my name as the primary author, no book goes to press without the assistance of many others. And so, I acknowledge them here for their help and contributions:

The publications staff at the American Dietetic Association for trusting me to be the voice of its nearly 70,000 members. Especially Laura Brown, my editor at ADA, whose enormous task it was to coax the copy from my computer, finesse and correct it, and then coordinate each deadline to get this manuscript to press on time.

Thanks also to Helen M. Seagle, MS, RD; Vicki I. Walker, MPH, RD; and Kathryn Brown, EdD, RD, who painstakingly reviewed the facts and opinions expressed in this book. Thanks also to Dr. Martin Graf, who reviewed the book's information about weight-loss drugs, bariatric surgery, and athletes.

A round of thanks for Acquisitions Editor Natasha Graf, Project Editor Allyson Grove, and Copy Editor Esmeralda St. Clair of Wiley Publishing, Inc., whose help shaped me from a serviceable magazine writer to a proficient book author. Like all good editors, their contributions were unmistakable during the writing process but are invisible now.

And plenty of credit is due to Mary Anne Kyburz-Ladue, RD, CDE, CD, my neighbor, friend, and researcher extraordinaire.

Thank you, too, to dearest Dad and beloved Mara and Liddy — fellow dieters all — for their applause and confidence. A thousand kisses for Jimmy, who taught me that healthy living is so much more than the miles walked and the meals eaten. And hugs to Jacob, who eats when he's hungry and stops when he's not, for teaching me to do the same.

## Publisher's Acknowledgments

We're proud of this book; please send us your comments through our Dummies online registration form located at www.dummies.com/register/.

Some of the people who helped bring this book to market include the following:

***Acquisitions, Editorial, and Media Development***

**Project Editor:** Allyson Grove *(Previous Edition: Pam Mourouzis)*

**Acquisitions Editor:** Natasha Graf

**Copy Editor:** Esmeralda St. Clair *(Previous Edition: Susan Diane Smith)*

**Assistant Editor:** Holly Gastineau-Grimes

**Technical Editors:** Kathryn Brown, EdD, RD, LD; Helen M. Seagle, MS, RD; Vicki I. Walker, MPH, RD; Martin Graf, MD (information about bariatric surgery, weight-loss medications, and weight loss for athletes only)

**Editorial Manager:** Michelle Hacker

**Editorial Assistant:** Elizabeth Rea

**Cover Photos:** © Lee Frost/Image State

**Cartoons:** Rich Tennant, www.the5thwave.com

***Production***

**Project Coordinator:** Erin Smith

**Layout and Graphics:** Andrea Dahl, Joyce Haughey, Michael Kruzil, Brent Savage, Shae Lynn Wilson

**Proofreaders:** Brian H. Walls, TECHBOOKS Production Services

**Indexer:** Lynzee Elze

---

**Publishing and Editorial for Consumer Dummies**

**Diane Graves Steele,** Vice President and Publisher, Consumer Dummies

**Joyce Pepple,** Acquisitions Director, Consumer Dummies

**Kristin A. Cocks,** Product Development Director, Consumer Dummies

**Michael Spring,** Vice President and Publisher, Travel

**Brice Gosnell,** Associate Publisher, Travel

**Kelly Regan,** Editorial Director, Travel

**Publishing for Technology Dummies**

**Andy Cummings,** Vice President and Publisher, Dummies Technology/General User

**Composition Services**

**Gerry Fahey,** Vice President of Production Services

**Debbie Stailey,** Director of Composition Services

# Contents at a Glance

# Table of Contents

# Part IV: Shopping, Cooking, and Dining Out ............... 149

## Chapter 13: Healthy Grocery Shopping ......................... 151



## Chapter 14: Outfitting and Using Your Kitchen ................. 161



## Chapter 15: Eating Healthfully While Eating Out ................ 169



# Part V: Enlisting Outside Help .................................... 185

## Chapter 16: Getting Help from a Weight-Loss Professional ....... 187

# Introduction

Does the world really need another book on dieting? More important, do you? Plenty of diet books make promises that this one doesn't. Lots tell you that losing weight and keeping it off is easy and effortless when you know their secrets. Well, we have a secret to tell you that the other books won't: Dieting gimmicks, such as banning pasta, don't work. And that's precisely why you need this book. It's not about fad plans or take-it-off-quick schemes. It's about balancing healthful eating and exercise for a lifetime.

Another so-called *secret* that the other books don't tell you is that when you know the facts about how the exercise you do and the foods you eat regulate your weight, you can drop pounds and keep them off without ever eating another grapefruit — unless you like grapefruit, of course. We believe that knowledge is power: the power to *choose* to lose. That's what this book is all about.

## You Can Trust Us

We know about losing weight, and this is what we bring to the table:

**The American Dietetic Association** is the largest organization of food and nutrition professionals in the world, with nearly 70,000 members. In other words, you can look to us for the most scientifically sound food and nutrition information available. Our members, with their extensive educational background, apply their knowledge of food, nutrition, culinary arts, physiology, biochemistry, anatomy, and psychology to help you translate nutrition recommendations into practical, clear, and straightforward advice.

We can't offer you a magic bullet to melt your extra pounds away, but we *can* provide a weight-loss and exercise plan that's realistic enough to last a lifetime. Since 1917, we have been serving the public through the promotion of optimal nutrition, health, and well-being by emphasizing a diet that includes variety, balance, moderation, and *taste*.

**Jane Kirby** is a registered dietitian and a member of the ADA. She is the food and nutrition editor of *Real Simple* magazine. She was the nutrition editor at *Glamour* magazine for 15 years and the editor-in-chief of *Eating Well* magazine. She's interviewed Doctors Ornish, Sears, Pritikin, and Atkins over the years. And she confesses to having been on all their diets — plus others. As Jane puts it:

> You name it; I've tried it. I went on my first diet when I was about 12 years old; I drank Metracal (the 1960s version of Slim-Fast). By the time I got to college, I had a borderline case of anorexia nervosa. I dieted down to 98 pounds. (I'm 5 foot and 5 inches.) I weighed as much as 160 pounds after my son was born (and that was *after* the birth). I've gained and lost about 250 pounds over my 50 years and spent about 30 years on the dieting treadmill. But I haven't dieted since my son was weaned 11 years ago. Today, I weigh 135. I know that I will never weigh 118 pounds (the weight that I always thought would make me smarter, prettier, richer, and happier). I don't starve myself, obsess about calories, or berate myself when 'I fall off the wagon.' But my cholesterol level is well under the 200 cutoff, and my HDL level (that's the good cholesterol) puts me at extremely low risk for heart disease. I don't eat everything I want to whenever I want it. (I do eat carefully.) I walk for at least one hour over the course of a day. I no longer believe that what I called my ideal weight is reasonable or attainable. Feeling great, and therefore looking great, is the goal. And it's comforting to read the new research that supports what my personal experience has taught me.

# About This Book

Our experience as food and nutrition professionals (and former dieters) shows us that the key to successful weight loss doesn't require magic, grit and determination, or the moral character of a saint. Weight loss success also doesn't require that you read this book cover to cover. Some chapters definitely do not apply to everyone. Just remember that the most important info is in the beginning. Part I can help you set reasonable goals and expectations. From there, though, feel free to skip around to chapters or topics that are of particular interest to you.

Some of the text topics may be familiar to you if you regularly read health magazines. The book aims to appeal to people whose nutrition knowledge ranges from shallow to deep. So if you're looking to dive headfirst into the subject, you won't be disappointed. And if you just want to get your feet wet, you can do that, too.

# What You're Not to Read

Don't feel obliged to read every paragraph. Technical information, marked with a Technical Stuff icon can enrich your understanding but it's not critical to your understanding or weight-loss success. The sidebars (boxes of text shaded in gray) function the same way — they're skippable. We hope you won't skip them, but know that the crux of the subject matter is in the running text.

# Foolish Assumptions

This book is written for anyone who has eaten too much and wants to lose weight. The information presented here is appropriate for someone wanting to lose 10 pounds or 100 pounds. In fact, we hope you'll use it as a guide to eating healthfully, and not only a way to lose weight. Because, when you discover how to eat the healthy way, you *will* lose weight.

# How This Book Is Organized

This book contains 28 chapters organized into 7 parts. The material is grouped so that you don't have to start at the beginning — although that's a nice place to start. If you'd rather, you can flip right to the chapter that contains the information you need. What follows is an explanation of what you can find in each part of the book.

## Part I: So You Wanna Lose Weight?

This part defines what a healthy weight is and how to find yours. It contains a comprehensive chapter on the health hazards of being overweight and a chapter about all the reasons that people get fat. (It's not only from eating too many cupcakes.) Then you can read about the fine points, such as the difference between being overfat and being overweight — there is a difference, and it's important to know what it is. And you can find information about how to tell whether your weight, and where you wear it, is a health risk for you.

## Part II: Getting Over Overeating

We live in a modern culture that promotes bigger = better. We're bombarded with advertising messages, sales promotions, and super-size options for every thing that we eat, drink, wear, and drive. It's not surprising that being hungry enters your mind when you're at the supermarket, a restaurant, or settling into the easy chair to watch a good movie. So, we eat, and we eat frequently, and we eat plenty when we do.

We can't blame food manufacturers and restaurant operators for our girth — well not entirely. Emotions and sales pitches have fueled our appetites. This part helps you determine why you eat the way that you do. Personal preferences, emotions, hormones, and culture all influence your eating style. When you understand what turns on your appetite, you're better prepared to get over overeating.

## Part III: Formulating a Plan for Healthful Eating

Getting to and staying at a reasonable weight without sacrificing the enjoyment of great-tasting foods is what this part is all about. Healthful living is putting all the food and nutrition advice you read and hear about into practice. You can find scientifically sound nutrition and weight-loss recommendations translated into practical and useful advice. You can also find out how important exercise is to losing weight and creating a healthy environment for your new body. In addition, you find out about calories — what they are and where they come from — as well as how to calculate how many calories your body needs for weight loss and maintenance.

## Part IV: Shopping, Cooking, and Dining Out

This is where the information about navigating the grocery store is located. Part IV also has affordable suggestions for stocking and outfitting your kitchen to make eating low calorie easier. And when you're planning to dine out, read the recommendations given in this part before you go.

## Part V: Enlisting Outside Help

When you can't go it alone, Part V has help for finding and working with health-care professionals you can trust. Now that surgery for weight loss is becoming more common — it seems some celebrities are peeling off pounds between commercials — you should know what's involved, so we include a chapter that runs down the basics of bariatric surgery.

Medications are also a big part of weight-loss treatment today, and because you need to be well informed before you take a weight-loss aid — be it prescription or a standard over-the-counter issue — you'll want to read the information. And there's a chapter that covers the most popular diets you may try (or have already tried) and runs down their good and bad points.

## Part VI: Special Circumstances

We could've called this part the other side of dieting because it's the anti-diet part. Some people shouldn't diet, at least not the way adults do. So this is where we include advice for feeding an overweight child, as well as spotting and seeking help for an eating disorder. Some athletes fall for crazy diet advice hoping for the magic to improve performance *and* lose weight — no, not all athletes are lean and mean — so this is where we put special advice for the runner, the cycler, and the competitive trainer.

## Part VII: The Part of Tens

As do all the *For Dummies* books, this one has a Part of Tens, too. You can find lists of dieting myths, easy ways to cut calories, and tips for healthy living. Plus, we include ten of the world's best low-calorie recipes that you can call your own.

## Appendix

In the five years since the publication of the first edition of this book, the Web has spun wider and deeper. The number of sites offering solid information and useful advice has soared higher than the numbers of chocolate chips in a box of cookies. We capture the best Web sites and list them here. You can also find listings for books and organizations that can help you in your search for more information about weight loss. All of them offer credible, useful, and trustworthy information.

# Icons Used in This Book

We include icons in the margins of this book to help you find the information that you're looking for more quickly. The following is a list of the icons and what they mean:

This icon points to a tip that can make the dieting process easier.

When you see this icon, you know that you're getting an important piece of information that's worth remembering.

This icon warns you of dieting myths and dangers. Be wary!

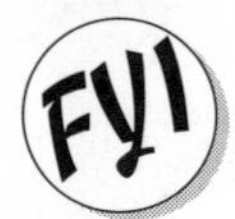


Because the dieting industry perpetuates many falsehoods, we use this icon to point out information that you can count on — and some fun facts, too.

When we get a little technical and talk about scientific research, we use this icon. You can skip this stuff if it seems too far over your head, but it's good to know.

This icon demystifies the diet lingo that you so often hear. Find out what these terms mean, and you'll sound like a pro in no time.

# Where to Go from Here

People come in a wide range of heights, weights, and girths. One is not better than another. But staying within *your* healthiest weight range can help you achieve optimal health and well-being. Join us in this book, starting at whatever point you like, and you'll see through the fog of fads and myths. Read on and find out how to stop dieting and start living healthfully.

# Part I
# So You Wanna Lose Weight?

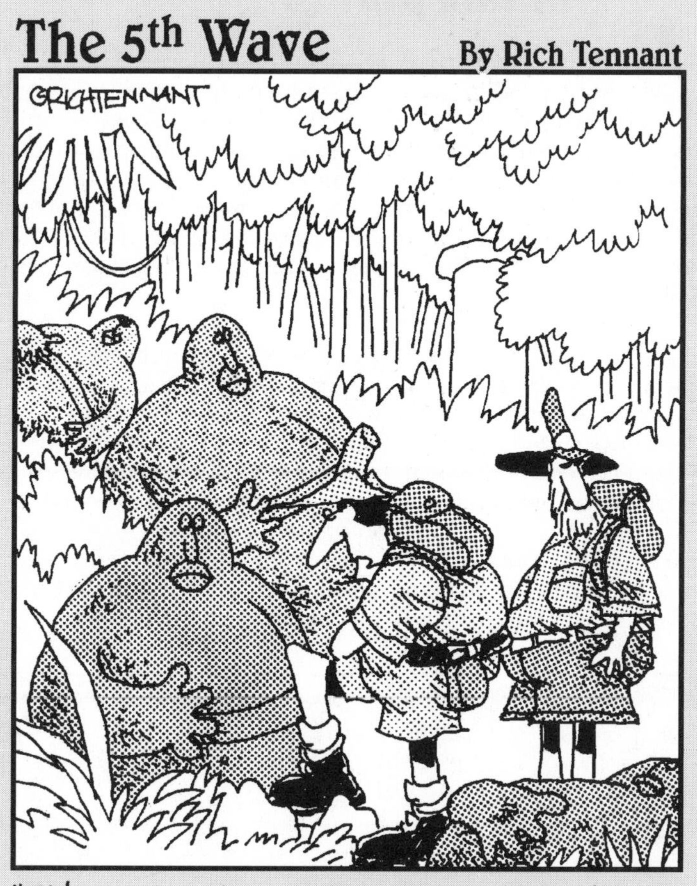


"It's a mystery why this ancient race of people died out so soon. They had an abundance of food available. The jungle here is filled with cookie bushes and the streams are full of bacon fish."

## In this part . . .

Before you even think about cutting calories, you need to understand how your weight affects your health. If you keep in mind that the point of losing weight is to make yourself feel better and improve your quality of life, then staying motivated is much easier. As your weight comes down, you'll find that you have more energy, more vitality, and more motivation. This part helps you see the weight–health connection and use it as a basis for your diet.

This part also helps you determine what weight range will bring you optimal health. You may be surprised to find out that you can enjoy terrific health at a weight that's higher than what you consider *ideal.* And if you feel at all discouraged about the amount of weight that you have to lose or you begin to lose hope in your ability to succeed this time, you'll find the last chapter in this part a source of encouragement. Genetics, past dieting history, current social situations, and your age may stack the deck against you, but we show you how to cut the deck in your favor.

# Chapter 1

# Getting Started

### In This Chapter

- Understanding how weight affects health
- Tailoring a diet to suit you
- Recognizing the particulars

The first edition of *Dieting For Dummies* was published in 1999, only five years ago. Since then, however, the number of people who need to lose weight has exploded faster than a tub of popcorn at the Cineplex. The science of weight loss has grown as well. We now have a better understanding of how our bodies store fat, how hunger is controlled, and why some people gain more easily than others. And we know more about applying the technical knowledge into practical how-to steps to help you lose weight and keep it off. That's what this book is all about. Translating the science of weight loss into an actionable weight-loss program that you can use.

## Weighing In on Your Health

The statistics from the Centers of Disease Control are startling: Sixty-four percent of adult Americans are overweight or obese. It's an historic high. That's why this book starts with an analysis of the health aspects of being overweight in Chapter 2. We didn't plan it that way to scare you. Although it's scary when you realize that death as a result of being obese is closing in fast on the death rates from smoking. We started the book with health, because we think it's the most important reason to lose weight. It takes the emphasis off short-term goals — the vacation to the beach, for example — that promote the use of fad diets and gimmicks.

And, while we're on the subject, we should mention that we hate the idea of "going on a diet," because it means, eventually, going off the diet. But more important, diets are about denial. Humans are programmed for pleasure. We are wired to enjoy plenty of flavors and textures. Denying any one of the sensory aspects of food means that you'll eventually go off the diet. See Chapter 6 for an explanation of your relationship with the foods that you eat.

The external messages and signals that bombard you are designed to make you eat, eat, eat. Unfortunately, those messages aren't about eating healthy foods. Portions are huge at restaurants; the ingredients and cooking methods that most affordable restaurants use and the items they serve all conspire against your health. Chapter 7 gives the details about what we've called the *Conspiracy to Consume.* Chapters 13 and 15 discuss in detail the ways you can spot the healthiest foods (in grocery stores and at restaurants) amid a tsunami of marketing terms, techniques, and tricks. And in Chapter 14, you'll find easy ways to turn the foods you love — that may not get the highest marks nutritionally speaking — into foods that can fit, easily and healthfully, into a lifelong eating plan.

## Getting motivated

Have you promised yourself that you'll get back to your senior-year weight before your 25th reunion? Or maybe you've vowed to lose weight before your wedding or your daughter's wedding. Everyone has set deadlines. And, unfortunately, most everyone has busted them. Losing weight to look better is one place to find your incentive. Many successful dieters get started with external motivators like appearance. Then as they progress on their weight-loss plan and start feeling healthier, their motivation internalizes.

Chapter 12 can help you internalize your motivation. When you start moving, not only will you start losing weight, but also you'll sleep better, be in a better mood, and have more energy than you've had in years.

## Finding support

And as you read through this book, you'll come across references to many studies that we've included to illustrate and support the ideas we're giving you. Most of them involve *successful losers* — people who lost weight and kept it off. We think that hearing their experiences can help you reach your goals, too. If we didn't think that the information in this book could help you to reach your goals, we wouldn't have written it. We may not have met face to face, but please know that we're rooting for you.

### Setting goals

To figure out where you're headed, you need to know where you are. Part I and especially Chapter 3 can help you to examine your current weight and help you determine your healthiest weight — you may not have as much to lose as you think.

And Chapter 4 can help you understand some of the reasons that you became overweight in the first place. We know that you'll find those reasons supportive, not punitive. And, we know that they can motivate you to reach your goal weight.

## Understanding Conflicting Advice

"Eat pasta." "Don't eat pasta." "Diets don't work." "*This* diet does work." "Wine is good." "Alcohol can kill you." For every health claim, a counterclaim comes right back at ya. We understand that you're bombarded with information about eating right. In fact, if you rely on news reports to decipher nutrition advice, it may appear that recommendations change as often as a traffic light. Remember that news is news because it flies in the face of convention.

Despite the headlines, no one food or food group is better — or worse — than another. (See Chapter 24 for an explanation of some of the most frequently circulated diet myths.) Folks today tend to remember the sound bite, not the big picture. This book gives you the big picture, because it's a summary of many studies, opinions, and recommendations and offers you the knowledge to understand the science. Specifically, Chapter 20 takes a critical look at the many diet plans that you often hear about on those news programs and lets you know which ones may help you and which ones are just bunk. Chapter 16 gives you details about getting guidance from a weight-loss professional — when to do so and who to trust, and Chapter 19 talks about the various weight-loss programs that you may consider trying and runs down the pros and cons of each.

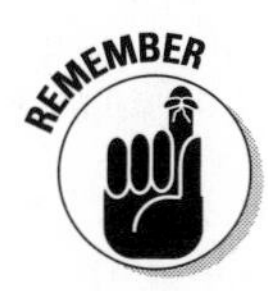


One of the objectives of this book is to decipher and review all sides of the eating-advice controversy when conflicting opinions arise. For example, many well-respected scientists from well-respected research universities have heavily criticized the venerable Food Guide Pyramid. We explain the issues in Chapter 9 and tell you how the conflicting advice may affect how you eat.

# Customizing Your Weight-Loss Plan

We promise you that this is the most personalized diet book you'll ever use, because it helps you write your own weight-loss plan. Chapter 10 has the specifics. The weight-loss plan that you find in these pages is based on changing the ration of calories stored and calories burned. Of course, to lose weight you must burn more calories than you take in. (See Chapter 8 for more information.)

Obviously, one way to do that is to eat fewer calories, and Chapter 25 gives you a quick list of the easiest ways to do that. However, we don't want you to live your life counting calories and grams of fat or minutes of exercise. Of course, keeping lists and tallying calories is a good place to start. But eventually, your weight-loss plan will evolve into a healthy lifestyle. Eating for pleasure may sound like a frightening proposition if you're a typical overweight American. But when weight loss is about eating the things that *you* like and making your health a priority instead of an afterthought, success is assured.

You may have forgotten how it feels to be satisfied after eating a meal rather than full or stuffed. In Chapter 5, we talk about hunger, how to turn it down, and how to get back in touch with its subtle signals. That's part of eating nutritiously, too. Our bodies are wired to send codes and signals before, during, and after eating to tell us when to eat and when to stop. It's all part of Mother Nature's insurance that we survive. It's a remarkable system, but it's a little antiquated when you figure that (luckily) famine is rare in our society.

## Being active

Eating is only half of a healthy weight-loss plan. We want to move you to move. So, we place a large emphasis on physical activity. Because we don't want to kid you into thinking that you can lose weight and keep it off without a little sweat, we show you how easy it is to incorporate exercise into your day without sucking yourself into a pair of spandex shorts or signing up for base-pounding Tae Bo classes — unless you like that kind of thing, of course.

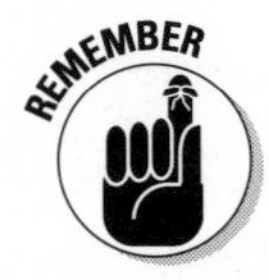


When an activity is fun, you're more likely to stick with it. The important thing is to find some form of exercise that you like to do.

Chapter 12 outlines an easy plan. Not only will it improve your self-esteem, it will help the weight come off easily. It's yet another part of Mother Nature's grand scheme: Exercise burns calories, but it also regulates your appetite and keeps hunger in check.

## Getting help for special circumstances

Simply cutting calories and adding physical activity isn't the whole weight-loss picture today. Some people need special help, because of their age, a unique medical problem, or because they're so active that the normal weight-loss advice doesn't apply.

For example, "wanting to lose a few pounds" may not accurately define your weight-loss goals, because you're one of the 30 percent of Americans who are obese. We give you details on drugs that have helped other obese people lose weight in Chapter 18. If you've tried diets and medication in the past and still haven't been able to keep your weight within healthy limits, surgery may be an option. Chapter 17 explains in detail the procedures available and everything you need to know, from cost to what to expect after the surgery, and how your eating plan will be changed.

Another group of overweight people who need carefully designed and prudent eating plans are children. Their nutrition requirements for growth and development can't be supported on the kind of weight-loss plan that an adult would follow. For them, that would mean too rapid a rate of weight loss. If you're the parent of a child who's overweight, turn to Chapter 22 for some advice. Likewise, athletes who are following a training schedule shouldn't cut calories dramatically or their performance suffers. Their diet prescription requires precision and balance. It's all outlined in Chapter 23.

And while we're talking about young people, tweens and teens are at high risk of taking dieting too far. We take a close look at anorexia and bulimia and other eating disorders in Chapter 21. If you suspect that you may have an eating disorder, or love someone who does, this chapter has many ideas and resources for support.

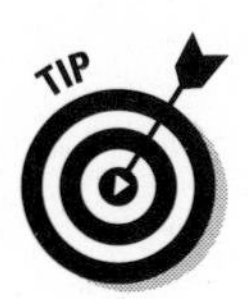


Above all, just remember to think of this book as a reference. It's not just a book about dieting; it's a manual for healthy living.

## Chapter 2

# Exploring the Connection between Weight and Health

### *In This Chapter*

- Running the great gamut of health risks
- Examining where you carry excess weight
- Making your health your first priority

If you've been trying to lose weight for much of your adult life, you're not alone. Excess weight is the number one nutrition problem. The statistics are alarming: Of the ten leading causes of death in the United States, being overweight is a risk factor for half; and the number of Americans who are overweight is increasing. It's estimated that 64 percent (or 130 million) American adults and about 15 percent of American children are overweight.

This chapter explains why being overweight is dangerous to your health and well-being. We hope that it puts your desire to lose weight in the proper perspective.

The medical community defines *overweight* as an excess amount of body weight, including fat, muscle, bone, and water. *Obesity* is defined as an excess amount of body fat. Athletes who have a large amount of muscle mass, such as professional football players, can be overweight without being obese. In reality, though, most people who are overweight are obese. That's why we, like most people, use these terms interchangeably in this book.

## The Health Risks of Being Overweight

Obesity isn't just a cosmetic problem; it's a health hazard. Being overweight puts excess stress on your body. Your lungs, heart, and skeleton need to work harder when you carry extra pounds of body fat. Try spending a few hours carrying around a 10-pound dumbbell. Tiring, isn't it?

Feeling okay now, you may be indifferent to health problems, but your extra weight strains all your body systems. The strain increases your risk for developing one or more of the following health problems:

- **Cancers:** Exactly why being overweight is associated with certain types of cancer is unclear, but statistics show a definite link. A postmenopausal woman doubles her risk for breast cancer if she gained as little as 20 pounds before menopause. Almost half of all breast cancer cases occur among obese women. The endometrial cancer risk among postmenopausal women also increases with weight gain, and being overweight increases the chances by one and a half times that a woman will die from her cancer. Although colon cancer isn't directly linked to obesity, where the weight is carried and the eating habits that lead to excess weight — high-fat, low-fiber diets — are.

  For more on the risks associated with where you wear your weight, see the section "Where You Carry Your Fat Matters," later in this chapter.

- **Diabetes:** Nearly 80 percent of people with type 2 diabetes are obese. This disease is particularly linked to weight gain after the age of 18. Even overweight children are getting the kind of diabetes that used to be associated only with overweight adults. (For more on the health risks for overweight children, see Chapter 22.)

  The medical evidence is clear: When you store excess weight around your middle, your risk of developing diabetes jumps. However, losing as little as 10 pounds can reduce your risk by 30 percent. And for those who already have type 2 diabetes, reducing body weight by as little as 5 percent can significantly improve blood glucose levels. Weight loss may also improve insulin sensitivity, which means that cells respond more efficiently to insulin. For some individuals, that means being freed from taking medication to control their disease.

- **Gallbladder disease:** The incidence of symptomatic gallstones soars as a person's body weight increases. A middle-aged woman who is more than 40 percent over her ideal body weight has a 33 percent greater chance of having gallstones than a lean woman of the same age.

- **Heart disease:** The American Heart Association classifies obesity as a major risk factor for heart disease. Nearly 70 percent of the diagnosed cases of heart disease is related to obesity. And it doesn't take much weight to put your health in danger. A weight gain of 20 pounds doubles your risk of heart disease. Fortunately, though, reducing your weight by only 5 to 10 percent increases your HDL levels (the kind of cholesterol that protects against heart disease) while reducing LDL and triglyceride levels, which are associated with increased risk when elevated.

- **Hypertension (high blood pressure):** Being obese more than doubles your chances of developing high blood pressure. Statistics show that approximately 70 percent of obese American men and women have high blood pressure. The good news is that you don't have to reach your ideal weight to get your blood pressure down. Many people see improvements within the first two to three weeks of a weight-loss program. Losing even 5 to 10 pounds can produce significant benefits and may even eliminate the need to take medication.
- **Respiratory problems:** Respiratory complications, such as sleep apnea, are linked to obesity. If you have *sleep apnea,* your breathing is halted briefly while you sleep, because your airways partially or totally collapse. In some extremely obese individuals, the condition is so severe that they fall asleep during the day — often while driving. Losing 10 to 15 percent of body weight can cure apnea.
- **Osteoarthritis:** Being overweight or obese increases your risk for getting this painful disease, causing the bone and cartilage in your joints to degenerate. One study reported that a weight gain of 9 to 13 pounds increased the pain in the knees of arthritis sufferers. On the flip side, losing the same amount decreases the odds of getting arthritis by 50 percent.
- **Psychological and social effects:** One of the most painful results of being overweight is the emotional suffering that it causes. Overweight people often face discrimination at work and in social settings. Many people assume that if you're overweight, you're gluttonous and lazy. Feelings of rejection, shame, or depression aren't uncommon. Also, American society equates thinness with attractiveness. The message, intended or not, makes overweight people feel unattractive.

But that's not all. Some of the other health hazards associated with being overweight and obese include

- Asthma
- Bladder control problems
- Depression
- Gout
- Increased risk of complications during surgery
- Menstrual irregularities
- Pregnancy complications
- Premature death
- Stroke

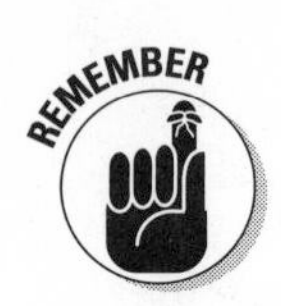


The benefits of trimming down aren't just cosmetic. Even a small reduction in your weight can improve many of the health problems associated with being overweight — not to mention boosting your self-esteem.

# Where You Carry Your Fat Matters

Your degree of risk for developing weight-related health problems depends not only on how overweight you are but also on where you store your excess fat. Body fat that accumulates around the stomach area poses a greater health risk than fat stored in the lower body. Typically prone to pot bellies, beer bellies, and apple shapes, men build up fat in the stomach area. Women are more prone to fat collecting around the hips, buttocks, and thighs, developing saddlebags or a pear shape. Figure 2-1 shows an example of each body type. People with apple shapes are more apt to develop diabetes, high blood pressure, heart disease, and certain types of cancer than are those who have pear shapes.

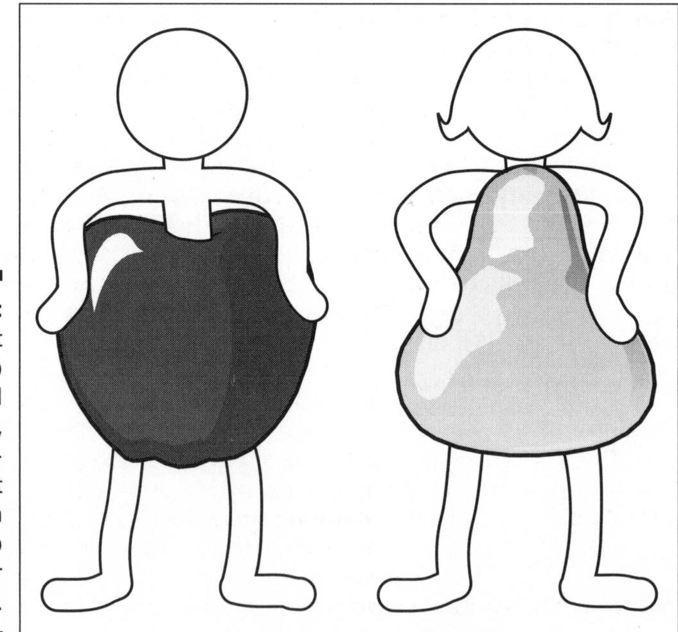

**Figure 2-1:** Overweight men tend to be shaped like apples, but overweight women tend to be pear shaped.

For the most part, becoming an apple or a pear when you gain weight is an inherited tendency. Women are naturally predisposed to store fat in their lower bodies for use as energy during pregnancy and breast-feeding. Yet, when women go through menopause, they tend to change from pears to apples. However, your gender and age may play only a partial role. Smoking and drinking too many alcoholic beverages seem to increase fat accumulation in the stomach area in both men and women.

# "You Look Mahvelous Dahling, Simply Maaahhhvelous!"

But, "It's not how you feeeel daaahhhling; it's how you look!" Sure, losing weight results in a slimmer and trimmer-looking you. But your motivation for losing weight should be your health, not only your appearance. When you feel good, you'll look good, too.

You'll be pleasantly surprised at how much better you feel — physically as well as mentally — after you lose weight. Walking up a flight of stairs or around the mall won't leave you breathless. Playing with your kids in the park will be a pleasure that won't exhaust you. You'll have more energy to do what you want to do, and you'll have fun doing it!

Maintaining a healthy weight is obviously important for good health. Going on a diet and off, and on, and off, and on is a pattern that often results from trying to lose weight for appearance's sake, not health. It comes from quick weight-loss gimmicks and fad diets where you drop a few pounds and then gain them back, plus a few more. If you repeatedly lose and gain, then changing your focus to maintaining a healthy weight may be the answer. Think long-term approach rather than fast results.

Long-term weight loss is a matter of attitude and conditioning. One of the reasons you bought this book is to find an answer to your weight problem. How many other diet books have you read? How many other books have you purchased? The diet book industry, which regularly has several books on best-seller lists, is built on the idea that diets are unsuccessful; otherwise, why would you need more than one book on the subject? Most diet books make promises that they can't deliver, because their concepts of dieting are based on the short-term. But successful weight losers and maintainers look at the long-term. This book encourages you to focus on weight-loss strategies that last rather than fads.

Consider the differences in Table 2-1.

**Table 2-1 Short-Term versus Long-Term Diets**

| ***Short-Term Diets*** | ***Long-Term Diets*** |
|---|---|
| Focus on the *don't* | Focus on the *do* |
| Swear off favorite foods | Concentrate on making healthier choices |
| Focus on denial | Focus on enjoying feeling better, healthier, and more energized |
| Describe eating plans with terms like *never, always, forever,* and *for the rest of your life* | Establish flexible, short-term, attain-able goals |
| Promise immediate results | Deliver success gradually |
| Allow no room for slips | Leave room for indulgences |
| Ban some foods altogether | Encourage variety |
| Emphasize food or foods as the cause of being overweight | Emphasize eating nutritiously and/or healthy exercise plans |
| Are extreme | Are gradual |

# Chapter 3

# Assessing Your Own Weight

### In This Chapter

- Calculating your healthy weight range
- Determining your weight-related risk factors
- Getting pinched all over to calculate body fat
- Figuring out what all the measurements mean

What exactly is a healthy weight? A healthy weight is a *range* that relates statistically to good health. Being overweight or obese is statistically related to weight-related health problems, such as heart disease and hypertension. (See Chapter 2.) Healthcare professionals use three key measurements to determine whether a person is at a healthy weight:

- **Body Mass Index (BMI):** A measure that correlates to how much fat is on your body.
- **Waist size:** A measure that helps to indicate whether the location of your body fat is a health hazard.
- **Risk factors for developing weight-related health problems:** For example, your cholesterol level, blood pressure, and family history.

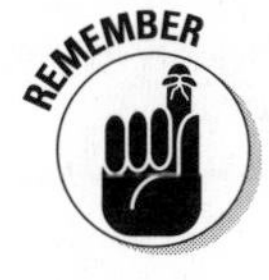


What *you* should weigh for optimal health may be quite different from what someone else should weigh, even if that someone is your same height, gender, and age. The information in this chapter can help you determine what weight is best for you — your *healthy weight,* not the lowest weight that you think you can reach.

## More Than Just a Number

When you step onto your bathroom scale, the number shows you how much your total body weighs. This total includes fat, muscle, bone, and water. Even though a healthy weight depends on more than the number on the scale, that number is a general starting point that you can use to assess your weight.

After you know your weight, you can compare it to the healthy weight ranges of the *quick estimate method* or use it to calculate your BMI. (See the "The Quick Estimate Method" section and the "Body Mass Index" section, both later in this chapter.) But what if your weight falls above these ranges? For most people, that's less healthy. The more that you weigh beyond and above the healthy weight range for your height, the greater your risk for weight-related health problems.

The information in this chapter is only for adults over 18 years old and should not be applied to children. For healthy weights for children, see Chapter 22.

## The Quick Estimate Method

To quickly estimate your healthy weight, you can use the following method. First, figure the median weight for your height by using the appropriate formula:

- **Men:** 106 pounds for 5 feet, plus 6 pounds per inch over 5 feet or minus 6 pounds per inch under 5 feet.
- **Women:** 100 pounds for 5 feet, plus 5 pounds per inch over 5 feet or minus 5 pounds per inch under 5 feet.

For example, if a man's height is 6 feet, then his median weight is 178 pounds [106 + (6 x 12) = 178]. If a woman measures 5 feet and 5 inches, then her median weight is 125 pounds [100 + (5 x 5) = 125].

After you find your particular median weight number, you can calculate your healthy weight range. First, subtract 10 percent from your median weight (for the lower number in your healthy weight range) and then add 10 percent to your median weight (to find the higher number in your range).

Okay. Go back to that 6-foot man. Ten percent of 178 pounds is 18 pounds, so 178 pounds minus 18 is 160 pounds, and 178 pounds plus 18 pounds is 196. So the healthy weight range for a 6-foot man is between 160 and 196 pounds. As for the woman who measures in at 5 feet and 5 inches, we'll spare you the math and just give you the answer: Her healthy weight range is 113 to 137 pounds.

## Body Mass Index

Now, you can use Body Mass Index (BMI) for determining whether you're at a healthy weight or overweight and therefore at a greater risk of developing weight-related health problems. BMI strongly correlates to the total fat on your body, and best of all, it's easy to determine and is applicable to all adults. (You can find BMI charts for children in Chapter 22.)

Follow these steps to calculate your BMI:

1. **Convert your weight from pounds to kilograms.**

   Your weight (in pounds) ÷ 2.2 = your weight (in kilograms). For example, 132 pounds ÷ 2.2 kilograms = 60 kilograms.

2. **Convert your height from inches to meters.**

   Your height (in inches) ÷ 39.37 = your height (in meters). For example, 65 inches ÷ 39.37 meters = 1.65 meters.

3. **Calculate your Body Mass Index.**

   Your weight (in kilograms) ÷ [your height (in meters) × your height (in meters)] = BMI. For example, 60 kilograms ÷ (1.65 meters × 1.65 meters) = 22.03.

BMI is usually calculated in kilograms and meters, but if you feel more comfortable using pounds and feet, this formula will work for you:

$$\frac{\text{your weight (in pounds)} \times 704.5}{\text{your height (in inches)} \times \text{your height (in inches)}} = \text{your BMI}$$

Table 3-1 enables you to determine your BMI without doing any math. Locate your height in inches in the left-hand column and follow the row across to your weight in pounds. Your BMI is at the top of the column at the intersection of your height and weight.

## No more growing fat gracefully with age

For many years, weight charts were the only standards against which people compared themselves. Insurance companies, the publishers of these charts, emphasized an ideal weight as opposed to a healthy weight and held to different height and weight recommendations depending on age — one set of recommendations for ages 19 to 34 and another for ages 35 and older.

Later, the 1995 edition of Dietary Guidelines for Americans printed revised weight tables. An improvement over the age-based tables, the new tables indicated that a person's healthy weight range was the same regardless of age. Experts realized that the 10 to 15 pounds that many people put on as they age, although common, aren't healthy.

**Table 3-1 BMI Chart**

| | *Normal* | | | | | | *Overweight* | | | | | *Obese* | | | | | | | | | | *Extreme Obesity* | | | | | | | | | | | | | | |
|---|---|---|---|---|---|---|---|---|---|---|---|---|---|---|---|---|---|---|---|---|---|---|---|---|---|---|---|---|---|---|---|---|---|---|---|---|
| ***BMI*** | ***19*** | ***20*** | ***21*** | ***22*** | ***23*** | ***24*** | ***25*** | ***26*** | ***27*** | ***28*** | ***29*** | ***30*** | ***31*** | ***32*** | ***33*** | ***34*** | ***35*** | ***36*** | ***37*** | ***38*** | ***39*** | ***40*** | ***41*** | ***42*** | ***43*** | ***44*** | ***45*** | ***46*** | ***47*** | ***48*** | ***49*** | ***50*** | ***51*** | ***52*** | ***53*** | ***54*** |
| ***Height (inches)*** | ***Body Weight (pounds)*** | | | | | | | | | | | | | | | | | | | | | | | | | | | | | | | | | | | |
| 58 | 91 | 96 | 100 | 105 | 110 | 115 | 119 | 124 | 129 | 134 | 138 | 143 | 148 | 153 | 158 | 162 | 167 | 172 | 177 | 181 | 186 | 191 | 196 | 201 | 205 | 210 | 215 | 220 | 224 | 229 | 234 | 239 | 244 | 248 | 253 | 258 |
| 59 | 94 | 99 | 104 | 109 | 114 | 119 | 124 | 128 | 133 | 138 | 143 | 148 | 153 | 158 | 163 | 168 | 173 | 178 | 183 | 188 | 193 | 198 | 203 | 208 | 212 | 217 | 222 | 227 | 232 | 237 | 242 | 247 | 252 | 257 | 262 | 267 |
| 60 | 97 | 102 | 107 | 112 | 118 | 123 | 128 | 133 | 138 | 143 | 148 | 153 | 158 | 136 | 168 | 174 | 179 | 184 | 189 | 194 | 199 | 204 | 209 | 215 | 220 | 225 | 230 | 235 | 240 | 245 | 250 | 255 | 261 | 266 | 271 | 276 |
| 61 | 100 | 106 | 111 | 116 | 122 | 127 | 132 | 137 | 143 | 148 | 153 | 158 | 164 | 169 | 174 | 180 | 185 | 190 | 195 | 201 | 206 | 211 | 217 | 222 | 227 | 232 | 238 | 243 | 248 | 254 | 259 | 264 | 269 | 275 | 280 | 285 |
| 62 | 104 | 109 | 115 | 120 | 126 | 131 | 136 | 142 | 147 | 153 | 158 | 164 | 169 | 175 | 180 | 186 | 191 | 196 | 202 | 207 | 213 | 218 | 224 | 229 | 235 | 240 | 246 | 251 | 256 | 262 | 267 | 273 | 278 | 284 | 289 | 295 |
| 63 | 107 | 113 | 118 | 124 | 130 | 135 | 141 | 146 | 152 | 158 | 163 | 169 | 175 | 180 | 186 | 191 | 197 | 203 | 208 | 214 | 220 | 225 | 231 | 237 | 242 | 248 | 254 | 259 | 265 | 270 | 278 | 282 | 287 | 293 | 299 | 304 |
| 64 | 110 | 116 | 122 | 128 | 134 | 140 | 145 | 151 | 157 | 163 | 169 | 174 | 180 | 186 | 192 | 197 | 204 | 209 | 215 | 221 | 227 | 232 | 238 | 244 | 250 | 256 | 262 | 267 | 273 | 279 | 285 | 291 | 296 | 302 | 308 | 314 |
| 65 | 114 | 120 | 126 | 132 | 138 | 144 | 150 | 156 | 162 | 168 | 174 | 180 | 186 | 192 | 198 | 204 | 210 | 216 | 222 | 228 | 234 | 240 | 246 | 252 | 258 | 264 | 270 | 276 | 282 | 288 | 294 | 300 | 306 | 312 | 318 | 324 |
| 66 | 118 | 124 | 130 | 136 | 142 | 148 | 155 | 161 | 167 | 173 | 179 | 186 | 192 | 198 | 204 | 210 | 216 | 223 | 229 | 235 | 241 | 247 | 253 | 260 | 266 | 272 | 278 | 284 | 291 | 297 | 303 | 309 | 315 | 322 | 328 | 334 |
| 67 | 121 | 127 | 134 | 140 | 146 | 153 | 159 | 166 | 172 | 178 | 185 | 191 | 198 | 204 | 211 | 217 | 223 | 230 | 236 | 242 | 249 | 255 | 261 | 268 | 274 | 280 | 287 | 293 | 299 | 306 | 312 | 319 | 325 | 331 | 338 | 344 |
| 68 | 125 | 131 | 138 | 144 | 151 | 158 | 164 | 171 | 177 | 184 | 190 | 197 | 203 | 210 | 216 | 223 | 230 | 236 | 243 | 249 | 256 | 262 | 269 | 276 | 282 | 289 | 295 | 302 | 308 | 315 | 322 | 328 | 335 | 341 | 348 | 354 |
| 69 | 128 | 135 | 142 | 149 | 155 | 162 | 169 | 176 | 182 | 189 | 196 | 203 | 209 | 216 | 223 | 230 | 236 | 243 | 250 | 257 | 263 | 270 | 277 | 284 | 291 | 297 | 304 | 311 | 318 | 324 | 331 | 338 | 345 | 351 | 358 | 365 |
| 70 | 132 | 139 | 146 | 153 | 160 | 167 | 174 | 181 | 188 | 195 | 202 | 209 | 216 | 222 | 229 | 236 | 243 | 250 | 257 | 264 | 271 | 278 | 285 | 292 | 299 | 306 | 313 | 320 | 327 | 334 | 341 | 348 | 355 | 362 | 369 | 376 |
| 71 | 136 | 143 | 150 | 157 | 165 | 172 | 179 | 186 | 193 | 200 | 208 | 215 | 222 | 229 | 236 | 243 | 250 | 257 | 265 | 272 | 279 | 286 | 293 | 301 | 308 | 315 | 322 | 329 | 338 | 343 | 351 | 358 | 365 | 372 | 379 | 386 |
| 72 | 140 | 147 | 154 | 162 | 169 | 177 | 184 | 191 | 199 | 206 | 213 | 221 | 228 | 235 | 242 | 250 | 258 | 265 | 272 | 279 | 287 | 294 | 302 | 309 | 316 | 324 | 331 | 338 | 346 | 353 | 361 | 368 | 375 | 383 | 390 | 397 |
| 73 | 144 | 151 | 159 | 166 | 174 | 182 | 189 | 197 | 204 | 212 | 219 | 227 | 235 | 242 | 250 | 257 | 265 | 272 | 280 | 288 | 295 | 302 | 310 | 318 | 325 | 333 | 340 | 348 | 355 | 363 | 371 | 378 | 386 | 393 | 401 | 408 |
| 74 | 148 | 155 | 163 | 171 | 179 | 186 | 194 | 202 | 210 | 218 | 225 | 233 | 241 | 249 | 256 | 264 | 272 | 280 | 287 | 295 | 303 | 311 | 319 | 326 | 334 | 342 | 350 | 358 | 365 | 373 | 381 | 389 | 396 | 404 | 412 | 420 |
| 75 | 152 | 160 | 168 | 176 | 184 | 192 | 200 | 208 | 216 | 224 | 232 | 240 | 248 | 256 | 264 | 272 | 279 | 287 | 295 | 303 | 311 | 319 | 327 | 335 | 343 | 351 | 359 | 367 | 375 | 383 | 391 | 399 | 407 | 415 | 423 | 431 |
| 76 | 156 | 164 | 172 | 180 | 189 | 197 | 205 | 213 | 221 | 230 | 238 | 246 | 254 | 263 | 271 | 279 | 287 | 295 | 304 | 312 | 320 | 328 | 336 | 344 | 353 | 361 | 369 | 377 | 385 | 394 | 402 | 410 | 418 | 426 | 435 | 443 |

After calculating your BMI, you can determine whether you're at a healthy weight:

- **Healthy weight:** BMI of 19 to 24.9
- **Overweight:** BMI of 25 to 29.9
- **Obese:** BMI of 30 and above

BMI gives a more accurate assessment of body fat than weight alone, but it can overestimate body fat in people who are really muscular, such as linebackers or weightlifters, and it can underestimate fat in people who have lost plenty of muscle weight, such as your 100-year-old granny. And even if you have a normal BMI, you may not be at a healthy weight for you. Therefore, you also need to measure your waistline.

## Waist circumference

Even if you've never stepped on a scale or measured your height, you can use your waist measurement as an indicator of your health status.

You can't use your waist size to get an absolute percentage of body fat, but it does provide information regarding the *location* of your body fat. And knowing where your fat is located, along with your BMI, enables you to determine whether you're overweight and therefore need to lose weight. As we explain in Chapter 2, fat that accumulates around your stomach area makes you more susceptible to a variety of health problems. People who accumulate fat around their waists (known as *apples*) are at greater risk for developing serious chronic illness than are people who collect fat on their hips and buttocks, known as *pears.*

Follow these steps to get your waist circumference:

1. **Relax your shoulders and stand naturally.**
2. **With a tape measure, measure your waist at the point below your rib cage but above your belly button.**

   Make sure the tape is snug but doesn't pinch your skin and is parallel to the floor.
3. **Breathe out.**
4. **Read the number.**

   If your BMI is 25 to 34.9 and your waist size is more than 40 inches if you're a man or more than 35 inches if you're a woman, you're at an increased risk of developing serious weight-related health problems. Even if your BMI falls into the healthy weight range of 19 to 25, you're at a greater health risk if your waist size is larger than your hips. Table 3-2 illustrates how waist circumference coupled with BMI increases your health risk for diabetes, high blood pressure, and heart disease.

**Table 3-2 Health Risk of High Waist Circumference**

| *BMI* | *Less Than 40 Inches Men/ Less Than 35 Inches Women* | *More Than 40 Inches Men/ More Than 35 Inches Women* |
|---|---|---|
| 25.0 – 29.9 | Increased | High |
| 30.0 – 34.9 | High | Very High |
| 35.0 – 39.9 | Very High | Very High |
| over 40.0 | Extremely High | Extremely High |

# Factoring In Your Personal Risk

You may decide to lose weight based solely on the size of your waist or by comparing your BMI to the BMI chart. But healthcare professionals use more than these measurements to analyze your weight. They also look at weight-related risk factors before determining whether the weight you're at is healthy.

The risk factors that healthcare professionals look for include:

- Age (older than 45 years old for males or 55 [or postmenopausal] for females)
- Arthritis in the knees or hips
- Family medical history of weight-related health problems
- Family history of early death (younger than 55 for males and 65 for females) from heart disease
- High blood pressure
- High blood cholesterol
- High blood sugar
- Respiratory problems
- Smoking

If you have any of the risk factors that I mention in the previous list, even if you're in the healthy weight range, many healthcare professionals may suggest that you lose 5 to 10 percent of your body weight to improve or lessen these risk factors. If you are overweight, getting to your healthy weight is all the more urgent.

Do not even think about losing weight if you're pregnant or breast-feeding or are less than 18 years old.

# Using the Latest High-Tech Methods

BMI and waist size allow you to quickly compare your weight to the healthy weight range for your height and judge your relative "fatness." But other, high-tech ways are available to determine how much fat you have, which is often referred to as your *percent body fat.* You may read about these methods in magazine articles and weight-loss books or see that health clubs, commercial weight-loss programs, or even local university research facilities are offering them. But you should know that they're not the methods of choice because of impracticality or impreciseness issues. So keep reading to take a closer look at these various methods and their limitations.

## Underwater weighing

Underwater weighing is the most accurate method for determining your percent body fat, but it's the least practical, because it's done with sophisticated equipment at university research facilities. This method is based on the premise that fat floats — think of how oil rises to the top in a bottle of salad dressing. Therefore, you can determine how much of your body is lean and how much is not if you submerge your body in a large tub of water.

To determine your percent body fat in this manner, you sit in a large tank or tub full of water in a special chair with a weight belt around your waist. (If you're thinking that this sounds more like a job for an escape artist cut from the same cloth as the great Houdini, try another method, because it gets worse — keep reading.) A trained technician then submerges you beneath the surface of the water as you force all the air out of your lungs. You must remain underwater for about 10 seconds so that the technician can record your weight. The technician repeats this procedure eight to ten times to determine an average. (See what we mean?)

To measure your body's volume, the technician computes the difference between your body's weight measured in air and its weight underwater. The technician then calculates your body density by dividing your body mass by the volume of the water that it displaces, minus any air left in your lungs. After computing density, the technician uses another formula to determine your percent body fat.

## Skin-fold thickness

You've probably reacted negatively to being pinched in the past. It's not a *nice* thing to do to someone. But put your preconceived notions away for now and open up that mind of yours, because measuring *skin-fold thickness* (the amount of fat just under the skin) is a simpler method for determining percent body fat. When an experienced practitioner does the measuring, it's an accurate calculation of total body fat.

However, this method can yield inaccurate results if a less-than-skilled individual takes the measurements or if performed on an older person or on someone who is severely overweight. Given that the results can vary greatly depending on the practitioner, you should view the results skeptically.

To find out your percent body fat using the skin-fold test, a person trained to take a skin-fold measurement, such as a doctor, dietitian, or health club staffer, measures your skin-fold thickness using skin-fold calipers at the upper arm, upper back, lower back, stomach, and upper thigh. The technician takes two sets of measurements and obtains an average at each site. Then he converts the millimeters that the calipers measure and places those numbers in a formula to arrive at the percent body fat of your entire body.

Now you know where the expression "pinch an inch" comes from. It may not be scientifically precise, but if you can pinch a 1-inch-thick (or more) fold of skin on the back of your upper arm, you're probably overfat.

## Bioelectrical impedance

Okay. So the name *bioelectrical impedance* may sound like so much razzmatazz, but this method is legit and relatively easy to undergo. So quit rolling your peepers and keep reading.

Bioelectrical impedance is another relatively simple method for determining percent body fat, but it can produce inaccurate results if a person is dehydrated, overhydrated, severely overweight, or older with little muscle mass.

Using bioelectrical impedance, a trained technician takes readings from a machine that delivers a harmless amount of electrical current through your body to estimate total body water, which reflects the amount of muscle or lean tissue you have. (Muscle contains water, and fat contains little water.) To determine the amount of body fat you have, the technician finds the difference between your body weight and your lean tissue.

# Putting It All Together

Look back at your BMI, your waist size, and your percent body fat (if you have access to this measurement). Compare your numbers to the numbers in Table 3-3. Which column do you fit into?

**Table 3-3 Healthy Weight or Overweight?**

| | | *Healthy Weight* | *Overweight* |
|---|---|---|---|
| BMI | | 19 to 24.9 | Over 25 |
| Percent body fat | Women | 15 to 25 | Over 25 |
| | Men | 10 to 20 | Over 20 |
| Waist size | Women | Varies | Over 35 inches (increased health risk when coupled with a BMI of over 25) |
| | Men | Varies | Over 40 inches (increased health risk when coupled with a BMI of over 25) |

You probably don't need to lose weight if your weight is within the healthy range, if you've gained less than 10 pounds since you reached your adult height, and if you're otherwise healthy. However, you *can* benefit from losing weight if you're overweight and you

- Carry excess body fat around your waist
- Have weight-related risk factors
- Have a family history of weight-related health problems

Your doctor may even suggest that you lose a few pounds even if you're within a healthy weight range because of the increased risk if you have health problems such as diabetes, high blood pressure, or arthritis.

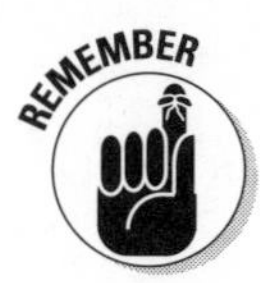


The bottom line: Achieving and maintaining a healthy weight reduces your health risks. It also makes you feel better, increases your energy level, and boosts your confidence.

## Assessing your weight based on percent body fat

If you ever have the opportunity to get your specific percent body fat measured by underwater weighing, skin-fold caliper, or bioelectrical impedance, use these estimated guidelines to assess your weight.

| | ***Percent Body Fat*** | |
|---|---|---|
| | ***Women*** | ***Men*** |
| Normal (optimal) | 15 to 25 percent | 10 to 20 percent |
| Overweight | 25.1 to 29.9 percent | 20.1 to 24.4 percent |
| Obese | Over 30 percent | Over 25 percent |

# Chapter 4

# Are You Destined to Be Overweight?

### *In This Chapter*

- Eat, drink, and be merry, for tomorrow . . .
- Determining your genetic predisposition
- Combating the factors that affect your weight

Eating too much and not exercising enough are the fundamental reasons people gain weight. But genetics, metabolism, and environmental factors explain how large your appetite is and how efficiently your body uses the food you eat. However, don't let the scientific studies and statistics in this chapter overwhelm you, such that you throw in the towel at the onset of your diet. It's true that some of the reasons that you gain weight are beyond your control, but that doesn't mean that you can resign yourself to life in the fat lane — slurping up soda pop and inhaling the chips while channel-surfing for your fave TV reruns.

This chapter helps you figure out your own genetic predisposition and helps you manage those factors you *can* control. You can take inspiration from the fact that many people who suffer with being overweight for most of their lives have been able to lose weight and keep it off.

## Evaluating Your Chances

Take this quiz to uncover your risk of gaining weight. Answer *yes* or *no* to the following statements and then read on to find out more about the factors that are especially relevant to you.

- Are you under 25 years old?
- Were you an overweight child or adolescent?
- Is one or both of your parents overweight?
- Do you sit or relax more often than you move around?
- Do you believe that eating fat-free or lowfat food means that you can eat more of it?
- Do you eat out often — especially at fast-food places?
- Have you quit smoking in the last year?
- Are you taking antidepressants or steroids?

If you're female:

- Did you start menstruating earlier than age 11?
- Have you never had a child?
- Do you have more than three children?
- If you have had a child, did you gain the bulk of your pregnancy weight in the first trimester?
- If you have had a child, did you gain more than 35 pounds during pregnancy?

A *yes* answer to any of these questions indicates that you may be at risk of weight gain. Keep reading to find out why.

## Your age affects your weight

If you're an average American and you're under 25, it's likely that you're going to gain weight over the course of your lifetime. And if you're female, you'll gain weight for a longer period of time than a male will.

A June 2002 study reported in *The Annals of Internal Medicine* confirmed earlier studies published in the *Archives of Internal Medicine* 150, 1990, that showed women gain an average of 16 pounds from age 25 to age 54, and then their weight starts to decline at about age 55. Men gain an average of 10 pounds starting at age 25 and stabilize at about age 45. They also begin to lose weight at about age 55. For both men and women, weight gain is highest in people aged 25 to 34 years.

### Early dieters are big gainers

In a 1994 *Glamour* magazine survey of overweight women who started dieting when they were young, half the women reported that their adult weights are unhealthfully high. The younger the woman was when she started dieting, the higher her current weight is now. The study also found that those who dieted as children weigh more than women who first started dieting as teenagers or adults. But even those who dieted later in childhood didn't escape — these women still described themselves at the high end of normal weight.

## Big children are often bigger adults

Children's health specialist William Dietz, Jr., MD, PhD, has determined that three critical periods may exist for the development of obesity: the prenatal period, childhood between the ages of 5 and 7, and adolescence.

- **The prenatal period:** Although more research is needed to fully understand the relationship between nutrition during gestation and birth weight to the onset of obesity later in life, several studies suggest a connection. For example, research shows that a greater prevalence of adult obesity exists in babies born to diabetic mothers who tend to gain an above-average amount of weight during pregnancy and have large babies. Another study suggests that babies who are undernourished during the first two trimesters *in utero* have an increased risk of obesity as they age.
- **Between ages 5 and 7:** In normal development during the first year of life, an infant's body weight — specifically the amount of fat *(adipose tissue)* — is higher in proportion to the baby's height. Gradually, the weight-to-height ratio declines. Then, between the ages of 5 and 7, children naturally increase their fat stores. Nutritionists call this stage *adiposity rebound.* Some longitudinal studies suggest that children whose adiposity rebound occurs earlier (before the age of 5½) are heavier and fatter adolescents and adults than children whose rebound is average (age 6 to 6½) or even later. The hypothesis is that children who rebound earlier grow fatter for a longer period of time.
- **Adolescence:** Other studies show that 80 percent of children who are obese during adolescence (ages 10 to 13) remain obese as adults. Girls have a greater risk than boys for getting and staying overweight; in fact, several studies show that 30 percent of all obese adult women were obese in early adolescence.

See Chapter 22 for more information about helping children grow into healthy, non-obese adults.

## Nature or nurture?

Studies show that 80 percent of children born to two obese parents become obese. Contrast that with the fact that only 14 percent of children born to normal-weight parents become obese. But studies on adopted children show that genetics account for only about 33 percent of a child's weight. Lifestyle factors, such as whether the family is active and their eating habits, are more important. Heredity controls only your metabolism — how quickly or slowly that you use calories.

## The set point theory

Although the exact mechanism isn't clear, many health experts believe that each person is born with a genetically predetermined weight range that the body strives to maintain. Human bodies used this system to protect them from starvation when access to food wasn't as easy as a trip to the drive-through or a dash to the corner mini-mart. *Set point* is the weight a body naturally and easily maintains and is generally within a healthy weight range for most people. Unfortunately, this level is generally higher than most people like, cosmetically speaking, and may explain why reaching a desired weight goal — especially those pesky 5 or 10 pounds — can be so difficult. Set points aren't set in stone; they may change from time to time, but then new set points tend to stay as fixed as the old one.

## If you don't move it, you won't lose it

A study conducted by the Centers for Disease Control found that 37 percent of obese people engage in no physical activity whatsoever. Whereas an athlete may burn up to 5,000 calories a day, a sedentary individual may begin to gain weight on as few as 1,800 calories. Regular exercise not only burns calories, but it also helps to build lean muscle, which in turn, burns more calories. (See the discussion of body fat in Chapter 3.)

Studies of children show that the more television they watch, the more they weigh. Experts credit this dubious honor to the fact that TV cuts down on physical movement, and the nonstop food cues that it delivers may prompt overeating.

## In your genes

Laboratories do plenty of research on mice genes. The research is promising and fast developing. For example, a gene called *ob* is responsible for the production of *leptin,* a hormonelike substance that helps the brain regulate appetite. Leptin, which is made in fat cells, travels to the brain, signaling to the brain that the cells have enough fat so that the appetite mechanism can be turned off. Another gene, known as *db,* also regulates leptin to reduce appetite, but it cranks up metabolism as well to control how fast or slowly calories are used.

Another family of genes called FOX has been found in mice that don't gain weight, regardless of how much they pig out. The PPARd gene that's activated in thin mice helps them burn calories faster than mice whose PPARd wasn't active. Scientists have found only *similar* genetic material in human DNA; unfortunately, they haven't yet found exactly the combination of genes or their structure that leads to obesity in humans — but they're working on it. Researchers suspect that the cells of obese people have diminished gene activity in much the same way that people with diabetes have reduced sensitivities to insulin.

Adult TV watchers suffer a similar fate. In fact, a 2002 study in the Journal of the American Medical Association of 50,000 women demonstrated that for every two hours in front of the TV each day, obesity increased 23 percent. Strangely, watching television is more fattening than other sedentary activities, such as reading, sewing, driving a car, or sitting at a desk. The flip side is encouraging. The antidote seems to be one hour of brisk walking, because that's all it takes to reduce your risk of obesity by 24 percent. Researchers recommend that you limit your TV watching to 10 hours a week. Americans watch about 30 hours a week.

## Faux food is a faux pas

Nutritionists call it the *Snack-Well syndrome* after the line of nonfat food products that people gobble up with abandon. It's believed that these kinds of products — which are fat free but still contain substantial numbers of calories — are at least in part responsible for the increasing numbers of calories that Americans are eating — and in turn, America's expanding waistline. People have discovered that fat-containing foods are fattening. But simply because a food has zero fat doesn't mean that it's a *free* food and that you can eat as much of it as you want. Yes, fat content is important, but when it comes to weight loss, total calories are even more important.

Some examples of how fat-free foods can be dangerous to a diet:

- A serving of Lite Cool Whip has the same number of calories as the regular kind: 25 per 2 tablespoons.
- A cup of nonfat vanilla yogurt has 223 calories, whereas the whole-milk version has a mere 24 calories more.
- Replacing a tablespoon of butter on a bagel with 2 tablespoons of jelly eliminates the fat but doesn't change the number of calories.
- A lowfat blueberry muffin has 131 calories but a regular blueberry muffin has only 7 more calories, 138.

## Fast food = fast fat

Eating out frequently, especially in fast-food restaurants, means that you're probably eating more fat and calories than you want or need.

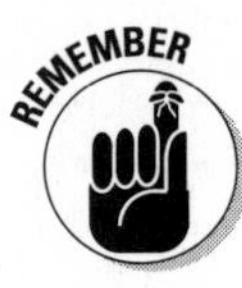


Fast food has several problems.

- **Although low-calorie choices are available, most people don't order them.** A typical fast-food meal averages 700 to 1,200 calories. Part of the blame rests on the fact that portion sizes are out of control. *Super-sizing* an order of fries or a soda may cost only a few cents more and seem like a bargain, but it comes at a big caloric price. A super-size order of fries has a whopping 540 calories and 26 grams of fat; in comparison, a small order has 210 calories and 10 grams of fat. A large 32-ounce cola has 310 calories, but a small cola has 150 calories.

  Everyone eats more when given more to eat. Barbara Rolls and her fellow researchers at Pennsylvania State University confirmed what most people know from experience. The study in the *American Journal of Clinical Nutrition,* published in December 2002, showed that when served large portions of macaroni and cheese for lunch, test subjects ate 30 percent more than when given small sizes. Thirty percent in this study translated to about 675 extra calories. Do that for five days in a row and you'll gain more than a pound!

- **Whether you eat in the restaurant or in your car, you're probably eating quickly — much too quickly.** One of the best ways to moderate how much you eat is to relax, eat slowly, and focus on your meal. People dining in restaurants at booths and benches that offer only about ten minutes of comfort — or worse yet, eat while driving — aren't focusing on enjoyable eating. They're wolfing down their meals, so they can head off on their next errand or rush back to work. It takes about 20 minutes for the body to register that it has received food; so often they're back at their desk long before they feel how much they ate.

Particularly when it comes to fast-food chains, people tend to eat in response to outside cues, such as advertising, bargain prices, convenience, and speed — rarely for health or pleasure.

- **Eating fast food more than twice a week increases your chances of becoming obese by 50 percent, because you eat fewer fresh fruits, vegetables, whole grains, and fiber.** That's what researcher Mark Pereira, PhD of the Harvard Medical School told attendees at the American Heart Association's 43rd annual meeting in March 2003. He examined the diets of almost 4,000 people for 15 years to draw his conclusions. It makes sense.

## Up in (stead of) smoke

You may gain up to 10 pounds when you quit smoking, but most people return to their normal weights at the end of a year. The gain, according to research conducted at Kaiser Permanente in California and published in the *Journal of the American Dietetic Association* (1996; 11:1150–1155), seems to be due to eating extra calories in the first month after you quit and peaks at about six months. Although it's not clear why quitting smoking leads to weight gain, it's likely that nicotine somehow increases metabolic rate and quitting smoking lowers it.

Canadian researchers from Université Laval in Quebec explain it another way in their 2002 study reported in the August edition of *Physiology and Behavior.* Nicotine, whether from smoking or a patch, lowers a body's set point. Remove the nicotine and a person will eat until the new, and unfortunately higher, set point is reached. See the section, "The set point theory" earlier in the chapter for more details.

A study published in the *American Journal of Public Health* (1996; Volume 86, Number 7) offers a solution. When researchers followed 9,000 women for two years, they found that smokers who quit and added one to two hours of vigorous physical activity each week averaged a 4-pound weight gain; former smokers who did not exercise averaged a gain of 8½ pounds. Even more beneficial was exercising two or more hours per week. Light smokers had an average gain of just 3 pounds, and heavy smokers gained 6 pounds. By comparison, light smokers who quit but did not change their activity level gained 5 pounds on average, and heavy smokers nearly 9½ pounds. Meanwhile, women who continued to smoke still gained, too: about one pound during the study.

## Drug-induced gains

If you find that you're gaining weight on a long-term medication that your doctor has prescribed for you, discuss the possibility of switching to a different brand. Medications have different side effects, even if they're in the same class or family, so your doctor may be able to find one that works better for you. The drugs listed in Table 4-1 are strongly associated with weight gain.

**Table 4-1 Drugs That Cause Weight Gain**

| *Type of Medication* | *Brand Names* | *Used to Treat* |
|---|---|---|
| MAO inhibitors | Marplan, Nardil, Parnate | Depression |
| SSRIs | Prozac, Zoloft, Paxil | Depression |
| Tricyclic antidepressants (amitriptyline, imipramine, desipramine, clomipramine, and so on) | Elavil, Tofranil, Norpramin, Anafranil, and others | Depression, urinary incontinence |
| Mirtazapine | Remeron | Depression |
| Lithium carbonate | Eskalith, Lithobid, Lithonate, Lithotabs | Mood disorders, seizures |
| Valproic acid | Depakene | Seizures |
| Carbamazepine | Carbatrol, Epitol, Tegretol, Tegretol XR | Seizures |
| Olanzapine | Zyprexa | Psychotic disorders |
| Clozapine | Clozaril | Schizophrenia |
| Corticosteroids | Prednisone, Vanceril, Flovent | Asthma |
| Sulfonylurea derivatives | Glucotrol, Orinase, Diabinese, Amaryl, Avandia, | Noninsulin dependent (type 2) diabetes |
| Antineoplastic agents | Tamoxifen | Breast cancer |

## For women only

If you're a woman, you gain weight more easily than a man for several inherent reasons.

### Early puberty

According to research performed by Stanley Garn and his associates and reported in the *American Journal of Clinical Nutrition* (1986; 43:879–883), the earlier a girl reaches *menarche* (her first period), the heavier she's apt to be as an adult. Research indicates that if you had your first period at age 11 or younger, by age 30 you'll weigh between 9 and 11 pounds more than a woman who started after age 14. The study also found that more than 26 percent of early maturers were obese by age 30, compared to only 15 percent of girls who started their periods later in life.

### Menopause

By the time women hit their 50s, two-thirds of them are overweight. That coincides with menopause, but research can't explain why. It may be the reduction in estrogen at midlife. The manufacturing of estrogen requires fat. As estrogen drops, fat stores may rise to cushion the fall. But women who've taken hormone replacement therapy (HRT) experience similar weight gain. The difference is where the weight goes on. Natural menopause turns women into apples with the bulk of their weight around their waists. Women on HRT stay pears (carrying their weight around their hips) longer.

### Pregnancy

Many women hold on to 5 pounds or more following pregnancy, which they often never lose. That's especially true if you gain more than 35 pounds. However, this disheartening piece of news *doesn't* mean that pregnant women should severely limit their weight gain during pregnancy. (The optimum maternal weight gain for a healthy 6½- to 8-pound baby is between 25 and 35 pounds.) Rather, pregnant women should try to control the *rate* at which they gain weight.

If you gain most of your pregnancy weight early on (during the first 20 weeks or about the first trimester) rather than during the last part of your pregnancy, you may have more trouble getting back to prepregnancy size. In the first trimester, the fetus needs little energy, so any large weight gain — in excess of 5 to 7 pounds — goes to the mother's fat stores, not to the infant. During the first three months of pregnancy, you can expect a weight gain of 2 to 4 pounds. After that, the gain should be about 1 pound per week. Recommendations are different if you begin your pregnancy at an unhealthy weight. For some obese women, the 1-pound-per-week rule is too much.

Many women lose about 10 pounds immediately following delivery and another 5 pounds in the first month or two. The rest of the weight usually continues to drop slowly over the next 6 to 12 months. How quickly you shed the weight depends upon several factors, including your calorie intake, your activity level, and whether you're breast-feeding. A strict weight-loss plan isn't recommended while you're nursing, because your body needs extra calories to produce milk. Losing 2 to 4 pounds a month won't affect your ability to nurse, but a loss of more than 4 or 5 pounds after the first month isn't recommended until you stop nursing.

# Beating the Odds

Does weight loss seem harder than you thought? Don't despair. More than a third of the people followed by The National Registry of Weight Control (NRWC) reported that they had been obese since childhood. The NRWC is a database of more than 4,000 individuals who have maintained a loss of at least 66 pounds for 5½ years. Seventy-three percent of these individuals had at least one overweight parent. Yet even though the obesity cards were stacked against them, they were able to lose weight and keep it off. Almost all of them said that to lose or maintain their weight, they changed *both* their eating habits *and* their activity habits.

Their words of weight wisdom:

- Choose meals that are lower in fat and calories and watch portion sizes.
- Keep track of what you eat and stay within your calorie limits.
- Discover how to recognize and manage the cues that tell you to eat even when you're not hungry.
- Get physically active and stick with it.

Losing weight and keeping it off isn't necessarily easy. But the benefits of living at a healthy weight are worth it. Not only do you lower your risk for many diseases, including diabetes, high blood pressure, high cholesterol levels, heart disease, stroke, some forms of cancer, and arthritis, but you feel better, too — both mentally and physically.

# Part II
# Getting Over Overeating

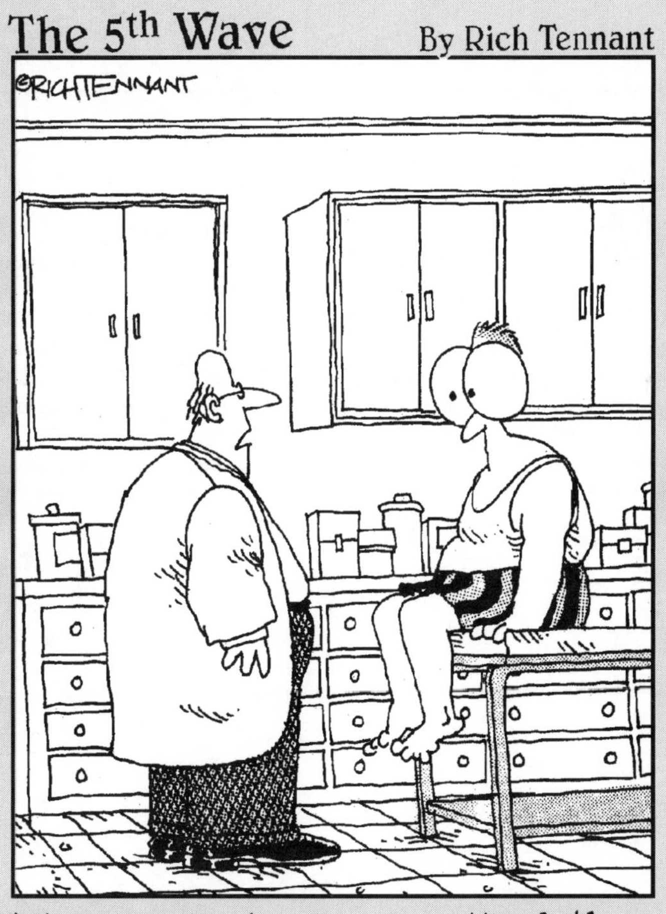


"I'm surprised no one's noticed this before, but your weight gain appears to be a result of your eyes simply being bigger than your stomach."

## In this part . . .

One of the most difficult weight management concerns is controlling all the reasons you eat that have nothing to do with being hungry. You may eat because you're anxious, depressed, stressed, or because you're celebrating. This part gives you tips for improving your relationship with the refrigerator, helping you to control your eating by identifying when you're really hungry and when you're not.

# Chapter 5

# Turning Down Your Hunger Alarm

### In This Chapter

- Understanding that it's all in your head
- Tuning in to your hunger signals
- Watching out for cravings versus hunger

How much you eat isn't a matter of willpower or lack of it. It's an inborn, powerful biological drive to assure human survival. Trying to override the system with diet and food restriction is counterproductive, because it triggers the body's chemicals to turn on your appetite and increase hunger. Every time you under eat or deny your body's need for food, you actually crank into high gear a complex system of chemical reactions that tells you to eat. A vicious cycle? You bet. This chapter discusses some ways to get back in touch with your natural hunger cues — not the external or emotional cues that sometimes call you to eat whether or not you're actually hungry.

## Recognizing How Hunger Works

You may think that your hunger alarm is all in your stomach and that dieting is all in your head. But the truth is that hunger is regulated by a complex system of chemicals that communicates with all the systems of the body. Signals are sent back and forth from your brain to your body. What starts hunger depends on whether the signals come from sensory or mechanical origins.

### The brain

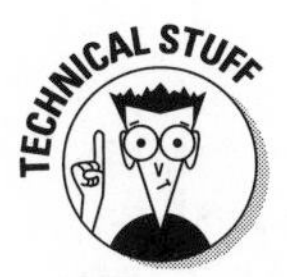


Scientists have identified that specific areas in the brain, primarily the hypothalamus, are in part responsible for processing eating behavior. The *hypothalamus* is one of the glands that controls the endocrine or hormone system in the body. The cells in the hypothalamus communicate with cells in other parts of the brain to coordinate the release and uptake of chemicals forming the feedback system that helps regulate how much and what you eat. What starts the chemical chain? Food can be the trigger that stimulates the brain to turn the desire to eat into the actual act of eating. How a food smells, what it looks like, how you remember it tasting — in short, its sensory appeal — excites chemicals within the brain.

The breakdown products of foods — amino acids from protein, fatty acids from fat, and glucose from carbohydrates — regulate hormones such as insulin, which affect the process at a cellular level. They send messages to the brain telling it that fuel is needed and that it's time to eat.

When the body needs nourishment, *neurotransmitters* (chemicals that transmit information to the neurons or brain cells) are released. Although more research is needed to explain the exact mechanisms, one neurotransmitter called *Neuropeptide Y* (NPY) is thought to relay "Eat" signals or "You can stop now" messages to various parts of the brain.

Scientists have recently identified two chemicals circulating in the blood that communicate with NPY:

- **Ghrelin:** From the Indo-European root meaning *growth, ghrelin* is the newest compound, and it's secreted in the lining of the stomach.
- **Leptin:** From the Greek word for *thin, leptin* is secreted by fat cells throughout the body. Not only do they "talk" to the brain's NPY, but they may also communicate directly with each other and cut out the middleman, the hypothalamus.

### Ghrelin and glucose

According to the theory, low levels of glycogen (carbohydrate in storage form in your body) and low blood sugar (glucose) levels stimulate a spike in ghrelin and NPY's activity in the hypothalamus. As NPY is stimulated, your desire for sweet and starchy foods goes up. And when ghrelin rises, so does appetite. While you sleep, your glycogen and blood sugar stores are used up, and they send a message to the brain to release NPY. It's no coincidence that the favorite morning foods are rich in carbohydrates — cereal, breads, bagels, and fruit. Skipping breakfast increases NPY levels so that by afternoon, you're set up for a carbohydrate binge. This craving for carbs is not the result of a lack of willpower; it's an innate biological urge at work. Stress and dieting are thought to trigger NPY production as well.

### The leptin link

Leptin works the opposite way. After eating, leptin levels increase and inhibit the firing of NPY, so you feel full. It follows then, that if it's been a while since you've eaten, say when you got up in the morning, your blood levels of glucose are low and therefore leptin is low, and ghrelin is high.

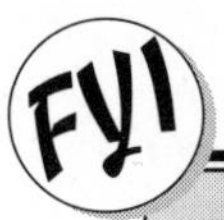

### Your stomach is talking

The role that ghrelin plays in appetite regulation was identified when obesity surgeons noticed that patients who had a type of gastric surgery that bypassed the stomach, lost their appetite. In contrast, patients who had another type of operation that reduced stomach size, but left the stomach intact continued to be plagued by hunger pains. Eventually, they were able to "stretch" their smaller stomachs to accommodate increasing amounts of food and eventually regained their lost weight. For more on weight-loss surgery, see Chapter 17.

This doesn't mean that you're at the mercy of your chemical make up — at least not entirely. The circulating levels of ghrelin, for example, peak at different times depending on when you have your heaviest meal. People who eat big lunches show ghrelin peaks at a different time than people whose main meal is at night.

### The galanin-fat connection

Another neurotransmitter called *galanin* is released when fat stores need filling up. Research on galanin indicates that galanin is responsible for the human appetite for fat as opposed to carbohydrates. How galanin works within individuals may help explain why some people store more fat than others do. In the evening, galanin levels tend to rise, which may be nature's way of making sure that people have enough calories to last them through the night without taking in more food.

Eating late at night has been associated with increased weight — not because the body processes calories differently after dark — but because hunger and fatigue late in the day can cause you to overeat. The type of foods most people like to eat at night is also a contributing factor. Just think about it: Do you crave celery sticks while watching your favorite prime-time TV shows? Reaching for high-fat and high-sugar foods is more likely.

## CCK: The appetite control chemical

Another way that appetite is regulated is by how much food the stomach holds. When you eat, food enters and fills your stomach and then travels to the intestinal tract. As the food is digested and the body's cells are fed, a chemical called *cholecystokinin* (CCK) is released. CCK sends signals to the brain to say "enough" by turning on feelings of fullness and turning off the appetite.

However, this chemical reaction doesn't work properly in some people. Researchers think that certain conditions, such as excessive dieting, *anorexia* (a form of self-starvation), and *bulimia* (a condition in which a person binges on huge amounts of food and then purges to get rid of what was overeaten) may affect many appetite-control body chemicals, including CCK. In bulimics, for example, researchers think that either the CCK mechanism doesn't work properly (so their brains never get the signal to stop eating) or the body's chemical systems become so desensitized that the person eats huge quantities of food quicker than the brain is able to signal satisfaction and fullness. The opposite effect may occur in anorexics — the CCK mechanism is so *over*sensitized that they feel full after only a few bites of food. When bulimics start eating normally, their CCK systems usually normalize. In a person with anorexia, the CCK hunger-satiety system also tends to normalize after he gains weight.

For more information about anorexia and bulimia, see Chapter 21.

Most people who have trouble with creeping weight gain eat because of appetite — not because they're hungry. What's the difference? Would you dig up a turnip and eat it dirty and raw? Or would you rather have a dish of double chocolate fudge brownie ice cream? Hunger would force you to do the former; appetite is at work in the latter. But both have their origins in the brain, and both affect a series of chemical and hormonal reactions, which ultimately results in the physical act of eating. The key is to get back in touch with your natural hunger signals so that you eat when you're hungry, not just because you have an appetite.

# Realizing How Dieting Makes You Hungry

Dieting experts and researchers Peter Herman and Janet Polivy have looked thoroughly at the biology and psychology of eating. (See *Current Concepts in Nutrition* 16, 1988.) They have found that people who have a long history of dieting lose their ability to recognize subtle hunger clues, having suppressed them for so long that they feel hunger only when they're drop-dead ravenous. And when they eat, they overeat because they're no longer able to recognize subtle feelings of fullness. Their "biological indifference," as it has been called, is so ingrained that chronic dieters eat or don't eat based only on outside influences such as time of day, thoughts, and beliefs . . . not on what their bodies are actually telling them.

On a biochemical level, excessive dieting may trigger the leptin-ghrelin mechanism discussed in the previous section and is nature's way of ensuring that you stay well fed. Remember, your body is programmed to survive and one way is to make sure you maintain weight. That's why humans have an infinite capacity to store fat. In times of famine, this came in handy, but today, it's a burden.

## Getting back in touch with your hunger

Arbitrary portion sizes and years of parental instruction to "clean your plate" have conditioned people to ignore their innate ability to tell when they've had enough to eat. Cleaning the plate right down to the china pattern, they finish the whole portion simply because it's there, not because they really need to. Re-learning to recognize and respect your hunger and satisfaction signals takes time. These techniques can help:

- **Eat slowly.** Your brain needs up to 20 minutes to get the message that your body has had enough to eat.
- **Don't wait until you're famished to eat.** Plan ahead. You're apt to overeat when you're absolutely flat-out starving. People who skip meals or eat skimpy meals often eat when they're ready to drop. Eating three meals and two or three small snacks is one way to make sure that you're never too hungry or too full. Remember, what counts is the total number of calories that you consume each day, not how often you eat.
- **Pay attention to how you feel, and eat mindfully.** You need to eat slowly to recognize the sometimes-vague signals that you've had enough to eat. The goal is to internalize those feelings. Until you can hear and heed the conversations that your brain and stomach are having, wear clothing with waistbands. Loose clothing may be more comfortable, but a waistband that's snug around your middle can serve as a reminder to stop eating when it feels tight.
- **Buy only single servings of foods that you crave, or you may find it difficult to stop eating even when you're full.** In the *Journal of Marketing* 60(3), 1996, marketing professor Brian Warsink, PhD, conducted research at the University of Pennsylvania that looked at the way people use different-size packages of cooking oil, spaghetti, M&M's, and other items. He found that many people use a product more freely when they aren't worried about running out, when price isn't important (larger packages are often cheaper than smaller ones), and when space is tight (larger packages take up plenty of room). So if ice cream in the freezer tempts you, don't buy it in gallons. Single-size servings, purchased one at a time, may be a wiser move.

  Similarly, at restaurants, think small. Super-sizing may seem like a value, but calorically speaking, it's a bad investment. In 2001, a new group of researchers at the University of Pennsylvania demonstrated what Dr. Warsink had in 1996: The larger the portion size, the larger the amount of food, and the greater number of calories that you eat. (For more on the push to eat, see Chapter 7.)

Full but not satisfied? That may be your body's way of telling you that the meal that you just ate wasn't well-balanced. Some researchers think that your body has a feedback system that tells your brain when it has enough carbohydrate, fat, and protein. When a meal is heavy in one nutrient and light in the others, you get little satisfaction from your meal.

Your body is sensitive to sensory fulfillment as well. Creamy textures and sweet flavors need to be balanced with crunchy and savory ones. That's one of the reasons that diets that eliminate an entire group of food are so frustrating: Besides being unbalanced nutritionally, they're unbalanced in flavor and texture. The Atkins diet (see Chapter 20) is an example of just such a diet.

### Why you eat more premenstrually

If you just can't say no to premenstrual cravings, you have a good reason: Your body doesn't want you to. A study at the University of British Columbia demonstrates what many women have suspected for some time: Women eat differently during the second half of their cycles — surprisingly, though, only if they've ovulated that month. Susan Barr, PhD, and her colleagues studied 42 women and compared their daily food intakes with their daily body temperatures. The women who had a rise in body temperature, signaling ovulation, had eaten more calories during the second half of their cycles. The women whose temperatures showed no change, and therefore had not ovulated, did not change their caloric intake. For the full report, see *The American Journal of Clinical Nutrition* 61(1), 1995.

When an egg is released but isn't fertilized, the body secretes progesterone to start the menstrual flow. If no egg is released, the surge in progesterone doesn't occur. Progesterone has a *thermogenic effect;* in other words, it makes heat. To produce the heat, energy — in the form of calories — is burned. The women did not know when *or if* they were ovulating, proving that women subconsciously and automatically eat more to make up for the calorie deficit. The average increase was about 260 calories, but some women ate up to 500 extra calories a day. Women on birth control pills don't ovulate, so they don't experience progesterone's fuel burn.

### What time is dinner?

Often, people eat not because they're hungry, but because it's time to eat — another way of ignoring your body's messages. Eating based on time rather than hunger is one of the problems with the three-meals-a-day tradition. Sure, it's practical, but consider that on the three-squares plan, a body is expected to run for 5 hours between breakfast and lunch, 6 to 7 hours between lunch and dinner, and then 11 to 12 hours until breakfast (figuring that your breakfast is at 7 a.m., lunch is at noon, and dinner is between 6 and 7 p.m.). If you're a breakfast skipper, you're hoping to go for about 16 hours without eating. But the human body needs to be fueled every 3 to 4 hours to prevent energy dips, metabolism slowdowns, crankiness, and cravings from interfering with life.

To help quell what may be legitimate hunger pangs, many people pick or graze on food throughout the day, not counting those mini-snacks as part of their food intake. A handful of popcorn here, a few pieces of candy there, half a piece of office birthday cake — you get the picture. The calories add up and keep people from being physically hungry, because they've been eating all morning. But that doesn't stop most folks from sitting down to eat a full lunch when the clock strikes noon.

This doesn't mean that you should starve yourself all morning if you're hungry. Going past the point of hunger to ravenous can set the perfect scenario for overeating — eating beyond the point when hunger is satisfied. Retrain yourself to recognize feelings of hunger and respect them. Eat when you feel them and stop when they stop. Don't eat when you're not hungry. This approach starts with eating breakfast, planning snacks, or eating only part of your lunch and saving the rest for a snack later on in the afternoon. Eat regular meals but don't eat by the clock.

If you've been skipping meals or eating too infrequently, adjusting and recognizing your hunger signals will take some time. When you recognize one, wait 10 to 15 minutes. If you still feel hunger, eat. If you don't, you may have mistaken a hunger signal for another sensation.

Some people are so conditioned that they miss the normal signals of hunger. The following signals are normal responses to hunger — not just appetite. You don't need to experience all of them to know it's time to eat. But feeling them can help you recognize how your body signals mealtime.

- Difficulty concentrating
- Feeling faint
- Headache
- Irritability
- Lightheadedness
- Mild gurgling or gnawing in the stomach
- Stomach "talking"

Feeling stressed? Ask yourself: Am I biologically hungry? If you can no longer recognize your hunger signals, you'll have to rely on outside clues for a while. Ask yourself if it has been more than five hours since your last meal? Was it substantial enough? If you decide that you're truly hungry, eat. Make sure that the snack has carbohydrate, protein, and some fat for greater staying power. (See Chapter 28 for well-balanced, calorie-controlled snacks.)

If what you feel is not physical hunger, try to label the emotion or feeling and honor it with an appropriate action. For example, if you're feeling angry, list the reasons that you feel that way and take appropriate actions to resolve the anger. Chapter 6 is all about labeling your emotions and not using food to numb your feelings.

## You call it dieting; your body calls it starving

When you go on a severe calorie-restricted diet, your body doesn't know whether your goal is to squeeze into a small pair of jeans or to protect yourself from death from starvation. So it reacts in the only way it can: It hoards the calories that you give it. The psychological results of extreme dieting and starvation are similar as well. People who are always on a diet exhibit psychological behaviors similar to those of people who are starving in prison camps.

A landmark study done during World War II (see the *Journal of Clinical Psychology* 4, 1948) clearly shows how similar the effects of dieting and starving are. Normal-weight men who were conscientious objectors to the war were asked to restrict their eating for 6 months to lose about 25 percent of their body weight so that the effects of starvation could be studied. The men reduced their normal intake by about 25 percent; if they stopped losing weight, their intake was restricted even more. While they were being starved on their diets, they became increasingly focused on food; they collected recipes and replaced pinup pictures of women with pictures of food. They were irritable, upset, and argumentative. They became apathetic and lethargic. When they were allowed to regain their weight, they gorged themselves and didn't feel in control of their eating. They continued to be obsessed with food.

### Chronic dieting

If you're a chronic dieter, you may be at risk of developing the same psychological characteristics of people who are starving: a tendency to eat excessively after you're "allowed" to eat, to become overly emotional, to have trouble concentrating, and to obsess about food and eating. How you answer the following question is a good indication of whether you're dieting too much: What would you do if the scale showed an extra five pounds?

If you're a dieter, you'd probably overeat. That's what researchers at the University of Toronto, Ontario, Canada, found when they weighed dieters and nondieters and told them that they weighed 5 pounds heavier or 5 pounds lighter than their actual weights. (See the *Journal of Abnormal Psychology* 107, 1998.) Dieters who believed that they were heavier experienced lowered self-worth and a worsening of mood that led them to relinquish their dietary restraint and overindulge in available food. Nondieters and dieters who were told that they weighed 5 pounds less weren't affected by the false weight feedback.

### The bottom line

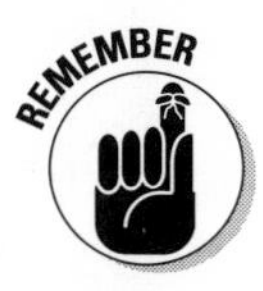


To get over overeating, you need to start listening to your body. As simple as it sounds, it's the only way to change your habits once and for all. One way to prepare to hear what your body is telling you is to plan your meals and snacks. Many overweight people eat chaotically and in response to outside cues (advertising) and sensual cues (the smell of food). In addition, they often use food to tame emotions. Knowing what you're going to eat, when and where you'll eat, takes forethought and planning. It puts order to your diet. When you use the tools in this chapter and the menu-planning advice in Chapters 9 and 10, you'll hear your body talking to ya.

## Chapter 6

# Understanding Your Relationship with Food

### In This Chapter

- Taking a close look at your triggers
- Making an attitude adjustment

From the time your mother or father hands you a cookie to quiet your crying, food becomes more than just a way to nourish your body. It's a way to nourish your soul as well. Regardless of your weight and whether you realize it — you eat for different reasons. You may eat to celebrate, to calm, to feel comfort or joy, or when times are darkest, perhaps you eat to relieve loneliness and boredom. How you feel about yourself and your body is likely to be enmeshed in your relationship with food. Shame and guilt may also play a role in your range of emotions that affect how you deal with food.

In this chapter, we investigate the emotional reasons people have for eating, even when they're not hungry. We help you to understand why you eat when you do and offer you some suggestions for replacing emotion-driven food habits with healthier behaviors.

## Determining Whether You're an Emotional Eater

The first step to discovering how emotions affect your eating is to understand your relationship with food. Answer the questions in Table 6-1 as honestly as you can. Think about how frequently each question is true for you and put a check mark in the box that corresponds to your answers: *sometimes, often, always,* and *never.* By analyzing your responses, you can better understand your triggers — your strengths. Then refer to the sections that follow the table to find out what your responses mean and to understand how to deal with these issues.

**Table 6-1 Are You an Emotional Eater?**

| *Do You . . .* | *Sometimes* | *Often* | *Always* | *Never* |
|---|---|---|---|---|
| Eat even when you're not hungry? | | | | |
| Crave certain foods and have trouble controlling the amounts of them that you eat? | | | | |
| Always clean your plate? | | | | |
| Find yourself in the kitchen or at the snack machine when faced with a difficult task? | | | | |
| Eat when you're stressed, angry, lonely, or tired? | | | | |
| Splurge on favorite foods when you're alone? | | | | |
| Feel guilty or unworthy when you eat foods that you think you shouldn't — especially high-calorie foods, such as fried items or desserts? | | | | |

## Eating when you're not hungry

If you eat when you're not hungry, you're not alone. Many people do. Unfortunately, physical hunger is often low on the list of reasons to eat. Many people eat, because the clock says that it's time to, because people around them are eating, or because a food simply looks or smells good. The key is to recognize these triggers and deal with the emotions behind them in ways not related to food. (Of course, if you're hungry, then you should eat.)

## Craving favorite foods

If you can't resist your favorite foods, you're probably responding to a craving rather than hunger. What's the difference? A *craving* is based in emotions; *hunger* is rooted in biology. When you're hungry, any number of foods can satisfy you, but a craving is a highly specialized, very intense desire to eat a particular food or type of food. During a craving, the desire is sometimes so strong that you may go out of your way to get it. For example, when you crave potato chips, celery sticks just won't cut it.

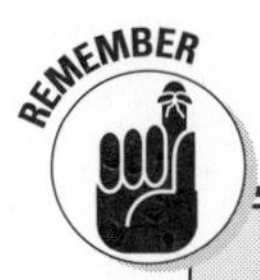


## Keeping a food journal

Most people don't make the connection between how they feel and how much they eat until they keep a food journal, which is nothing more than a record of the foods you eat, when you eat them, and how you're feeling when you eat. A small notebook or a few index cards that you can clip together and fit into a pocket or purse will work. Record three weekdays and one weekend day, because you probably eat differently on weekends and for different reasons. Just remember to do the following:

- **Record everything you eat.** That includes the swipe your finger made through the brownie batter. If you eat crackers, record how many. (Check out Chapter 9 for suggestions on estimating portion sizes.)
- **Record where you're eating.** In your car, watching TV, while preparing dinner, in your office, at a party.
- **Record your feelings.** What were you thinking or feeling when you ate? Were you angry, sad, or happy? Or just hungry?
- **Record information immediately after eating a food.** You don't want to forget anything or filter your emotions; your feelings may change later in the day. You're looking for clues to why you eat, not only to what you eat.
- **Don't edit.** Try to be as accurate and honest as possible. This information is for your eyes only. It's a journal, not a newsletter. No one else needs to see it.
- **Analyze your journal at the end of the day and determine where improvements are needed.** Calculate the number of servings from each of the food groups in the pyramid. (See Chapter 9.) Determine the intensity of your emotions and how they affected your eating.

According to a survey conducted by H. P. Weingarten, PhD, at McMaster's University in Ontario, Canada, (published in the December 1991 issue of *Appetite*), 97 percent of women and 68 percent of men experience food cravings. Researchers believe that older people are generally less driven by cravings, particularly older men. The time of day also dictates food cravings — late afternoon or early evening is the prime time when cravings tend to occur. Hormones are thought to play a role as well. For example, during pregnancy and during certain times of a woman's menstrual cycle, food cravings are quite common. But dieters, especially those who frequently go on and off diets, tend to experience cravings most often. And their cravings tend to be the strongest at the beginning of their diets.

How best to deal with food cravings? Nothing can stop a craving cold, and you can't come up with a one-size-fits-all solution. Experiment with a few of the following tips to figure out what works best for you:

- **Substitute foods.** For example, try a glass of lowfat chocolate milk or a Fudgsicle instead of a chocolate candy bar.
- **Use portion control.** Buy smaller, single-size servings of favorite foods, such as ice cream, to satisfy the craving and quell the instinct to go overboard.
- **Give into the craving.** Don't eat around your craving in the hopes that it will go away. You'll probably end up eating more food and calories than you would have if you simply gave in to your craving to begin with. Many people end up eating the craved food anyway after attempting to eat around it, because they still aren't satisfied.

## Always cleaning your plate

Do you always feel compelled to clean your plate? Whether this mentality comes from well-meaning parents or a fear that you'll never eat a meal this good again, it's a particular problem for dieters and most overweight people. This kind of conditioning means that you probably lost track of your hunger mechanism and can no longer recognize when you're no longer hungry. Membership in the Clean Plate Club can be especially hazardous for people who eat out often, because restaurant portions can be gigantic and arbitrary. Restaurants plan their menus for economics and customer expectations, not health. (See Chapter 15 for more on eating out.) A solution is to order only from the kid's menu or appetizer portions. And don't ask for super-size portions at fast-food places.

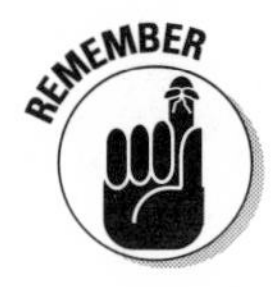


If finishing the bag of chips or the entire burger is your pattern, buy smaller sizes. Counter the fear-of-famine mentality by remembering that more is always available and that, yes, you *will* have a meal that good again. See Chapter 5 for ways to get back in touch with your hunger signals.

## Eating instead of working

Procrastination and boredom are common reasons for eating. It's a way to kill time and put off doing tasks that need to be done. Classic research on dieters and nondieters performed at California State University (*Addictive Behaviors* 2, 1977) showed that when faced with monotonous tasks — in this case, writing the same letter over and over again — dieters and nondieters alike ate more crackers. When they engaged in a stimulating mental activity, such as a creative writing project, they ate fewer crackers.

A more recent study, April 2002, published in *Psychology of Medicine* illustrated that dieters are easily distracted from their work. So if a boring project or a big job is headed your way, be sure that you eat a well-balanced breakfast, lunch, and dinner, and plan some snacks. If you restrict your calories too much, eating is all you'll think about. And if you find yourself at the fridge, try reaching for some ice water, raw veggies, or fruit before digging into the cookie jar. Or take a walk around the block or around the office to help clear your head.

## Eating when you're stressed, angry, lonely, or tired

Eating to distract yourself from difficult emotions isn't a constructive or healthy way to deal with your problems. The more deeply you feel the effects of your emotions, particularly the negative ones, the more you're apt to eat. For overweight people, this reaction may be especially problematic.

A study conducted by Michael Lowe of Rutgers University and Edwin Fisher, Jr., of Washington University [*Journal of Behavioral Medicine* 6(2), 1983] compared the emotional reactivity and emotional eating of normal and overweight female college students. For 12 days, the women kept track of how they were feeling just before eating and recorded what and how much they ate. The results showed that the obese women were more emotionally reactive and more likely to engage in emotional eating than women of normal weight — but only at snack time, not at meals. The more emotional that the women were feeling, the more they ate, and the heaviest women were the most emotional. However, the two groups did not differ in their reactions to positive, happy feelings, nor did they eat in response to good emotions.

If you're keeping a food journal (see the sidebar, "Keeping a food journal" in this chapter for details), see how many times you used words that signal stress, sadness, anger, loneliness, or exhaustion. Try one of these nonfood coping strategies if emotion, not hunger, triggered you to eat:

- Talk with a friend.
- Go for a walk, play with your pet, or ask someone for a hug.
- Release anger by pounding your fist into a pillow or just go ahead and scream!
- Confront the person who is making you angry.
- Cry if you need to.
- Practice breathing exercises, breathing in and out deeply, to help center yourself.
- Ask for time out or help on a project, if needed.

- Take a yoga or meditation class.
- Schedule time for yourself.
- Get a good night's sleep or take a nap.

## Eating healthfully around others but splurging alone

Overeating only when you're alone is usually the result of buying into the diet industry propaganda that you hear from television, well-meaning friends, and your own inner voice: "Don't eat too many calories," "You shouldn't eat that," "That cake is too fattening." Foods get labeled, and if you eat these *good* or *bad* foods, *you* become good or bad. These thoughts can make you restrict your eating so severely that when you're calm, alone, and not afraid of being judged, you splurge and enjoy all the foods that you otherwise think you shouldn't eat.

This kind of restrictive eating keeps the diet treadmill rolling. Cognitive therapists know that when a negative thought ("I shouldn't eat that dessert" or "It's just going to end up on my thighs") leads to negative feelings ("I'm so fat; what a failure I am"); negative behavior (eating too much of the dessert and continuing to overeat) is sure to follow. Perception becomes reality.

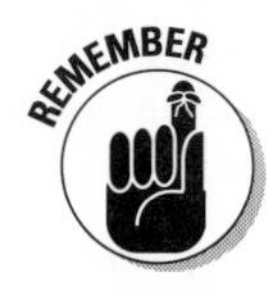


You need to replace negative, irrational thoughts with positive, rational ones. One way is to get away from all-or-nothing thinking. Pull back from the extremes and stay moderate. Get rid of *should* and *shouldn't.* No food is all good or all bad, and neither are you. Quiet your own internal *food police* by listening to your sympathetic, caring, and loving voices. The conversation may sound something like this: "That cake sure looks good. I'd love to try it. My weight loss may slow down if I eat a big piece. So I'm going to have just a small slice. Yum, I sure will enjoy that. I will feel satisfied, and I won't have to forage for sweets later."

## Feeling unworthy to eat or guilty about eating

Feeling unworthy to eat or guilty about eating also comes from the food police at work. And it's classic diet-think. Eating is not a moral issue, and neither is food. Eating and hunger are part of the human condition — you have to eat in order to live. You can squelch the food police by letting your nurturing voices be heard. Instead of thinking, "Do I deserve this?" ask yourself, "Am I hungry?" If your answer is "Yes," then eat.

### Name that mood

People who belong to 12-step programs, such as Alcoholics Anonymous, use techniques to keep from engaging in their addictive behaviors. One method is called HALT, which stands for Hungry, Angry, Lonely, and Tired. These physical and emotional feelings can masquerade as cravings for substances or behaviors. So if a 12-stepper feels the need to return to his self-destructive behavior, a quick inventory reveals what needs to be done. For example, you can relieve feelings of loneliness with a call to a friend or cure tiredness with a nap. The point is to recognize the triggers and deal with them rather than substitute unhealthy behaviors.

Psychologists know that giving your emotions a name makes them easier to deal with. Labeling makes feelings concrete, and therefore, you can cope with them. If you engage in emotional eating, labeling what you're feeling when you eat may be the secret to eating less.

# Adjusting Your Attitude

That society discriminates against overweight people is a fact of life. It starts in school, and anyone who has been larger than his classmates can tell tales of the rejection and ridicule that come out from the mouths of thinner peers. That the prejudice is widespread in the business world, too, is well documented. And countless men and women can tell you that their weights and their dissatisfaction with their bodies keep them from getting close to other people or sometimes even enjoying sex with their spouses.

Being overweight takes a toll on your self-esteem and the way you relate to others. Self-esteem is key to your relationship with food, too. If you don't feel good about your body, you may not feel good about the food you put into it. And without a healthy relationship with food, your body image will plummet. It's a Catch-22 situation.

This section is about body image: finding out how to feel good about who you are, regardless of your body size or shape.

## Just whose ideal are you anyway?

According to research conducted by the Kellogg's Corporation (published by the Opinion Research Corporation), women in the United States determine their ideal body size and shape from the way models in television ads and fashion magazines look, not from the way women look in real life. Women are obsessed about their weight, fueled by a society that sets an artificial standard for beauty based on the way models look. Women also believe that how they're described by men and by each other promotes the notion of an ideal woman, whom they will never be able to match.

The Kellogg's survey found that women tend to focus on the specific body parts they don't like, not on their bodies as a whole. They may like their hair color and think that they're tall enough, but only 14 percent of the women surveyed were happy with their weights. Almost a third of the women surveyed said that a woman's ideal weight is between 110 and 125 pounds, and half said that a weight between 126 and 145 is ideal. But in reality, there is no such thing as an *ideal* weight, because people are genetically programmed to be different shapes and sizes.

That so many women are confused about what they should look like isn't surprising. The role models look nothing like the average woman. In fact, if you think about it, it's the fashion models who don't conform to the standards of the average adult, not the other way around. Only 1 in 40,000 women has a supermodel-like body — 40,000! That ratio means that out of the entire population of Indiana, a state with more than 6 million residents, only 152 women have model-perfect bodies!

Table 6-2 compares the average American woman to the media's and society's ideals, demonstrating that when it comes to selling clothes, life doesn't imitate art. In fact, it's getting farther away from it. Marilyn Monroe, the pinup girl of the 1950s, wore a size 14 dress — the same size that many women in the United States wear today. This isn't to say that a size 14 is healthy for all women. It depends on your height and other factors. If you're 5 feet tall and you wear a size 14, then you're probably unhealthy. But if you're 5 feet 6 inches tall, a size 14 may be okay, even though you'd still be considered on the large side by society's standards. The scary thing is that today's models, who are usually at least 5 feet 8 inches or taller, typically wear only a size 6. And between 1955 and 1998, the measurements of a *Playboy* centerfold dropped by 35 percent.

**Table 6-2 Female Role Models**

| | *Average Woman* | *Mannequin* | *Model* |
|---|---|---|---|
| Dress size | 12 | 6 | 6 |
| Weight | 152 | — | 120 |
| Height | 5'4" | 5'10" | 5'8" to 5'11" |
| Body measurements | 37-34-40 | 34-25-34 | 34-25-34 |
| Percent body fat | 34 | — | 18 |
| BMI (Body Mass Index) | 26.1 | — | 17.2 |

This phenomenon isn't unique to women. Even male models and mannequins are smaller than the average American male. Table 6-3 illustrates the differences.

**Table 6-3 Male Role Models**

| | *Average Man* | *Mannequin* | *Model* |
|---|---|---|---|
| Pant size | 37 | 30 | 30 |
| Suit size | 42 regular | 40 regular | 40 regular |
| Weight | 180 | — | 145–150 |
| Height | 5'9" | 6' | 6' |
| Body measurements | 41 chest | 39 chest | 39 chest |
| | 37 waist | 30 waist | 30 waist |
| Percent body fat | 22 | — | 15 |
| BMI (Body Mass Index) | 26.6 | — | 20.5 |

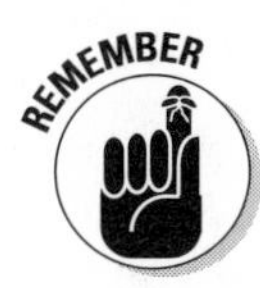


The important point to take away from these tables is that you need to stop comparing yourself and your weight to unrealistic numbers. Even if you diet religiously, you probably won't end up with the body of a supermodel. Stop beating yourself up for not meeting standards that are clearly unrealistic and concentrate on the things you can do to make your body healthy. And begin to feel good about your progress, too.

One study of obese women — their average weight was about 218 pounds — conducted by Foster and others at the University of Pennsylvania did just that [see the *Journal of Consulting and Clinical Psychology* 65(1), 1997]. The women were asked to write down their goal weights and then the weight-loss amounts that they would consider "acceptable" and "disappointing." Most women set their goals 32 percent lower than their starting points (about 72 pounds). "Acceptable" was about a 25 percent loss (55 pounds), and the women considered a weight loss of only 17 percent of their starting weights (38 pounds) to be "disappointing."

After 6 months of dieting, exercising, and behavior modification and 6 months of maintenance, the average weight loss that these women were able to maintain was only 16 percent of their defined starting weights (or 36 pounds). They hadn't even reached their "disappointing" weight. Did they fail? No. These women can be called successful for several reasons: A weight loss of just 10 percent is enough to bring down high blood pressure, lower cholesterol and triglycerides, and improve overall health. And these women beat that goal by 6 percentage points.

More important, all the women were happy with their losses and were surprised to find that even though they hadn't reached the weight loss they initially called disappointing, they felt better physically and emotionally than they had expected.

The lesson is that accepting a weight loss that doesn't match the number you dreamed of is healthier than writing off the success as a failure and then giving in and gaining the loss back — plus a few more pounds. A healthier weight strategy is to maintain the loss for a few months and then reach for another 10 to 15 percent loss. Think of weight loss as moving down a flight of stairs — not a ramp — with landings to stop and evaluate your progress.

Unfortunately, most people don't give themselves credit for progress. They strive for perfection. Actually, most dieters who consider themselves successful at maintaining weight loss lose about half the weight between their beginning weight and the ideal that they think they *should* weigh.

## Is your body image accurate?

Society shouldn't dictate how people look. But in reality, it does. About 95 percent of females and 30 percent of males have issues about the way their bodies look. The thing is, it's the only body you have. So if you're not happy with your body, make the commitment to start taking better care of it.

Exercise and stretch your body, fill it with the foods it needs to help keep you healthy and strong, and remember all the good that your body does for you. You may never look like a supermodel, but that's okay — virtually no one will. However, everybody can be healthy. When you start taking care of your body, you'll feel better about your body and about yourself. So get started today.

Check out some techniques to try if your body image needs improving:

- **Remember that your perception of your body is a thought ("I hate my jelly belly"), but you feel it like an emotion ("I'm unlovable").** So if you can change the thought ("My stomach stayed round after the children were born"), you can change the emotion ("I'm happy that my body can give life").
- **Use your body.** It functions. Any woman who has breast-fed her child, for example, can explain the shift in thinking about her breasts as functioning entities rather than as sexual objects. Use your thighs to carry you through the woods, up a mountain, or down the street. Give them something to do rather than thinking of them as something to hide.

- **Know that body images wax and wane.** Some days, you may like your shape; other days, you may feel woefully inadequate. Think of times when you were not disappointed with your body. What were you doing? Do that activity more often.
- **Figure out how you perceive your body image.** Either alone in front of a mirror or with a kind, loving, and trustworthy friend, stand up straight and close your eyes. If you're a woman, stretch your arms out in front of you and indicate the width of your hips. If you're a man, do the same to indicate how thick you think your middle is. Now open your eyes and compare. Were you accurate? Many women with distorted body images think that their hips are much wider than they are. And many men may think that their bellies are larger than they really are, too.
- **Try not to play the mix-and-match, pick-and-compare body parts game with other people.** You know, you'd like to have one woman's thighs, another's bust, or if you're a guy, one man's biceps and another's flat stomach. Remember that every body has great parts and not-so-great parts, and begin to appreciate your body for what it is. It's the only one you have!
- **Give yourself credit for the physical attributes you do like, such as good teeth, great hair, sexy feet, a pretty belly button, or a lovely voice!**

# Chapter 7

# Marketing to the Masses: The Conspiracy to Consume

### *In This Chapter*

- Conning you into buying unhealthy edibles
- Marketing larger food portions and more
- Eating for health and convenience, too

No doubt about it, folks today do more than ever. Between working longer hours, shuttling kids to more activities, or even having more than one job, it may feel like the demands on your time squeeze out the preparation of your own food. So getting a cheap, quick meal without going to the grocery store or spending more than a few minutes in the kitchen seems like a good thing. However, the problem with that thinking is that, in many cases, portion sizes are too large. Sophisticated (even sneaky) marketing tricks deceive you into eating more than you know you should.

Of course, no one would claim that the goal of restaurants and food manufacturers is to make America the fattest nation in the world, but that's what's happened. Americans buy and eat larger portions of food and consume more of them on a daily basis than ever before. As a dieter (or someone contemplating a diet), that's not a comforting thought. So in this chapter, we help you identity some of the most common marketing techniques and show you how to avoid falling prey to them.

## Luring You into Buying

We try to control our appetites, but we can't get away from food. It's available in places that never used to sell it, such as drugstores, gas stations, and health clubs. Not only is food more available, it's marketed aggressively. Make no mistake. The size of soft-drink cups, the pricing of super sizes, and the aromas from the bakery department at the supermarket are all strategically calculated to get you to buy.

## Selling point: The power of advertising

How many commercial jingles can you hum? How often do you use advertising slogans in your everyday speech? C'mon, 'fess up: When was the last time that you said: "Try it; you'll like it" or "Where's the beef?" Probably not too long ago, right?

The fact is that advertising and promotions work, and they're especially effective when it comes to food. Advertising drives brand awareness. Unfortunately, healthy and naturally grown foods, such as bunches of broccoli and spinach aren't generally branded, but the most highly processed foods are.

## Value marketing: Help or hindrance to the consumer?

Most people respond to marketing cues when shopping. That means that your buying decisions are usually not based on need but rather in response to specific triggers. So after you're lured into the store or restaurant through advertising, you'll get bombarded with other kinds of marketing.

For example, the fast food industry uses a technique that encourages customers to part with a little extra cash and, at the same time, feel like they're getting a huge deal. We call it *super-sizing.* They call it *value marketing.*

On average, larger portions don't cost manufacturers too much more.

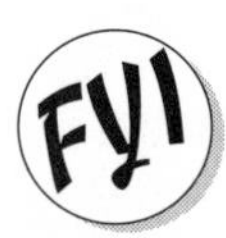


Generally, at most restaurants, only 20 percent of the retail price goes toward the food itself. Overhead, employee costs, advertising, and promotions make up the bulk of their operating expenses.

So by offering value meals or super-size deals, restaurants give patrons more food (and calories and fat) for a bargain price. And to sell customers on the idea, don't forget all the placemats, signs, menu cards, label pins, and other point-of-purchase materials encouraging you to up-size. If you're the restaurant owner, this tactic means more profits. As a consumer, value marketing is clearly a penny wise and a pound foolish.

Table 7-1 illustrates the caloric and financial costs of value meals. Look at the out-of-pocket expenses that the calories buy. It's pennies. Now consider the real price of the extra calories — how many diet books, diet foods, larger clothing sizes, medical bills, weight-loss programs you'll eventually buy if you eat those extra calories?

**Table 7-1 The Real Cost of Super Sizing**

| *Menu Item* | *Up Size* | *Increase Cost to Restaurant* | *Extra Calories* |
|---|---|---|---|
| Movie popcorn | Small to medium | 0.71 | 500 |
| Cola | Small to super size | 0.60 | 260 |
| Fries | Small to large | 0.64 | 330 |
| Cheeseburger | Quarter pound cheeseburger to value meal | 1.41 | 660 |
| Tuna sub | 6-inch to 12-inch | 1.53 | 420 |
| Chocolate chip ice cream | Kid's size to double scoop | 1.62 | 390 |

**Adapted from From Wallet to Waistline, the National Alliance for Nutrition and Activity, June 2002.*

## More is better but not for health

Like value marketing, the more items you see on a menu or in a store, the more you want to buy — and eat.

Perceived variety is another marketing gimmick that restaurants, particularly fast-food outlets use frequently. The next time that you go to a fast-food restaurant, count how many times that *fries* show up on the menu. Not only are there usually three or four sizes of fries, but they're also *bundled* in several places with the value meals as well as the extensive children's meals. But it's still the same food item. Now notice all the other menu items that are repeated the same way, and you can see why you get the impression that the restaurant is offering variety in abundance. When in reality, the menu is quite limited. When you can see through this marketing gimmick, you may realize that there aren't really so many items that you want to buy (and eat) after all.

Likewise, you see variety marketing every time you grocery shop. The more *shelf facings* (the trade term for rows of product) that a product gets, the more you're apt to buy. Take salad dressing, for example. Offering more variety or getting you to believe that plenty of variety is being made available to you is one of the reasons that manufacturers bottle a single flavor in so many different bottle sizes and shapes not to mention the actual number of flavors within one brand.

## Chaos theory: Messy equals more

A study published in July 2003 by Barbara Kahn, Professor of Marketing at the Wharton School, demonstrated the success of variety marketing. She showed that if consumers only *think* they have plenty of variety to chose from, they buy more. Seeing huge displays of jelly beans at movie theaters and candy shops and observing the way people "gobbled" up the goodies inspired her research.

Plenty of studies have shown that variety induces people to buy more, but Kahn and co-researchers demonstrated that even perceived variety can lead to real profits. In one of the experiments, test subjects were given only six different jelly bean flavors, either arranged neatly or all mixed up. When scrambled, it appears that there are more kinds than there are. And as expected, the test subjects ate more of the randomly organized jelly beans than the neatly arranged ones.

Large portions are the other half of *more-is-better marketing.* When people started eating more meals at restaurant, from takeout, and the supermarket's prepared-foods departments, portion sizes began to increase as well. For example, in 1970, 34 percent of food dollars were spent on foods eaten out. But by the late 1990s, 47 percent of food budgets went to foods that someone else prepared. Through the 1980's when eating out became a habit, the size of portions really took off, and they're still showing no sign of moderating. Table 7-2 shows the enormous growth in portion sizes that Marion Nestle, PhD, MPH, reported in the *American Journal of Public Health* in February 2002. (See Chapter 9 for more on portion sizes.)

Not only do large sizes mean more calories per serving, but they also encourage people to eat more as well. Researcher Barbara Rolls and her colleagues at Pennsylvania State University gave subjects one of four different-size portions of macaroni and cheese and told the diners to eat as much as they liked. The test subjects ate 30 percent more when they were served the largest portions. (If you want to read more about Rolls's study, check out the *Journal of Clinical Nutrition* from December of 2002.)

**Table 7-2 Increase in Portion Sizes**

| *Food* | *USDA Standard Size* | *Restaurant Portion % Larger* |
|---|---|---|
| Cookie | 0.5 ounce | 700 |
| Cooked pasta | 1 cup | 480 |
| Muffin | 1.5 ounces | 333 |
| Steak | 3 ounces | 224 |
| Bagel | 2 ounces | 195 |

# Having It Their Weigh: Ingredient Realities

Food manufacturing today relies on ingredients and cooking techniques that can undermine your health and weight-loss efforts if you're not careful, which is another reason to find ways to prepare more meals at home.

## Fattening up menus

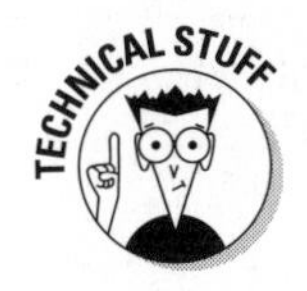


*Hydrogenation* is a process that adds hydrogen to an oil under heat and pressure to extend shelf life and improve the texture of foods that are made with it.

Unfortunately, the kind of fat that's used in many restaurants is partially hydrogenated, which means it contains *trans fatty acids.* That's the kind of fat that lowers your good cholesterol and raises the bad. French fries, fried onion rings, taco shells, and salad dressing are among some of the many items that contain hydrogenated fats, and therefore trans fatty acids. Some researchers speculate that we have a threshold for trans fatty acids, because they rarely occur in nature. According to their theories, large amounts of trans fatty acids can't be metabolized for energy. Instead, they're stored as fatty acids — permanently. For more on the trans fat issue, see Chapter 10.

Prepared foods that you buy from the supermarket are another source of hydrogenated fats and therefore, trans fatty acids. For example, for pizza crust to crisp in the oven, fries to brown without a deep-fat fryer, chicken nuggets to brown in the microwave, and toaster pastries to pop hot from the toaster, hydrogenated fats are used. You may be surprised at how often they appear on ingredient labels. In 2006, the FDA will demand that the total amount of trans fat appears on the Nutrition Facts panel. Until then, check ingredient labels for hydrogenated or partially hydrogenated fats and oils. The earlier they're listed, the more the product has.

## Sweetening the bottom line

*High-fructose corn syrup* (HFCS) is another ingredient that's being pegged to the obesity crisis. Food manufacturers use HFCS in abundance. In the 1970s, sugar prices soared, making the cost of foods that depended on sugar cane almost unaffordable. As a result, food technologists found a way to make a cheaper, sweeter sweetener by transforming corn into HFCS. When HFCS was first introduced, few scientists questioned the effect that so much fructose would have on people's health.

## Catering to convenience

Convenience sells. It's a trend that's been building up for a while, and grocery stores, takeout places, and restaurants are offering simple ways to deliver dinner faster. The statistics that follow illustrate how important convenience is to the health of the food industry. Unfortunately, easy access to food has made staying healthy more difficult.

- A Market Research Institute study done in the spring of 2003 on behalf of Stouffer's foods revealed that Americans feel that the greatest source of stress at home is cooking dinner, and the top two factors guiding meal plans are taste and convenience. Nutrition is in third place.
- Starting in 1993, the percent of all consumers who think that convenience is important in the foods they eat reached 50 percent according to a National Eating Trends Survey.
- According to a 2003 Food Marketing Institute study, 97 percent of food retailers have deli departments, and 93 percent offer fresh, prepared foods. (The Food Marketing Institute, or FMI, is a trade association for the supermarket industry.)
- A USDA group crunched the numbers in 1999 and found that compared to meals at home, restaurant meals are higher in saturated fats and total fat but lower in calcium, iron, and fiber.
- Because Americans want nutrition to be convenient too, food manufacturers introduced more than 5,400 lower fat versions of foods between 1995 and 1997. Unfortunately, many of those products did not substantially lower total calories.

The most dramatic result of HFCS entering the food supply was its effect on the soft-drink industry. The availability of a low-priced sweetener meant that the cost of ingredients was so minimal that soft-drink manufacturers could practically give the stuff away. That's what happened at many fast-food restaurants and movie theatres. For pennies, restaurants could up-size your soda order to a pound-size serving. This kind of *value marketing* brings traffic to the establishments and, unfortunately, additional calories to the American diet. But are additional calories all that you have to worry about when it comes to HFCS?

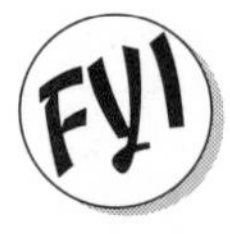


The fructose in high fructose corn syrup is metabolized just like the fructose in fruit, but with some significant differences. The first is that fruit is packed with additional nutrients, such as vitamins, minerals, and fiber. Fiber regulates digestion and metabolism. Soda, which is sweetened with HFCS, has no fiber or any other nutrient contribution other than calories. And a soda that is sweetened with 100 percent HFCS delivers far more fructose than a piece of fruit: A 2½ inch peach has 13 grams of sugar, of which only 2.4 grams are fructose. A 20-ounce bottle of soda contains about 33 grams of fructose.

In addition to soft drinks, HFCS is in candy, popsicles, pancake syrup, fruit-flavored yogurt, sweetened cereals, some pasta sauces, and apple juice. The enormous amount of HFCS in the American diet is worrying health scientists, because fructose has a unique metabolic response. It's clear in animal studies, but less so in humans, that fructose induces high blood pressure, high triglycerides (a form of fat in the blood associated with heart disease), impaired glucose tolerance (precursor to diabetes), and insulin resistance.

Some evidence suggests that fructose may cause weight gain and fat storage in humans, because it's metabolized into fat in the liver, rather than absorbed and processed into glucose the way that table sugar or other carbohydrates are. Additionally, because fructose doesn't stimulate insulin production, and therefore, *leptin* (hormone that increases after eating, turning off any feeling of hunger) concentrations remain low, you may still feel hungry even after consuming hundreds of calories from a soda. (See Chapter 5 for more about leptin.)

HFCS has a carbohydrate profile similar to regular table sugar. Both contain about 50 percent glucose and 50 percent fructose.

# Making Nutrition Convenient

Through the power of advertising, some people may become convinced that they need someone else to cook for them. Unfortunately, your weight and health isn't at the top of the food producers' list. So how do you ensure that you eat healthfully while still maintaining that convenience factor that makes you crave the store-bought or restaurant meals in the first place? Try one of these ideas:

- **Enlist family to help.** Assign jobs to family members and distribute meal preparation tasks just like professional kitchens do. Put someone in charge of making the nightly salad and ask someone else to do the chopping. You can also use your supermarket's salad bar as your *sous chef.* Buy your onions, peppers, or other recipe ingredients there prewashed and already chopped.
- **Cook once, eat twice.** Instead of stocking your freezer with frozen dinners from the supermarket, make a double batch of dinner and put half away for instant meals later.
- **Buy ready-to-cook produce.** Take advantage of the offerings in the produce section that include prewashed vegetables in ready-to-microwave packages.

- **Think variety in the kind of restaurants you visit as well as in the foods you order.** Add a salad or fresh cooked vegetables to round out the meal.
- **Read a good (cook) book.** Healthy, easy-to-prepare meals are one of the biggest trends in cookbooks. Fresh, minimally processed ingredients can be quickly tossed together to make a healthy meal — often requiring fewer ingredients than most fast checkout lines allow.

## Settling for fat

A sales and marketing organization known as NPD (formally known as National Purchase Diary) took a survey in 2002 that showed that 75 percent of the 8,000 people they asked thought that being fat is okay. In 1985, only 45 percent thought so. Food portions aren't the only things growing along with our girth. Sales of all kinds of plus-size products have increased, making it more comfortable to ignore our size and the health risks that come with being overweight.

- Wide-bodied SUVs and other light trucks outsold passenger cars in 2002.
- Compact cars have widened their seats by shrinking the center consoles.
- Between 1997 and 2001, the sales of queen-size mattresses went from 31 to 34 percent of bed sales and king-size went from 6 to 8 percent.
- Half of U.S. women wear a size 12 or larger, up from size 8 in 1985.
- Loose-fitting clothes and elastic waist-bands are the norm.
- Plus-size clothing accounts for 20 percent of all women's clothing.

# Part III

# Formulating a Plan for Healthful Eating

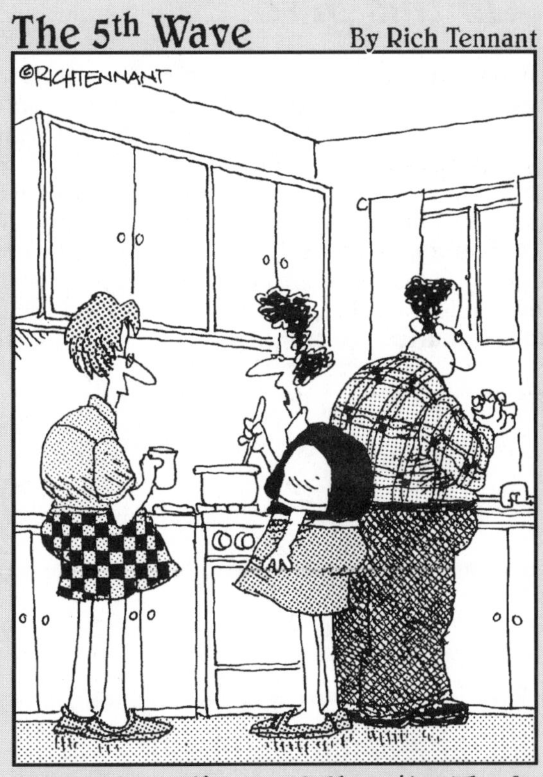


"Nutritionally, we follow the Food Guide Pyramid. When I first met Philip, he ate from the Food Guide Stonehenge. It was a mysterious diet and no one's sure what its purpose was."

## *In this part . . .*

When you understand how your weight affects your health, how your body processes calories, and how other factors besides hunger can affect your eating habits, you're ready to put a dieting plan in place. This part tells you how to set up a healthful eating plan, work physical activity into your lifestyle, and maintain your healthy weight for a lifetime. It also talks about the growing array of fat substitutes and artificial sweeteners and how they fit into your diet, separating the truth from the "too good to be true."

# Chapter 8

# Calorie Basics

### In This Chapter

- Measuring the energy in the food you eat
- Finding out about the big kahuna calories
- Figuring out just how many calories you need
- Being honest about potential weight loss

You eat calories. You count them. You shave them. You hate them. You've memorized the number of calories in your favorite foods. You know that eating too many calories makes you gain weight, and that you lose weight when you eat fewer. But more than simply reading the numbers on food labels, calorie know-how means knowing *why* some foods have more calories than others and figuring out the number of calories that your body needs to survive and thrive are the first steps to getting started on a healthy weight-loss plan. This chapter explains all about calories and tells you how to manage them.

## Defining Calories

Although the technically correct name is *kilocalorie,* everyone, including dietitians, uses the shorter *calorie.*

Calories are simply a way to measure energy — the energy in food as well as the energy released in the body. Technically speaking, 1 calorie is the amount of energy necessary to raise the temperature of 1 gram of water by 1 degree Centigrade. You expend about 1 calorie per minute when sitting relaxed. That's about the same amount of heat released by a candle or a 75-watt light bulb.

# Revealing Where Calories Come From

A calorie isn't a nutrient, but certain nutrients provide calories. Protein, carbohydrate, and fat make up the calorie contents of various foods. Although not considered a nutrient, alcohol also provides calories. In fact, one gram of

- **Protein** contains 4 calories
- **Carbohydrate** contains 4 calories
- **Fat** contains 9 calories
- **Alcohol** contains 7 calories

The remaining nutrients — water, minerals, and vitamins — do not provide calories, nor does fiber or cholesterol.

Few foods and beverages are 100 percent of any one nutrient. Most foods and beverages are a *combination* of protein, fat, and carbohydrate (and sometimes alcohol), so a food's calorie count is the sum of the calories provided by each nutrient. See how it works:

A bowl of chicken noodle soup contains 3 grams of protein, 7 grams of carbohydrate, and 2 grams of fat for a total of 58 calories:

| | | |
|---|---|---|
| 3 grams protein x 4 calories/gram | = | 12 calories |
| 7 grams carbohydrate x 4 calories/gram | = | 28 calories |
| 2 grams fat x 9 calories/gram | = | 18 calories |
| **Total** | = | 58 calories |

Even though most foods are made up of two or more nutrients, foods are categorized by their predominant nutrient. For example, a bagel and a bowl of cereal are considered carbohydrate foods even though they also contain protein and, sometimes, fat. Even though a chicken breast is considered a protein food, not all of its calories come from protein. Chicken also contains fat, which contributes calories.

Not all calories are created equal. Foods that are considered *empty-calorie foods* really have nothing in them as far as nutrition goes, except for calories. Sugary foods, such as candy, are prime examples. When you're restricting calories, you can make some room for empty-calorie foods but don't build your diet on them. If you do, you'll miss out on valuable minerals, fiber, and vitamins.

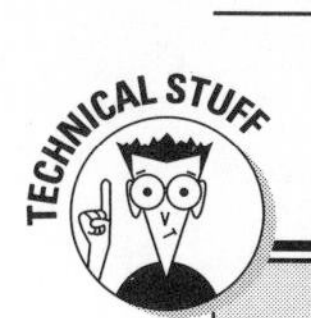


## Calorie counts

Calories are rounded on food labels, so when you multiply the grams of protein, carbohydrate, or fat, you may come out with a different value than appears on the label. Foods that contain 50 calories or fewer are rounded to the nearest 5-calorie increment; foods with more than 50 calories are rounded to the nearest 10-calorie increment. And foods that have fewer than 5 calories can be listed as having 0 calories. Although you may think that this rounding seems misleading or inaccurate, keep in mind that a 10-calorie difference is actually negligible in the grand scheme of things.

The opposite of empty-calorie foods are *nutrient-dense* foods. Calorie for calorie, they pack a solid nutrition punch by providing a good amount of vitamins, minerals, and/or fiber in comparison to the number of calories they provide. In other words, you get a big nutrition bang for your caloric buck. An example of a nutrient-dense food is an orange. For a mere 60 calories, you get about 3 grams of fiber, 100 percent of your daily vitamin C requirement, and a good amount of folic acid plus a spectrum of other micronutrients and phytochemicals, such as antioxidants.

# Tracking How Many Calories You Eat

Unfortunately, a magic formula for figuring out how many calories you eat is unavailable as yet — you simply have to track it. If you're keeping a food journal as we suggest in Chapter 6, dig it out now. If you didn't, or can't find it, you can catch up: Buy a small notebook and write down *everything* you eat for two days during the week and one weekend day — including that handful of M&M's, the dressing you put on your salad, and the pat of butter you put on your potato. Don't forget to include beverages, too. People tend to eat differently on weekends than on weekdays, so including a Saturday or Sunday in your tracking is important.

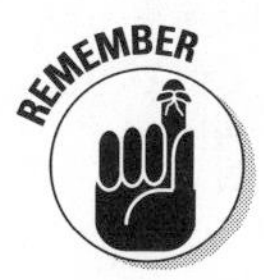


Make sure, too, to accurately estimate the amount of each food that you eat. Studies show that most people grossly underestimate their portion sizes — and can't figure out why they don't lose weight on their "diets"! The problem, of course, is that most people just eat too much.

The best way to determine how much you're eating is to weigh and measure your food. Fill your plate with the typical amount of food that you eat and then use a measuring cup, spoon, or scale to determine your serving size. Most people find it easiest to write down what they ate immediately following each meal; otherwise, they tend to forget about the incidentals, such as the glass of wine or soda, or the butter on the bread, and the amounts.

At the end of each day, go back and record the calories for each food you ate by using food labels or a book of calorie counts. (You can usually find pocket-size calorie count books in the grocery store checkout line — and more expanded versions in bookstores — that list hundreds of foods.) Then simply tally the number of calories for each food based on the amount you ate, and total up for the day. After your three-day recording period, add the total calorie counts together and divide by 3. This gives you the approximate number of calories (give or take a few) that you eat on average each day.

# Determining How Many Calories You Need

After you figure out how many calories you typically eat, the next step is to figure out how many calories you actually *need.* Not surprising, many people eat more calories than they truly need, resulting in excess weight.

## Taking key factors into account

Your calorie needs are unique to you and depend on a number of factors, including your age, sex, metabolism, activity level, and body size. The following list talks about the factors that affect your calorie needs in more detail.

To get a quick idea of your total calorie needs, multiply your current weight by 15 if you're moderately active or by 13 if you're not.

- **Your age:** Calorie needs peak at about age 25 and then begin to decline by about 2 percent every 10 years. So if you're 25 years old and need 2,200 calories to maintain your weight, you'll need only 2,156 by the time you're 35; 2,113 at age 45; 2,071 at age 55; and so on. One of the reasons for the reduced need is that an aging body replaces muscle with fat, which (unfortunately) burns fewer calories than muscle does. Yet, staying active and doing muscle-strengthening exercises keeps muscle mass in tact. And even recent work with seniors proves that you can build muscle at any age.

## A burning issue: Measuring calories in food

Where do they get the calorie counts on food labels and in diet books? The old-fashioned way: They burn it.

The scientists who measure calories in foods call this method *direct calorimetry.* They use an instrument called a *bomb calorimeter,* essentially a highly insulated box containing a special oxygen-rich chamber surrounded by water. A food sample is placed inside the chamber and is burned completely. The heat released raises the temperature of the water in the box. How high the water temperature rises determines how many calories are in the food. If the temperature of the water increases by 10 degrees Centigrade, for example, the food has 10 calories.

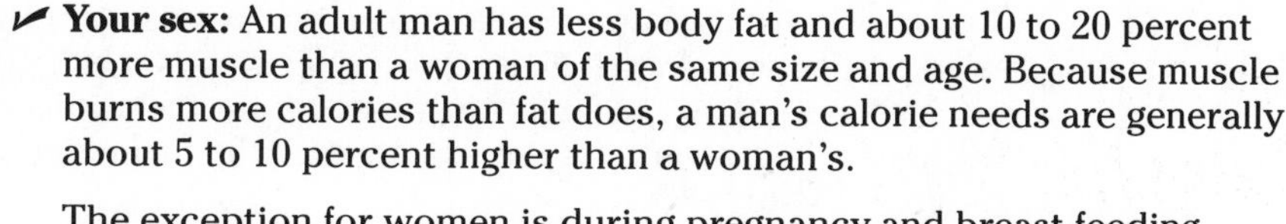

- **Your sex:** An adult man has less body fat and about 10 to 20 percent more muscle than a woman of the same size and age. Because muscle burns more calories than fat does, a man's calorie needs are generally about 5 to 10 percent higher than a woman's.

  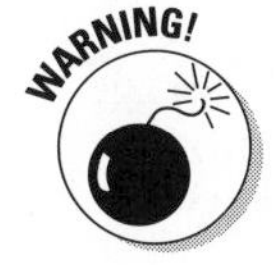
  

  The exception for women is during pregnancy and breast-feeding. During these times in your life, you definitely should *not* cut calories. In fact, you need to eat *more* calories — an extra 300 calories a day while pregnant and an extra 500 calories a day when breast-feeding.

  If you're overweight when you become pregnant, talk with your doctor about an appropriate calorie level for you. Contrary to the old adage, pregnancy is *not* an excuse to eat for two (or three or more!), but you do need to be sure that you're taking in an adequate number of calories. The same goes for while you're breast-feeding.

- **Your metabolism:** A living body needs a minimum number of calories to maintain vital functions, such as breathing and keeping its heart beating. This minimum number is called Basal Metabolic Rate (BMR). It's what most people are referring to when they talk about metabolism.

  You can compare your body to a car's engine: Some run efficiently, and others take plenty of fuel to keep them moving. Researchers can predict BMR accurately by conducting a special test that measures how much oxygen the body uses within a set amount of time.

  A quick and easy way to approximate your BMR without checking into a laboratory is to multiply your current weight by 10 if you're a woman or by 11 if you're a man. Your body needs about 10 to 11 calories, depending on your sex, for every pound you weigh to meet its basic needs. Therefore, a 150-pound woman needs about 1,500 calories a day; a 175-pound man needs about 1,925 calories. Additional calories are needed for digestion and activity. However, be aware that the more you weigh, the higher your calorie need will *appear* to be. You can find another, more accurate, way to determine your BMR that factors in your age in Table 8-1.

- **Your genetic blueprint:** The metabolic rate that you inherit from your family in part determines the number of calories that your body needs to function, and you can't change this factor. That's why your friend who is at the same height, weight, and activity level as you are may be able to eat more calories than you and never gain weight. Metabolic diseases that tend to be inherited, specifically those that affect your thyroid, can cause you to burn calories very quickly or very slowly. Though not as common as some people think, a malfunctioning thyroid gland can sabotage your best weight-loss efforts. Your physician can perform tests to determine your thyroid function.

- **Your body shape and the shape you're in:** Your body shape and size affect the number of calories you need. As explained earlier, muscle burns more calories than body fat does. So if you're solid and have a greater proportion of muscle to fat, your metabolism is higher. Likewise, if you have more body fat and less muscle, your metabolism is lower, and you have a greater tendency to store fat than someone who is tall and thin.

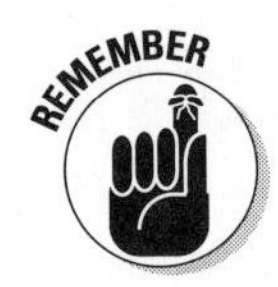


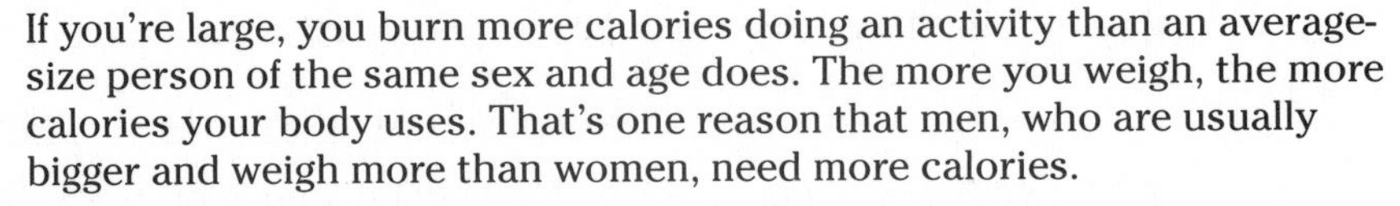

  If you're large, you burn more calories doing an activity than an average-size person of the same sex and age does. The more you weigh, the more calories your body uses. That's one reason that men, who are usually bigger and weigh more than women, need more calories.

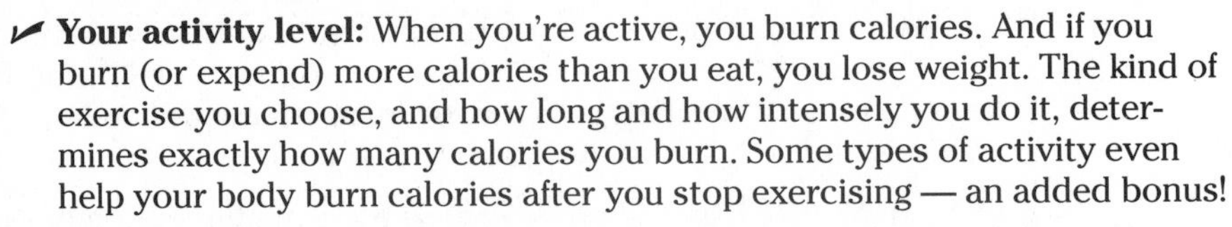

- **Your activity level:** When you're active, you burn calories. And if you burn (or expend) more calories than you eat, you lose weight. The kind of exercise you choose, and how long and how intensely you do it, determines exactly how many calories you burn. Some types of activity even help your body burn calories after you stop exercising — an added bonus!

  Exercise, particularly resistance training, is also important to help minimize muscle loss that naturally occurs as you get older and during weight loss. See Chapter 12 for more on how exercise helps you lose weight.

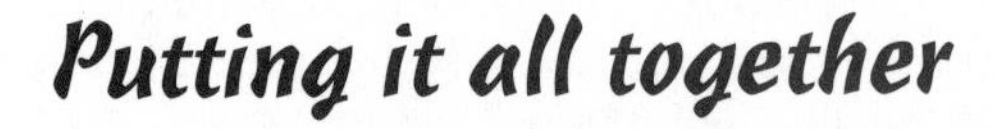

## Putting it all together

Determining your body's total energy needs takes a bit of math — so grab a calculator and go figure. (Don't let the prospect of a little math scare you away. This method is easier than, and almost as accurate, as checking into a research lab and submitting yourself to scientific scrutiny by a white-coated nerd with a clipboard and a stopwatch. And, if precision isn't your thing, flip to the end of this chapter for a shortcut version. It'll get you in the ballpark, but without a specifically assigned seat.) Follow these steps:

1. **Estimate your basic energy needs.**

   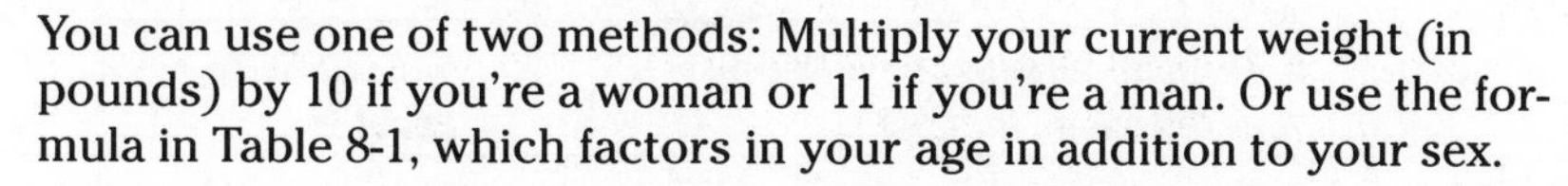

   You can use one of two methods: Multiply your current weight (in pounds) by 10 if you're a woman or 11 if you're a man. Or use the formula in Table 8-1, which factors in your age in addition to your sex.

   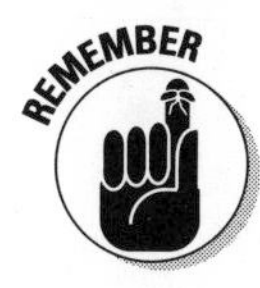
   

   In the formula, *weight* represents your weight in kilograms, so translate your weight into kilograms by dividing the number of pounds you weigh by 2.2.

**Table 8-1 How Many Calories Your Body Needs Per Day for Basic Energy Needs**

| *Age* | *Use This Equation to Calculate Your BMR* |
|---|---|
| **Men** | |
| 18 to 30 | [15.3 x weight (in kilograms)] + 679 |
| 30 to 60 | [11.6 x weight (in kilograms)] + 879 |
| Older than 60 | [13.5 x weight (in kilograms)] + 487 |
| **Women** | |
| 18 to 30 | [14.7 x weight (in kilograms)] + 496 |
| 30 to 60 | [8.7 x weight (in kilograms)] + 829 |
| Older than 60 | [10.5 x weight (in kilograms)] + 596 |

   For example: Sue is a 45-year-old female who weighs 155 pounds. She calculates her BMR like this:

   155 pounds ÷ 2.2 = 70.45 kilograms

   70.45 kilograms x 8.7 = 612.92 calories

   612.92 calories + 829 calories = 1,441.92 calories

   So, Sue's BMR — or the number of calories that her body needs at complete rest to function — is roughly 1,442 calories.

   If you figure Sue's BMR by using the shortcut method, her needs are about 1,550 (155 pounds x 10 = 1,550) — a bit higher than the full calculation, but still in the same ballpark.

2. **Determine your activity factor value.**

   How active are you? Find the description in Table 8-2 that best matches your lifestyle. If you have a desk job but fit in a dose of daily exercise (at least 30 minutes), consider yourself in the light or moderate category.

**Table 8-2 How Active Are You?**

| *If, Throughout Most of Your Day, Your Activities Include* | *Your Activity Level Is* | *Your Activity Factor Is* |
|---|---|---|
| Sitting or standing; driving; painting; doing laboratory work; sewing, ironing, or cooking; playing cards or a musical instrument; sleeping or lying down; reading; typing | Very light | 0.2 |
| Doing garage, electrical, carpentry, or restaurant work; house-cleaning; caring for children; playing golf; sailing; light exercise, such as walking, for no more than 2 miles | Light | 0.3 |
| Heavy gardening or housework, cycling, playing tennis, skiing, or dancing; very little sitting | Moderate | 0.4 |
| Heavy manual labor such as construction work or digging; playing sports such as basketball, football, or soccer; climbing | Heavy | 0.5 |

3. **Multiply your basic energy needs by the activity factor value that you determined in Step 2:**

   ____________ × ____________ = ________________

   BMR Activity factor Calories for activity

   Using Sue as an example, she multiplies her BMR of 1,442 by 0.3 because her activity level is light — running around after her kids, taking care of the house, and fitting in a 2-mile morning walk with her neighbors every other day. Sue needs 432.6 calories for her activity level.

   1,442 x 0.3 = 432.6 calories

4. **Determine the number of calories that you need for digestion and absorption of nutrients.**

   Eating food actually burns calories. Digesting food and absorbing nutrients uses about 10 percent of your daily energy needs. Add together your BMR and activity calories and then multiply the total by 10 percent.

   (____________ + ____________) × 10% = ________________

   BMR calories Activity calories Calories for digestion/absorption

The calculation for Sue's calorie needs for digestion and absorption looks like this:

1,442 calories + 432.6 calories = 1874.6 x 10% = 187.5 calories

5. **Total your calorie needs.**

   Add together your BMR, activity, and digestion/absorption calorie needs to get your total calorie needs — that is, the number of calories that you need to maintain your current weight.

| ________ | × | ________ | + | ________ | = | ________ |
|---|---|---|---|---|---|---|
| BMR calories | | Activity calories | | Digestion/ absorption calories | | Total calories |

   To maintain her current weight of 155 pounds, Sue calculates her total calorie needs like this:

   1,442 calories + 432.6 calories + 187.5 calories = 2,062 total calories

# Setting a Reasonable Calorie Level for Weight Loss

To lose weight, you have to cut down on how much you eat — but not too much. If you try to cut too many calories, you may not lose any weight at all. When you cut calories severely, your metabolic rate slows to adjust to the lower calorie level. In addition, you probably won't be able to stick to your plan for very long, because you'll be hungry all the time. This section can help you find the right balance of calories for you.

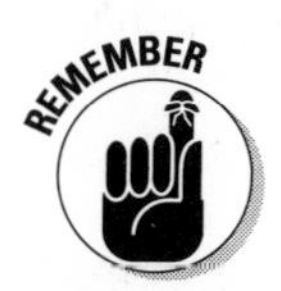


Too much food isn't the only cause of obesity; lack of exercise is also part of the formula. So when you think about dieting, you need to redefine your definition to mean cutting calories *and* upping exercise. See Chapter 12 for more information about adding exercise to your daily routine.

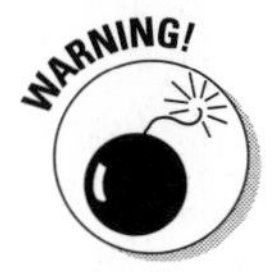


Don't cut your calorie level drastically when trying to lose weight; this strategy will backfire. Your body is programmed to defend your usual weight, so when calories are cut severely — to fewer than 800 to 1,000 a day — your metabolic rate adjusts to conserve the few calories you do give your body. You won't lose weight any faster than if you allowed yourself to enjoy 1,200 to 1,500 a day. Fortunately, when you overeat occasionally, your metabolism speeds up to burn the extra calories, too — ever striving to maintain your normal weight.

## Knowing how many calories to cut

Because there are 3,500 calories in a pound and 7 days in a week, you can cut your daily calorie intake by 500 to lose 1 pound a week (3,500 ÷ 7 = 500). To lose 1½ pounds, you need to cut 750 calories a day. A 2-pound-a-week loss means eliminating 1,000 calories a day. A faster rate of weight loss is generally associated with weight regain and yo-yo dieting. Remember the tortoise and the hare: Slow and steady wins the race.

Look at how these guidelines affect Mary's weight-loss plans. After determining how many calories she needs each day to maintain her present weight, she knows that her present calorie level is about 2,472 calories each day. To lose 1 pound per week, Mary needs to cut 500 calories a day, bringing her weight-loss calorie level to 1,972. To lose 1½ pounds a week, her new calorie level would be 1,722 (2,472 – 750 = 1,722). Attempting to lose 2 pounds per week means that Mary's calorie allotment would drop to 1,472 calories. This amount, while still safe, may be too low for Mary's personal needs.

## Using the 20 percent rule

If you're not eating many calories now and a reduction of 500 to 750 calories per day would put your calorie intake below 800 to 1,000 a day and, therefore, put your metabolism into low gear, use the 20 percent rule. It's a healthier way to lose weight.

First, figure out the average number of calories you eat now. To do so, see the section, "Tracking How Many Calories You Eat" earlier in this chapter.

After you determine the average number of calories you consume, simply subtract 20 percent. We'll use Maureen as an example. According to Maureen's food records, she eats about 1,800 calories a day and would like to lose 20 pounds. Her calculations are as follows:

1,800 calories x 0.20 = 360 calories

1,800 calories – 360 calories = 1,440 calories

If Maureen cuts her calorie consumption by about 360 calories to 1,440 calories, she can lose between ½ and ¾ pound a week — a healthy rate of loss that won't leave her starving. In about seven months, Maureen should reach her goal. Slow and steady, but she's more likely to keep it off than if she tried to lose it in half that time.

# Chapter 9

# Putting Healthful Eating Guidelines into Practice

### *In This Chapter*

- Letting the Food Guide Pyramid guide you
- Checking out food groups and portions
- Charting the course for weight loss
- Planning low-calorie meals

The United States Department of Agriculture's Food Guide Pyramid, although widely criticized and reworked by some health groups, is the main tool that we recommend to help plan your diet. In this chapter, we fill you in on the controversies and suggest how you can use this information to make your diet the healthiest it can be. Look for paragraphs marked with the FYI icon that highlight the topics and recommendations under debate.

## Glimpsing the Food Guide Pyramid

The Food Guide Pyramid (shown in Figure 9-1) is considered the mother of all pyramids. The Vegetarian, Mediterranean, and the Asian Pyramid among others were modeled after this one. It's flexible, practical, and visual, so no matter what your eating preferences are, you can make it fit your lifestyle.

The Food Guide Pyramid contains the building blocks for a healthy diet. If you follow the recommended servings listed for each food group in the pyramid each day and eat lowfat, low-sugar, and low-sodium choices within each group, you're sure to get enough protein, vitamins, minerals, and dietary fiber without getting excessive amounts of calories, fat, saturated fat, cholesterol, sodium, added sugars, or alcohol.

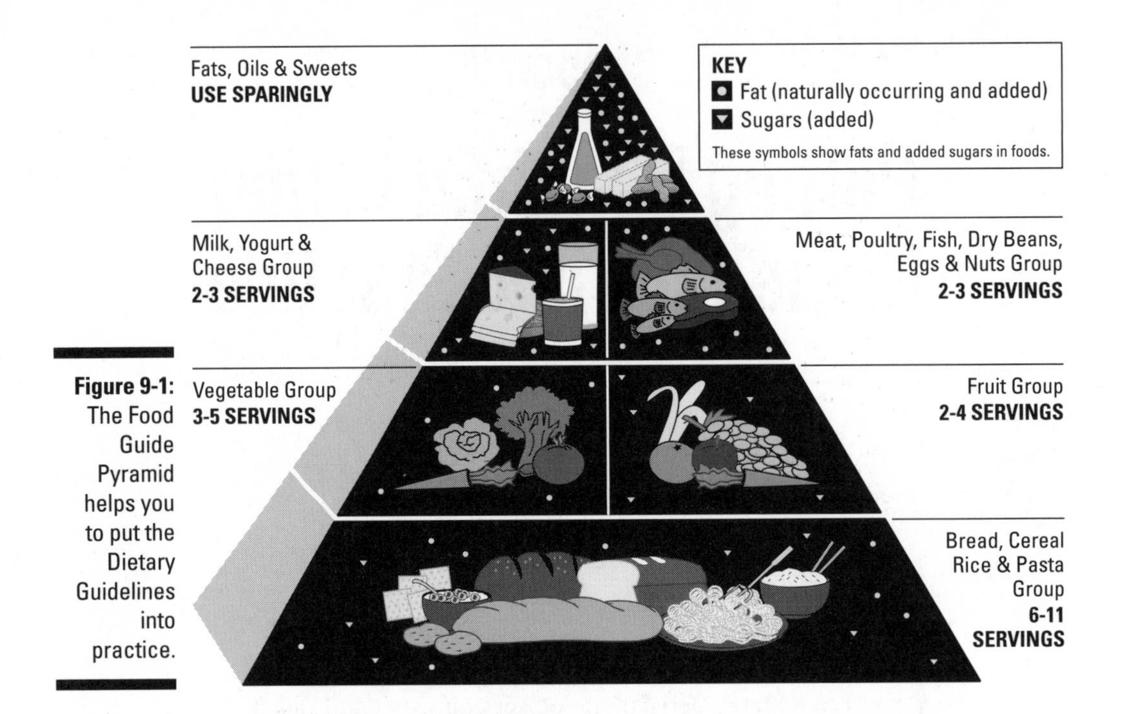


**Figure 9-1:** The Food Guide Pyramid helps you to put the Dietary Guidelines into practice.

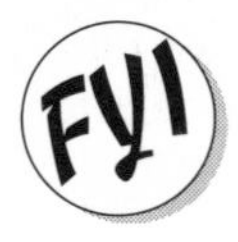

The USDA folks figured that the pyramid illustrated proportion as well as balance, variety, and moderation — the key features of a healthy diet. In focus group tests, the pyramid was easiest for most people to understand. However, not everyone agrees that the shape works. Though several countries have adopted the pyramid, China and Korea use a pagoda, Canada uses a rainbow, Great Britain and Mexico use a plate, and Australia, Sweden, and most of Europe use a pie chart. Sure, they may look different, but all recommend that consumers eat plenty of grains, vegetables, and fruits, and moderate amounts of meat and dairy.

Notice that a range of servings is given for each block, or food group, of the pyramid. The serving sizes are designed to help people maintain their weights depending on how active they are. The lower number is intended to provide adequate nutrition for sedentary women, and the upper limit is for active teenage boys. Individuals who want to lose weight need to stick to the lower number of servings and sometimes go lower still.

Hate the idea of counting calories? If you use the lower range of servings suggested in the pyramid, you'd be eating about 1,600 calories; the large number of servings totals 2,800 calories.

Fats and added sugars are concentrated in foods located at the tip of the pyramid. But they're also in foods found in the other food groups. When you choose foods for a healthy weight-loss diet, take the amount of fat and added sugars in those foods into consideration.

Remember:

- Choose lowfat foods from each of the food groups.
- Go easy on fats and sugars added to foods in cooking and at the table.
- Choose fewer foods that are high in sugars — candy, soft drinks, and sweet desserts.

Using the pyramid can help you identify where the bulk of your calories are coming from. Unfortunately, many people create a top-heavy pyramid by eating too much fat and sugar and not enough grains, fruits, and vegetables, as shown in the Actual Consumption Pyramid in Figure 9-2.

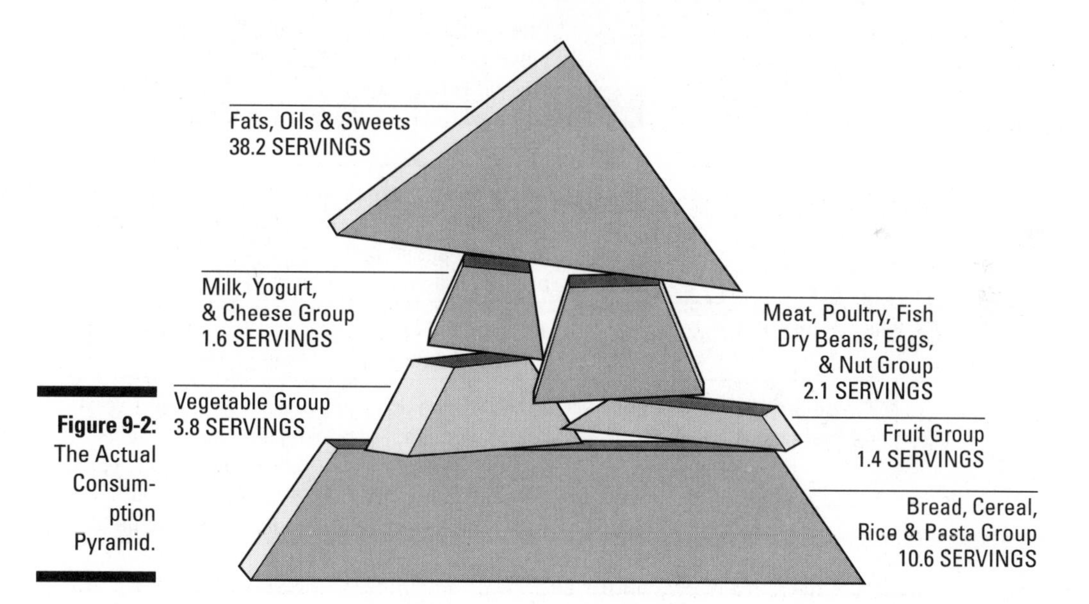


**Figure 9-2:** The Actual Consumption Pyramid.

# Understanding What Makes a Serving

Of course, few people eat foods that fit neatly into one of the pyramid blocks. Pizza, for example, can be counted as dairy, grain, and depending on the topping, either meat or vegetables or both. A cheeseburger piled high with lettuce and tomato and a bit of mayonnaise counts as a serving from each group.

Table 9-1 lists the sizes of many foods that constitute one serving. You can find an extensive list of servings sizes, detailed in the food group discussions that follow.

**Table 9-1 What Counts as a Serving**

| *Food Group* | *One Serving Is . . .* |
|---|---|
| Bread, cereal, rice, and pasta | 1 slice of bread; half a hamburger bun or English muffin; 1 small roll, biscuit, or muffin; 5 to 6 small or 3 to 4 large crackers; ½ cup cooked cereal, rice, or pasta; 1 ounce ready-to-eat cereal |
| Fruit | One whole fruit, such as a medium apple, banana, or orange; half a grapefruit; a melon wedge; ¾ cup fruit juice; ½ cup berries; ½ cup chopped fresh, cooked, or canned fruit; ¼ cup dried fruit |
| Vegetable | ½ cup cooked vegetables; ½ cup chopped raw vegetables; 1 cup leafy raw vegetables, such as lettuce or spinach; ½ cup cooked beans, peas, or other legumes*; ¾ cup vegetable juice |
| Milk, yogurt, and cheese | 1 cup milk, 8 ounces yogurt, 1½ ounces natural cheese, 2 ounces processed cheese |
| Meat, poultry, fish, dry beans, eggs, and nuts | Amounts should total 2 to 3 servings (for a total of 5 to 7 ounces) of cooked lean meat, poultry without skin, or fish per day. Count 1 egg; ½ cup cooked beans, peas, or other legumes*; or 2 tablespoons peanut butter as 1 ounce of meat |
| Fats, oils, and sweets | Use sparingly |

**Note that you can count dry beans, peas, and other legumes as a serving of vegetables or a serving of meat, but the same bowl of beans can't count as a serving from both groups.*

You've heard it before: It's not only *what* you eat but also *how much* that's important. As people eat more foods from restaurants and convenience stores, it's difficult to remember how large a serving should be. Portions of takeout food are huge — much larger than the standard portion sizes defined in the Food Guide Pyramid. (See Chapter 7 to read more about how portion sizes affect your weight and health.) Even cookbooks are instructing people to serve larger portions. For example, the 1964 edition of *The Joy of Cooking* recommends cutting a 13-x-9-inch pan of brownies into 30 bars; the 1997 version is cut into 16 bars.

## Perception isn't necessarily reality

Table 9-2 illustrates a few discrepancies between what most people consider an "average" serving and the size that the USDA's pyramid recommends [see Young and Nestle in the *Journal of the American Dietetic Association* 98(4), 1998].

**Table 9-2 How Large Is Medium?**

| *Food* | *USDA (In Ounces)* | *Perceived as Average (In Ounces)* |
|---|---|---|
| Bagel | 2.0 | 4.0 |
| Cookies | 0.5 | 1.0 |
| Muffin | 1.5 | 5.5 |
| Potato | 3.9 | 6.5 |

## Taking measures into your own hand

A half-ounce of peanuts. An ounce of cheese. Two cups of popcorn. A quarter cup of sunflower seeds. A teaspoon of butter. A 3-ounce chicken breast. These are foods that you're apt to run into when you're eating on the run. After all, no one goes to a restaurant or movie theatre packing measuring spoons or cups — at least no one we care to know. So how are you going to know what a serving of these foods look like?

A deck of cards is about the size of a 3-ounce chicken breast, but if the cards you play are on your computer screen more often than in your hand, you may not recognize what a portion looks like. But you take something with you wherever you go that can help you with portion size. It's in the palm of your hand. In fact, it *is* the palm of your hand, and it's the perfect portion measurement. That is, if you're an average female. Gentlemen, hold your honey's hand more often to get a sense of size. Better still, make sure to take her to restaurants and movies with you. Figure 9-3 gives you some other "handy" measurements.

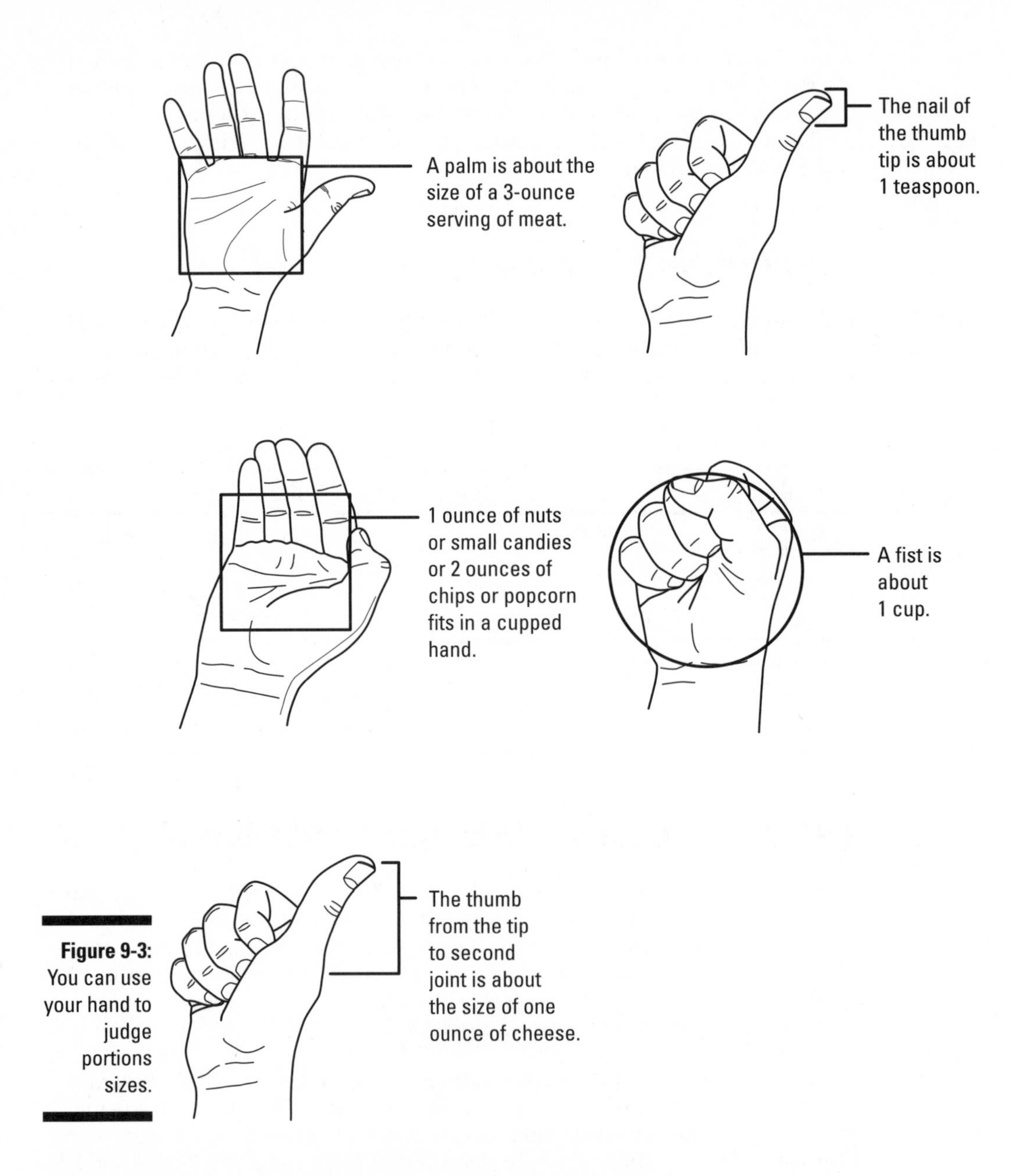


**Figure 9-3:** You can use your hand to judge portions sizes.

# Looking at the Food Groups

All your favorite (and not-so-favorite) foods have a place on the Food Guide Pyramid. Foods are grouped together because their nutrient content is similar. And each of the five food groups, which we describe in detail in the following sections, supplies your body with some of the nutrients that you need for good health. Remember, some of the foods in the various groups may be higher in fat or added sugars than others, so when you're watching calories, focus on the lower-fat options that contain less added sugar.

## The ground floor: Grains (6 to 11 servings)

Grains form the foundation of eating healthfully; they're low in fat and provide essential vitamins, minerals, and fiber. This group is the source of complex carbohydrates in your diet. But eating too many calories without getting beneficial nutrients is also common.

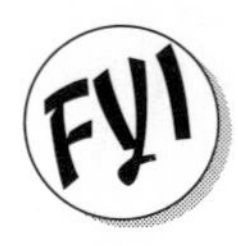


The grains group has been the source of the greatest controversy among health professionals. Critics think that too much emphasis is placed on carbohydrates as a foundation of a healthy diet and that the number of recommended servings is too high.

It's true that croissants, donuts, cookies, muffins, cake, and other high fat and sugar items are in this group because they can fit into a healthy diet — just not everyday, and probably not more than once a week if you're trying to lose weight. Because they provide more calories than nutrients, keep them to a minimum. The healthier choice is anything whole grain in a reasonable portion.

Make sure that at least three of your grain servings each day are whole grains — whole-wheat bread or cereal, for example. Use the ingredient labels to find the products with whole grains: You want whole wheat or other whole grain to be the first ingredient. Sugar, oil, and fats should be last on the list, if they appear at all.

Serving sizes for grains include the following:

- 1 slice of bread
- Half a hamburger or hot dog bun
- Half an English muffin or a 2½-inch bagel
- 1 small roll, biscuit, or muffin (about 1 ounce each)
- 1 ounce ready-to-eat cereal
- 5 to 6 small crackers (saltine size)
- 2 to 3 large crackers (graham cracker square size)
- 4-inch pita bread (white or wheat)
- 3 medium hard breadsticks, about 4¾ inches long
- 9 animal crackers

- ½ cup cooked cereal, pasta, or rice
- One 7-inch flour or corn tortilla
- 2 corn taco shells
- Nine 3-ring pretzels or 2 pretzel rods
- ⅕ of a 10-inch angel food cake
- 1⁄16 of a two-layer cake
- 3 rice or popcorn cakes
- 2 cups air-popped popcorn
- 12 tortilla chips

Fiber comes from the grains group, the fruit and vegetable group, legumes in the meat group and from nuts. Essentially, fiber is a carbohydrate that can't be digested. A healthy diet has 25 to 35 grams each day. High-fiber diets are associated with less heart disease and diabetes.

## Second tier: Fruits and vegetables

Fruits and vegetables form the next layer of the pyramid. Both provide important vitamins, minerals, and fiber. Without high-fat toppings, such as butter and whipped cream, they're also naturally low in fat with few exceptions.

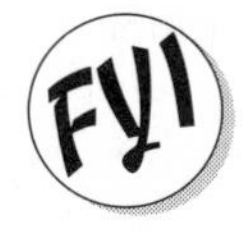


If you think that the number of servings of fruits and vegetables is impossible to consume each day, consider the fact that critics of the pyramid believe the recommendations are too low. For example, the Nurse's Health Study of more than 80,000 people demonstrated that people who ate more than eight servings a day had a 20 percent lower risk of heart disease than those who ate three or fewer servings. Further, their research showed that for each serving of fruits or vegetables, risk of heart disease decreased by 4 percent. Green leafy vegetables and vitamin C rich fruits had the greatest effect. For additional details from this study, see *Annals of Internal Medicine,* 2001, 134(12): 1106–14.

Most of the news in nutrition research is about the health benefits of a group of nutrients concentrated in vegetables and fruits called *antioxidants.* These nutrients help minimize the normal wear and tear that comes from living and can reduce the risk of cancer and stroke as well as heart disease. Vitamins, such as *folate* and *B6,* and the large family known as *carotinoids* — such as *lycopene* in tomatoes, *beta carotene* in mangos and carrots, *lutein* in spinach and collard greens, and *zeaxanthin* in greens and corn — are some of the antioxidants that have been identified. Yet researchers point out that so many other phytonutrients that haven't been isolated also factor in to the health benefits of eating more plant foods. Eating more fruits and vegetables, instead of popping supplements, ensures that you won't miss a single one.

### Fruits (2 to 4 servings)

Breakfast is a good place to begin building up fruit servings. You may already start your day with a glass of juice. Add a midmorning snack of fruit and have some for dessert at lunch or dinner, and you've made your goal of three to four servings a day.

Make at least one serving each day a citrus fruit. Orange and grapefruit juice are standard options, but don't forget about the many varieties of oranges (navel, temple, Valencia, blood, and mandarin) and grapefruits (Ruby Red, white, and pink) that are available, as well as tangerines, tangelos, kumquats, and Ugli fruit, which are also considered citrus fruits. When possible, select fresh fruit in season. In the Northern Hemisphere, you can buy fresh strawberries in February and apples in May. But because they aren't in season, the fruit must be flown into the market from other climates or put into storage. Out of season fruit tends to be grown for longevity rather than flavor. It's no wonder so many people are turned off by fruit when it means red but flavorless winter strawberries or mushy melons. Instead, choosing oranges and grapefruit in winter and berries in spring, means there's a better chance that the fruit was grown locally and will end up tasting juicy and fresh.

Canned or frozen fruit can be a good substitute when a recipe or your appetite demands an out of season fruit. Be sure to reach for ones packed without added sugar.

Experiment with new fruits that you haven't tried before — figs, guava, star fruit, or prickly pears, for example. Many supermarkets stock large varieties of fruits worth investigating. Or you may want to use a meal out for a taste test, which can also give you an idea of an appropriate and skilled way to prepare the new fruits. Try less-common varieties of favorite fruits, such as Winesap or Rome apples; Casaba, Persian, or Santa Claus melons; or Comice or Seckel pears. Blend fresh or frozen fruits together with a dollop of lowfat yogurt, a splash of orange juice, and a ripe banana for a scrumptious fruit smoothie. Toss citrus segments, grape halves, or strawberries in with mixed greens and add lowfat poppy-seed dressing for a pretty and nutritious salad. Or sprinkle fresh or dried fruits on cereal, on frozen or regular yogurt, into muffin batter, or into rice and stuffing dishes.

With so many fruitfully delicious options to choose from, you'll never have to eat the same fruit twice in a week. Use these guidelines to determine serving sizes for fruits:

- One whole fruit (a medium apple, banana, peach, or orange; or a small pear)
- ½ grapefruit
- Melon wedge (¼ medium cantaloupe or ⅛ medium honeydew)

- ¾ cup juice
- ½ cup mandarin or clementine orange sections
- ½ cup cut-up fresh fruit
- ½ cup cooked or canned fruit
- ½ cup frozen fruit
- ¼ cup dried fruit
- 5 large strawberries or 7 medium strawberries
- ½ cup raspberries, blueberries, or blackberries
- 11 large cherries
- 12 grapes
- 1½ medium plums
- 2 medium apricots or clementines
- ⅛ medium avocado (but beware of its high fat content!)
- 7 melon balls (or ½ cup melon)
- ½ cup fruit salad (made without mayonnaise)
- ½ medium mango
- ¼ medium papaya
- 1 large kiwi fruit
- 4 canned apricot halves, drained
- 14 canned cherries, drained
- 1½ canned peach halves, drained
- 2 canned pear halves, drained
- 2½ canned pineapple slices, drained
- 3 canned plums, drained
- 9 dried apricot halves
- 5 prunes

### Vegetables (3 to 5 servings)

If it weren't for French-fried potatoes and tomato sauce on pizza and pasta, many people wouldn't get any vegetables at all. Too bad, because vegetables are mostly water, so they're a great way for dieters to expand their meals. Vegetables are a great source of vitamin C, folate, beta carotene, minerals, and fiber — and practically no fat.

Use these guidelines to determine serving sizes for vegetables:

- ½ cup vegetables, cooked or chopped raw
- 1 cup leafy raw vegetables, such as lettuce or spinach
- 1 medium tomato or 5 cherry tomatoes
- Seven to eight 2½-inch carrot or celery sticks
- 3 broccoli florets
- ⅓ medium cucumber
- 10 medium green onions
- 13 medium radishes
- 9 snow or sugar peas
- 6 slices summer squash (yellow or zucchini)
- 1 cup mixed green salad
- ½ cup cole slaw or potato salad
- ½ cup leafy cooked greens, such as kale, Swiss chard, or spinach
- 2 spears broccoli
- 1 medium whole green or red pepper, or 8 rings
- 1 artichoke
- 6 asparagus spears
- 2 whole beets, about 2 inches in diameter
- 4 medium Brussels sprouts
- 1 medium ear of corn
- 7 medium mushrooms
- 8 okra pods
- 1 medium whole onion or 6 pearl onions
- 1 medium whole turnip
- 10 French fries
- 1 medium baked potato
- ¾ cup sweet potato
- ½ cup tomato or spaghetti sauce
- ¼ cup tomato paste
- ½ cup cooked dry beans (if not counted as a meat alternate)

- ¾ cup vegetable juice
- 1 cup bean soup
- 1 cup vegetable soup

Some vegetables are "starchy" and calorie dense; others are mostly water. If you're watching your weight, limit your starchy vegetables to one or two servings per day, and make the remainder of your veggie servings nonstarchy. Table 9-3 lists examples of starchy and nonstarchy vegetables.

**Table 9-3 Vegetable Variations**

| *Nonstarchy Vegetables* | *Starchy Vegetables* |
|---|---|
| Asparagus | Beets |
| Broccoli | Cassava (yuca) |
| Brussels sprouts | Corn |
| Cabbage | Lima Beans |
| Cauliflower | Peas |
| Celery | Potatoes |
| Chicory | Pumpkin |
| Cucumbers | Rutabaga |
| Eggplant | Sweet Potatoes |
| Escarole | Taro |
| Green beans | Turnips |
| Greens (such as collard, kale, mustard, and turnip) | Winter squash |
| Lettuce | Yams |
| Mushrooms | |
| Okra | |
| Peppers | |
| Radishes | |
| Sprouts | |
| Summer squash | |
| Tomatoes | |

Looking for ways to up your veggie intake? Try these delicious ideas:

- Pile a sandwich high with lettuce, tomato, and vegetables.
- Start every meal with a salad: a mix of dark green varieties of lettuce and colorful vegetables, drizzled with just a bit of low-calorie dressing.
- When you need a snack, reach for cherry tomatoes, celery, or sweet pepper strips. Many supermarkets carry small packages of celery or carrot sticks in their produce sections. They make good lunch box (or briefcase) snacks for kids of all ages.
- Toss pasta with steamed broccoli, carrots, and other veggies and top with a smidgen of Parmesan cheese for pasta primavera. Or add finely chopped veggies — such as carrots, onions, cooked eggplant, squash, or chopped spinach — to pasta sauce.
- Toss a can of veggie or tomato juice into your briefcase for a quick pick-me-up (and a serving of vegetables to boot!).
- Top a baked potato with thick vegetable salsa or stir-fried vegetables.

## Third tier: Animal foods and products

Moving up the pyramid, you find foods that come mostly from animals — the Dairy group and the Meat, Poultry, Fish, Dry Beans, Eggs, and Nuts group. Foods from this level contribute important nutrients, such as protein, calcium, iron, and zinc.

### Meat and meat alternates (2 to 3 servings equivalent to a total of 5 to 7 ounces)

Two to 3 ounces of meat, poultry, or fish (about the size of your palm) is an adequate amount of protein for a meal. Choose the select grades of beef, veal, and lamb to make sure that you get the least-marbled meats. Also, opt for lean cuts of meat, such as those from the round, loin, or leg (beef sirloin, ground round, or top round; pork tenderloin or loin chop; or leg of lamb). Select lean and extra-lean ground beef. Unless you're eating fat-free cold cuts, be extra cautious in the deli; many have more fat than lean meat per slice. Most fish are naturally lean.

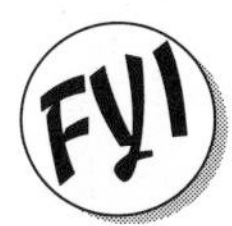


In the USDA view of the food world, meats, beans, nuts, and eggs are ganged together. They all do have higher amounts of protein than other foods in the pyramid, but that's where critics say the similarities end. Red meat has been associated with increased cancer risk, and some other meat, such as cold cuts, are particularly high in fat. New scientific evidence shows that nuts have vitamin E and beans have fiber that makes them more unique, not similar to meat. Plus, the fat in fish trumps the fat in red meat and chicken.

## Cruciferous vegetables

*Cruciferous vegetables* — bok choy, broccoli, Brussels sprouts, cabbage, cauliflower, kale, collards, kohlrabi, mustard greens, radishes, rutabaga, turnip, and watercress — are the cancer-fighters from the garden. They're called *cruciferous,* because their flowers or buds form a cross. Besides helping to protect against colon and rectal cancer, they're also good sources of calcium, iron, and folate.

When meat is your protein of choice, trim all visible fat before cooking and remove the skin from poultry before eating. And use lower-fat cooking methods, such as roasting, broiling, and grilling instead of frying, sautéing, or pan-frying. Have fish a minimum of one day a week, and make at least one meal meatless. Dried beans and peas (legumes) are a good substitute for meat in this group.

Check out these options to meet your protein needs:

**Meats (each counts as 1 serving):**

- 2 to 3 ounces cooked lean beef, pork, veal, or lamb without bone
- 2 to 3 ounces cooked poultry without skin or bone
- 2 to 3 ounces cooked fish without bone
- 2 to 3 ounces drained, canned fish

**Meat alternates (each counts as 1 ounce, about ⅓ serving):**

- 1 egg (yolk and white) or 2 egg whites
- ½ cup cooked dry beans (if not counted as a vegetable)
- 2 tablespoons peanut butter
- ¼ cup seeds, such as sunflower or pumpkin seeds
- ⅓ cup nuts, such as walnuts, pecans, or peanuts
- ½ cup baked beans
- ½ cup tofu

**Meat and fish products (each counts as 1 ounce, about ⅓ serving):**

- 1 ounce lean ham or Canadian bacon
- 1½ frankfurters (10 per pound)

- 1 frankfurter (8 per pound)
- ¼ cup drained canned salmon or tuna
- ⅓ cup drained canned clams or crabmeat
- 4 Pacific oysters or 11 Atlantic oysters
- 6 medium shrimp
- ¼ cup drained canned lobster or shrimp

### Dairy products (2 to 3 servings)

The Milk, Yogurt, and Cheese group shares the third tier of the pyramid with the Meat, Poultry, Fish, Dry Beans, Eggs, and Nuts group. Like foods in the meat group, dairy foods are a good source of protein. They're also some of the best sources of calcium and contribute vitamins A and D to your diet as well.

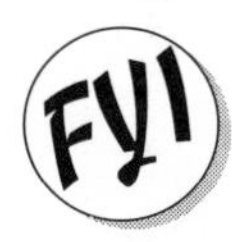


A word of caution: Dairy foods can be very high in fat, so reach for fat-free, lowfat, part-skim, or reduced-fat cheeses, ice cream, frozen yogurt, ice milk, and fluid milk products when you're watching your weight. If dairy products aren't your cup of tea, so to speak, make sure you're getting enough calcium by eating more dark leafy greens. A supplement may also add to your daily requirement. But keep in mind, recent evidence shows that dairy products can actually help you lose weight. There have been many studies that prove it. One intriguing body of work done at the University of Tennessee and published in the medical journal *Lipids* in February 2002 concluded that increasing dietary sources of calcium, especially from dairy products, reduced body fat even without calorie restriction and accelerated weight loss when calories were cut.

If you're lactose intolerant and can't eat dairy products without becoming ill, consider milk that has been treated to reduce the amount of lactose in it. You can find several brands on the market that are worth a try.

*Dairy* delicious ways to get calcium and protein in your diet include the following:

- 1 cup milk or buttermilk
- 1 cup yogurt
- 1½ ounces natural cheese
- 2 ounces processed cheese
- 2 cups cottage cheese (it's lower in calcium than most other cheeses)
- ½ cup ricotta cheese

## Alcohol in your diet

Although alcohol isn't technically part of the pyramid, keep in mind that like items from the pyramid's tip, you get calories but no nutrients in each and every glass. Limit your consumption to no more than two drinks per day if you're male and one drink per day if you're female. A serving of alcohol is defined as

- 12 ounces of beer
- 1½ ounces of hard or distilled spirits (80 proof)
- 5 ounces of wine

- ½ cup dry nonfat milk
- ½ cup evaporated milk
- 1 cup frozen yogurt or 1½ cups ice milk

Don't mistake cheese for the only ideal protein alternative to meat. Sure it delivers some protein, but it also comes with an abundance of fat. If you choose not to eat meat from the meat group, go for water-packed tuna, bean and bean spreads, such as hummus (made with a minimal amount of tahini paste), and soy products, such as tempeh and tofu. Or choose reduced-fat cheeses or lower-fat varieties, such as feta, baby Swiss, and part-skim mozzarella.

## *The tiny tier: Fats, oils, and sweets*

Just because this group is on the top of the pyramid doesn't mean that it's the best group. Instead, this placement means that, like a penthouse, few people can spend much time there. Scan the lists later in this section, and you'll see plenty of foods that you probably eat frequently. Most of these foods contribute practically no nutrients other than sugar, fat, and calories.

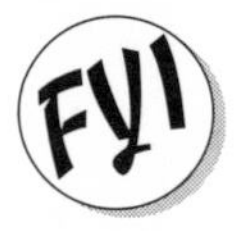


Grouping all fats with sugars riles some health groups. There's not much evidence to justify eating more sugar. However, critics say locking all fats and oils in the attic with sugar and sweets simply isn't fair. All fats have the same number of calories but consider the bigger picture: Trans fats, found in foods made with partially hydrogenated fat, such as some stick margarines and solid vegetable shortening, are as unhealthy as saturated fat — animal fat that's solid at room temperature. Both raise unhealthy LDL cholesterol and contribute to heart disease. Unsaturated fats, on the other hand, improve cholesterol levels and thus lower heart disease risk. The oils of nuts, seeds, and olives are unsaturated. The bottom line, use any fat sparingly; they're caloric. And when you do, make them unsaturated.

**Fats:**

- Bacon and salt pork
- Butter
- Cream (dairy or nondairy)
- Cream cheese
- Lard
- Margarine
- Mayonnaise
- Salad dressing
- Shortening
- Sour cream
- Vegetable oil

**Sugars:**

- Candy
- Corn syrup
- Frosting (icing)
- Fruit drinks (unfortified)
- Gelatin desserts
- Honey
- Jam or jelly
- Maple syrup
- Marmalade
- Molasses
- Popsicles and ices
- Sherbet

- Soft drinks
- Sugar (white and brown)

# Considering the Vegetarian Pyramid

If you don't eat meat, check out the Vegetarian Pyramid, shown in Figure 9-4. Because meat, poultry, and fish are not included in a vegetarian-eating plan, the foundation of this pyramid is divided equally among fruits and vegetables, legumes — such as soybeans and peanuts, and whole grains. Vegetarians should include foods from these three groups at every meal. Nuts and seeds, milk or soymilk, and oils should be consumed daily, and eggs and sugars only occasionally and in small quantities. But dieters should remember that servings of nuts, seeds, and oils should be small, because they're high in fat, and therefore, calories.

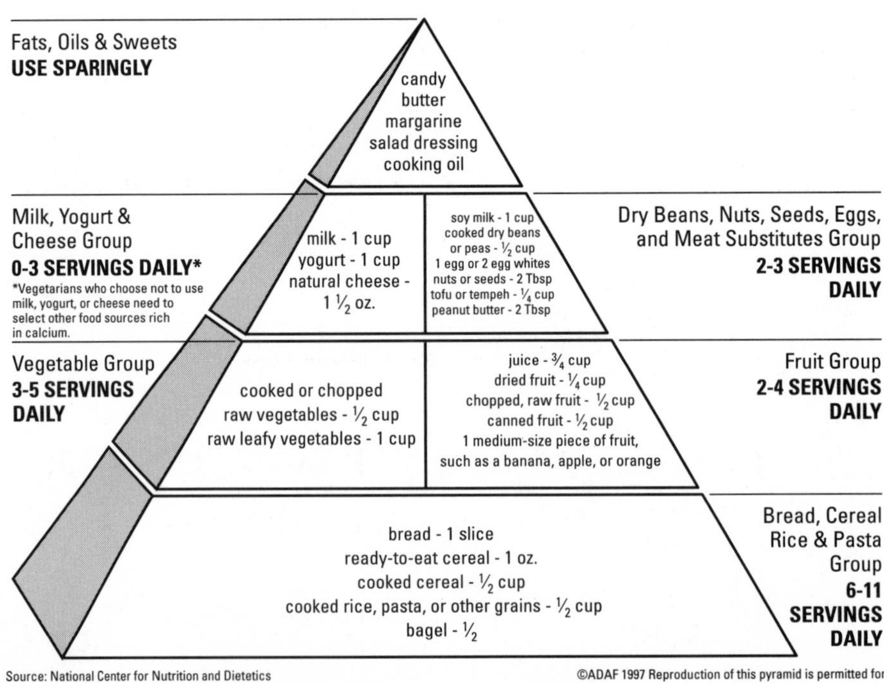


**Figure 9-4:** The Vegetarian Pyramid.

## Are vegetarian diets healthy?

There are varying degrees of vegetarianism. *Lacto-ovo vegetarians* eat dairy products and eggs and, as a group, usually meet their Daily Values for most nutrients.

*Vegans* eat only foods of plant origin. Because animal products are the only food sources of vitamin B12, vegans must use supplements or eat breakfast cereals, soymilk products, and vegetarian burger patties that are fortified with vitamin B12. In addition, vegan diets require care to ensure adequate amounts of vitamin D and calcium, which are found in dairy products. Iron and zinc are often in short supply, too, because meat is a primary source of these nutrients in most people's diets. Although there is some iron in many dark green vegetables, it is a form that is not readily absorbed. So, vegans must be especially diligent at making sure their choices include iron-rich foods.

Vegan sources of iron include

- Dry beans and peas, such as pinto beans, black-eyed peas, and canned baked beans
- Leafy greens of the cabbage family, such as broccoli, kale, turnip greens, and collard greens
- Lima beans and green peas
- Yeast-leavened whole wheat breads and rolls

Vegan sources of zinc include

- Black-eyed peas
- Miso (fermented soybean paste)
- Tofu
- Wheat germ and wheat bran
- Whole grains

Vegan sources of calcium include

- Leafy greens of the cabbage family, such as kale, mustard greens, and turnip tops; and bok choy (or pak choi)
- Tofu, if processed with calcium sulfate (read the labels)
- Tortillas made from lime-processed corn (read the labels)

Vegan sources of vitamin D include

- Fortified breakfast cereals and margarines
- Sunlight — your body makes vitamin D after sunlight (or ultraviolet light) hits your skin

# Using the Pyramid for Weight Loss

After you have a general idea of which foods belong in which food groups, you can start to plan your weight-loss diet. First, revisit the material in Chapter 8 to determine your calorie needs. Then, using the information in Table 9-4, determine the number of servings from each food group that you're allowed, based on your calorie level.

**Table 9-4 Food Group Servings for Various Calorie Levels**

| | *About 1,200* | *About 1,500* | *About 1,800* |
|---|---|---|---|
| Bread group servings | 5 | 6 | 8 |
| Vegetable group servings | 3 | 3 | 5 |
| Fruit group servings | 2 | 3 | 4 |
| Milk group servings | 2 | 2 | 2 |
| Meat group | 5 ounces | 6 ounces | 7 ounces |
| Fats, oils, and sweets | USE | VERY | SPARINGLY |

The Weight-Loss Pyramid, shown in Figure 9-5, is just like the Food Guide Pyramid, except that the number of servings from each group is decreased to the minimum amount needed for good health. When you're dieting and cutting calories, it's more important than ever to choose nutrient-dense foods and not waste calories on "extras" or high fat/sugar/calorie foods that provide little in the way of vitamins and minerals.

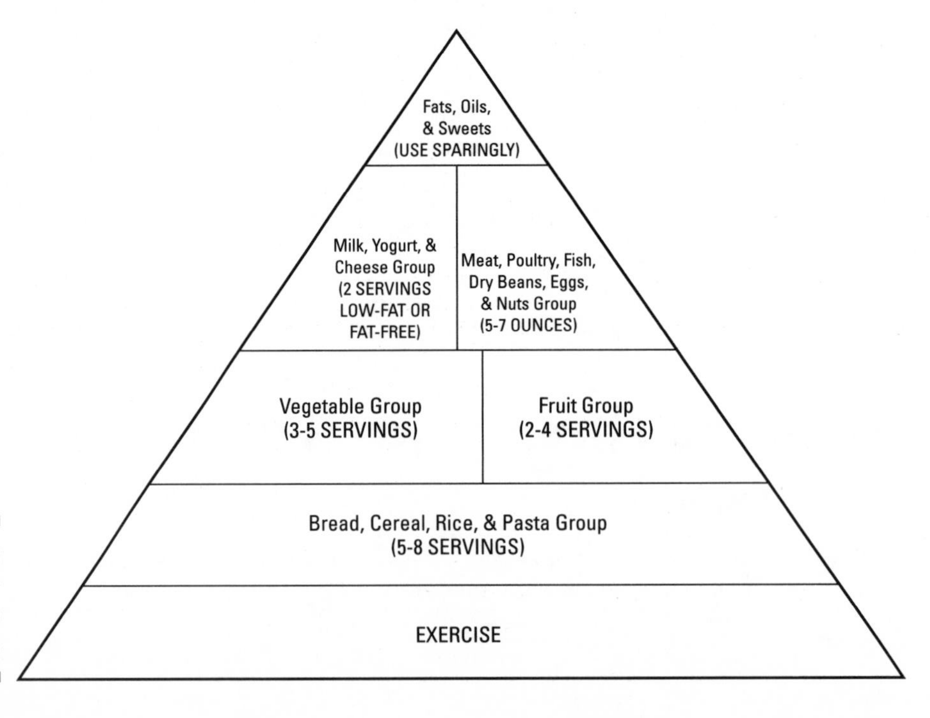


**Figure 9-5:** The Weight-Loss Pyramid.

For the 1,200 calorie diet, you may notice that the number of bread servings allowed is five — less than the usual minimum of six servings for the traditional Food Guide Pyramid. But don't worry; cutting back on a serving of bread won't put you at a loss for nutrients. You get plenty of the B vitamins and fiber that your body needs from five servings. Just make sure that your choices from this group are whole grain and high in fiber.

It's also sometimes difficult to get the 1,000 to 1,200 milligrams of calcium required from just two servings of dairy. To help boost your calcium intake from other food sources, include a serving of dark green, leafy vegetables; drink a glass of calcium-fortified orange juice as one of your fruit servings; and, for health insurance, include a calcium supplement.

Meeting all your nutrient requirements is difficult when drastically limiting calories. If your calorie intake is 1,200 calories or lower, be sure to take a multivitamin-mineral supplement.

# Planning Your Meals

How do you keep all these portion sizes and food groups straight? A simple sheet of paper can help. Make a grid like the one shown in Table 9-5, placing the days of the week across the top and the food groups down the side. Next to each food group, write the number of servings that your calorie level allows. Then, each day, make Xs in the appropriate columns until you reach your daily allotment. Not only is this chart a quick visual reference for you, but studies show that dieters who track what they eat each day are more successful in losing weight and keeping it off.

**Table 9-5 Sample Week at 1,200 Calories**

| *Food Group* | *M* | *T* | *W* | *T* | *F* | *S* | *S* |
|---|---|---|---|---|---|---|---|
| Bread (5) | xxxxx | | | | | | |
| Fruit (2) | xx | | | | | | |
| Vegetable (3) | xx | | | | | | |
| Meat (5 ounces) | xxx | | | | | | |
| Milk (2) | xx | | | | | | |
| Fats, oils, and sweets | x | | | | | | |

If you see that you've had all your meat and dairy for the day, for example, and you want something to snack on, try a piece of fruit or a few raw vegetables if you haven't had all your servings for the day.

A sample day may look like the following:

**Breakfast:**

- 6 ounces orange juice (fruit)
- 1 slice whole-wheat toast (bread)
- Hard-cooked egg (meat)
- Jelly (fats, oils, and sweets)

Don't skip breakfast. Your mother was right, and so are the 3,000 people in the National Weight Control Registry (NWCR). These people are losers! As in, on average each lost about 60 pounds and kept it off for about 6 years. A 2002 study in the journal Obesity Research reported that only 114 of the 3,000 didn't eat breakfast.

**Lunch:**

- Turkey sandwich made with 2 ounces of meat (2 bread, 2 meat)
- Lettuce and tomato (vegetable)
- 1 cup fat-free milk (milk)
- One-quarter cantaloupe (fruit)

**Snack:**

- 2 cups popcorn (bread)
- Diet soda (free)

**Dinner:**

- 2 ounces of broiled fish (meat)
- 1 small baked potato (vegetable)
- ½ cup broccoli (vegetable)

## "Free" foods may not be so free

Certain foods are considered "free" foods, because they provide almost no calories. Examples of free foods include sugar-free hard candies or chewing gum, diet soft drinks or drink mixes, club soda, sugar-free gelatin, and bouillon or broth. Using these free foods as extras throughout the day is fine, but don't overdo them. Although each one individually provides few calories, if you go overboard with some of them, the sodium can start to add up.

## Crunchy snacks

To lose weight, you know that you need to replace high-fat potato chips with lower-fat choices. But what do you eat when you need some crunch and you've had your fill of celery? Try one of these snacks (but don't forget to add them to your daily food group serving totals):

Lowfat crunchy snacks:

- 2 cups air-popped popcorn
- 4-inch pita cut into wedges and baked
- 10 baked tortilla chips
- 3 breadsticks
- ½ cup Cheerios
- 2 graham crackers
- 1 matzo
- Nine 3-ring pretzels or 2 rods
- 3 rice cakes
- 5 saltines
- 2 zwieback crackers

**Snack:**

- Apple (fruit)
- 1½ ounces lowfat cheese (dairy)
- 5 saltine crackers (grain)

# Tailoring Your Diet to Include Healthier Choices

To plan your diet, you can follow a printed diet sheet that offers no choice or variation regardless of your personal taste preferences. But what happens when you reach your goal weight? What have you discovered? Better to use the weight-loss process as a learning experience toward making healthier food choices. When you make those choices, keep these three points in mind:

- **Variety:** You can achieve a healthful, nutritious eating pattern with many combinations of foods. For the best variety, choose foods within and across food groups, because foods within the same group have different combinations of nutrients and other beneficial substances. For example, chicken, beef, pork, and fish all contain iron, but in varying amounts; pork has more B vitamins than other protein choices. Some vegetables and fruits are good sources of vitamin C or vitamin A, and others are high in folate; still others are good sources of calcium or iron. Choosing a variety of foods within each group also makes your meals more interesting from day to day.

- **Balance:** You need to balance the kinds and amounts of food on your plate as well as what you eat over the course of a day and over an entire week. The most satisfying meals are a combination of protein foods, grains, vegetables, and fruits. A lunch of only salad or a breakfast of only a bagel and coffee won't stay with you for long. But if you build balance into your meals, you'll feel satisfied longer.
- **Moderation:** Keeping portions moderate in size and content allows for flexibility. You may find room for a small or kiddie-size treat even on a weight-reduction diet but probably not a super-size treat.

# Chapter 10

# Using the Dietary Guidelines to Design Your Own Diet

### In This Chapter

- Making sure that you know healthy diet basics
- Huffing and puffing your way through to fitness
- Getting all the necessary nutrients and fiber, too
- Understanding how drinking alcohol affects health

Forgetting that you have many important reasons to eat is easy when you're dieting. Instead of calculating your calorie intake and expenditure with Scrooge-like precision, take the Tiny Tim approach and focus on all the goodies that foods give you — such as fiber, vitamins, minerals, and, of course, pleasure! Don't just concentrate on how many calories or how much fat is in a food — what you probably consider as negatives. In this chapter, you can find out how stepping back and looking at the big picture is what's best for your weight, as well as your general well-being.

Many kinds of dietary recommendations come from government-funded organizations and health associations. Some recommendations detail specific quantities of nutrients that you should consume daily, such as the Daily Values that you see on food labels and dietary supplement labels. Others, such as the Food Guide Pyramid and the Dietary Guidelines for Americans, are more general in nature, but they're hardly vague.

Both the Food Guide Pyramid and the Dietary Guidelines for Americans form the basis of good nutrition and health. Chapter 9 focuses on the Food Guide Pyramid and explains the different food groups and the number of servings that you need from each food group to stay healthy. This chapter examines the Dietary Guidelines for Americans and describes how to make food choices that help you get enough, but not too much, of the nutrients that your body needs for good health.

# Glimpsing the Basics of the Dietary Guidelines

Published in 2000 by the U.S. Department of Agriculture and the U.S. Department of Health and Human Services, the following list contains the ten Dietary Guidelines for Americans.

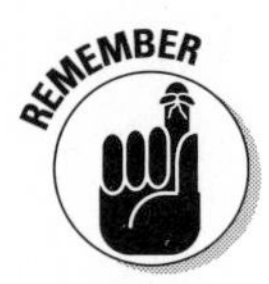


The 2000 edition of the Dietary Guidelines is a big departure from earlier versions. These are broader in tone and content and reflect a more international perspective. Though other nations' dietary advice may be worded differently, the international health community agrees that the following suggestions are essential to good health.

- **A**im for Fitness
  - Aim for a healthy weight
  - Be physically active each day
- **B**uild a Healthy Base
  - Let the Food Pyramid guide your food choices
  - Select a variety of grains daily, especially whole grains
  - Choose a variety of fruits and vegetables daily
  - Keep foods safe to eat
- **C**hoose Sensibly
  - Choose a diet that's low in saturated fat and cholesterol and moderate in total fat
  - Pick beverages and foods to moderate your intake of sugars
  - Choose and prepare foods with less salt
  - If you drink alcoholic beverages, do so in moderation

Notice that the guidelines are grouped into three categories (think A, B, and C). As you read them, you'll notice that the information in the third group, "choose sensibly" is much more specific than the general ideas in the first, "Aim for Fitness." This organization isn't meant as a hierarchy of importance. The idea is depth, meaning that the second group is more detailed than the first, and the third is ultra specific.

Be sure to remember that guidelines are just that — suggested steps that you can take to ensure good health. Remember, too, that these recommendations are for a healthy life, not for single meals or foods. For example, if you decide to eat a piece of birthday cake at your daughter's party, that's fine; you haven't ruined your diet or your eating habits. What counts is that over the course of time, you're striving to

- Be physically active
- Generally eat foods low in fat and high in fiber
- Include plenty of fruits, vegetables, and whole grains in your diet
- Be at an appropriate calorie level for you

The Dietary Guidelines apply to all healthy Americans ages 2 and over. They provide sound nutrition advice and are updated every five years to incorporate the most up-to-date nutrition knowledge. Keep reading to take a look at each of the guidelines in detail.

# Aiming for Fitness

For health, combining sensible eating with regular physical exercise is important. Fitness doesn't mean having a body like Vin Diesel, Jennifer Lopez, or even Jack LaLanne. Plenty of people don't have that kind of muscle definition but are considered fit. They engage in some kind of physical exercise on most days of the week and their weight is in the healthy range.

## Setting your sights on a healthy weight

Notice that the guideline is for a healthy weight — not a model-thin, impossible-to-maintain weight. See Chapter 3 for more information about finding a healthy weight for you. And if your weight is too much to be healthy, you have the solution in your hands — continue to read what's between these two yellow-and-black covers.

## Being physically active each day

This can be the easiest guideline to follow if you rethink your perception of physical activity. Think of it not as something that requires spandex and a gym membership, but as any activity that requires as much energy as walking at a brisk pace for 30 minutes. If you think that's too much time, wait until you hear this: You don't have to do it all at once. Got ten minutes? Sure you do — somewhere in your day. If you can find as little as ten minutes, three times a day, you've met the guideline.

Naturally, for weight loss, just meeting the guideline isn't enough. To burn calories, you have to get up and get moving! For more information about fun ways to get (and stay) active, see Chapter 12.

### When wheat bread isn't really what you think

You've decided to really focus on making sure that you get enough fiber in your diet. So you pick up a loaf of wheat bread instead of your usual white variety. But be careful — just because bread is brown in color or calls itself *wheat bread,* it doesn't mean that it's *whole* wheat bread.

All bread — white or wheat — is made with wheat flour. But in some bread, the flour is refined. These brown breads get their darker color from caramel coloring, not from the type of flour used. By law, any bread that's labeled *whole wheat* must be made from 100 percent whole-wheat flour, although the amount used can vary depending on the brand. The type of flour that's first in the ingredient list is the one present in the greatest amount.

To find high-fiber breads, read Nutrition Facts panels and ingredient lists. For maximum fiber impact, choose breads that list whole-wheat or whole-grain flour as their main ingredient.

# Building a Healthy Base

The middle part of the guidelines gets a little more specific by defining "sensible eating," but the advice is still pretty general. The overall message is one that's probably familiar to you: Eat a variety of foods.

## Letting the pyramid guide you

Chapter 9 is all about the Food Guide Pyramid; you may want to flip back and review it. But, for efficiency, the short course says that the foods in the pyramid are grouped by the nutrients that they contain. Foods with similar nutrient profiles are classified together. For example, milk, cheese, and yogurt are in the dairy group. Any food that you can think of can fit into at least one of the blocks of the pyramid. Some foods, such as pizza, fit into more than one block — dairy, grains, vegetables, and meat if we're talking about some of the toppings you may put on it.

The other important message that the pyramid is designed to convey is variety. By eating some of each food group each day and different foods within each food group, you can ensure that you're getting all the nutrients that you need. Even when the goal of a food plan is weight loss, variety is still important as the diet pyramid in Chapter 9 illustrates.

Lack of variety is one reason that single-food reduction diets, such as the grapefruit diet or a no-carbohydrate diet aren't a good idea. Besides being B-O-R-I-N-G, these diets are nutritionally unbalanced.

Serving sizes are key to using the pyramid as a guide to eating. Many people's perceptions of what constitutes a serving are way out of whack — usually much larger than recommended. We talk about serving sizes in more detail in Chapter 9.

## Choosing a variety of grains daily

Whole-grain breads and cereals, pasta, and rice, are key parts of a varied diet, because they provide vitamins, minerals, complex carbohydrates (starch and dietary fiber), and other substances that are important to good health. They're also low in fat — as long as you eat them without butter or creamy sauces. Few people eat enough of these foods, though, whether they're trying to lose weight or not.

## Packing a fiber punch

Dietary fiber, which is found only in plant foods, is one of the most important components in whole grains, fruits, and vegetables.

Eating enough fiber

- Helps the bowels function properly
- Can alleviate symptoms of chronic constipation, diverticular disease, and hemorrhoids
- May lower your risk for heart disease and some cancers

Because different foods contain different types of fiber, make sure to choose a variety of fiber-rich sources every day. And because other components of fiber-containing foods may be partly responsible for the health benefits of a high-fiber diet, make sure to get your fiber from foods as opposed to supplements.

There are two kinds of dietary fiber:

- **Soluble** fiber has been proven to help decrease blood cholesterol levels, thereby reducing the risk of heart disease. Soluble fiber slows the absorption of glucose, which may help to control blood sugar levels in people with diabetes. Soluble fiber is found in foods such as oats and oat bran, barley, brown rice, beans, and many vegetables and fruits, such as apples, oranges, and carrots.

- **Insoluble** fiber, also known as *roughage,* is mainly responsible for keeping things moving along your digestive tract. Good sources of insoluble fiber include whole-grain breads and cereals, wheat and corn bran, many vegetables, such as green beans and potatoes, and the skins of fruits and vegetables.

Most grains, fruits, and vegetables are two-thirds insoluble and one-third soluble. Fruit tends to be 50-50, and the fiber in oatmeal, barley, and legumes is about 65 percent soluble. Some manufacturers provide the amount of soluble or insoluble fiber on Nutrition Facts panels, but it's not required. Typically, you just see the total amount of dietary fiber provided. A quick tip: A food is considered to be a *good* source of fiber if it provides at least 2.5 grams per serving.

Oddly enough, until 2002 there wasn't a Recommended Dietary Allowance (RDA) for fiber, because it isn't considered a nutrient in the way that vitamins and minerals are. Unlike vitamins, minerals, and other nutrients, fiber can't be digested. But because fiber's relationship to good health and long life is so compelling, the National Academy of Science, the organization that writes the RDAs, has finally made a recommendation for adults, adolescents, and children.

The RDA is based on calorie intake and is set at 14 grams per 1,000 calories. To put it another way, a woman who eats 2,000 calories a day should include 28 grams of total fiber in her diet. You need a mix of soluble and insoluble — which is plenty, considering the amount that most Americans currently eat. On average, people consume only about 14 to 15 grams of fiber — about half the minimum amount recommended. If you don't eat enough fiber, find ways to get more into your diet. Just be sure to add it gradually to give your body time to adjust. And drink plenty of fluids, too, to help the fiber move easily through your digestive tract.

## Eating a variety of fruits and vegetables daily

You probably know that you don't eat enough fruits and vegetables, but you're not the only one. Most people don't eat the two to three servings of fruits and/or three to five vegetables a day recommended as a minimum by almost all health authorities. If it weren't for French fries and pizza, plenty of people wouldn't eat a single fruit or vegetable on most days of the week. Sure, eating some is better than eating none, but relying on the same fruits or vegetables week in and week out doesn't offer enough variety.

## Filling up with fiber

Looking for quick and easy ways to add fiber to your diet? Try some of these delicious tips:

- For a side dish, have ½ cup of any one of the following: lentils (5 grams), cooked dried beans (7 grams), cooked whole grains, such as wheat berries (2 grams) or cracked wheat (3 grams). Mix it with ½ cup of one of these vegetables: peas (3 grams), green beans (2 grams), or spinach (1 gram).
- Make an opened-face sandwich with a sliced tomato (1 gram) and a slice of whole-grain toast (2 grams). Top it with 1 ounce of low-fat mozzarella.
- Select your cereals wisely. You have tons of high-fiber cereals to choose from now — some offering up to 10 grams per serving. Look for cereals that provide at least 2 grams of fiber per serving.
- Reach for fiber-rich fruits and think of them as ingredients, not just as snacks — especially a pear (4 grams), an apple (3 grams), a couple of figs (3 grams), 1 cup of strawberries (3 grams), or a banana (2 grams). Add them to salads, cereal, and yogurt or use them as a topping for pancakes and waffles.
- Make short-grain brown rice a staple (4 grams of fiber per cup). It has a rich, nutty flavor and tastes much better than the long-grain variety. If you can't find it at your local supermarket, check health food stores or Asian supermarkets.
- Sneak vegetables in wherever you can — pizza, soups, stir-fries, rice, sandwiches, and pasta dishes. The sky's the limit!
- A surprising source of soluble fiber is reduced-fat foods. The guar gum that many reduced-fat foods contain in place of fats is soluble fiber. ***Caution:*** This doesn't give you license to replace fresh produce and whole-grain products with faux fats, but they do contribute a marginal amount of healthful fiber. For example, one piece of a brand-name fat-free chocolate loaf cake contains 1 gram of fiber, as does one fat-free oatmeal cookie, a full-fat one contains only ½ gram. Surprisingly, even 2 tablespoons of fat-free ranch dressing has ½ gram of fiber.

Mother Nature gave you the ability to enjoy the flavors and textures of hundreds of fruits and vegetables, and she sprinkled her nutrients among them. Make Mother happy and at least try to increase the variety of fruits and vegetables you do eat. In most cases, canned, frozen, and fresh have the same nutrient profile. Besides some mighty delicious flavors and textures, look at all the good stuff that she packed into her bounty:

- **Phytochemicals** — which include hundreds of naturally occurring, beneficial substances — are abundant in plant foods. Although the role of phytochemicals for promoting health isn't certain, researchers think that they may help protect against certain cancers and heart disease.

- **Plant foods** are among the best sources of *folate,* a B vitamin that, among its many functions, reduces the risk of a serious type of birth defect.
- **Minerals,** such as potassium, calcium, and magnesium, which are found in a wide variety of vegetables and fruits, may help to reduce the risk of high blood pressure.
- **Antioxidant nutrients,** such as vitamin C, beta carotene, which forms vitamin A, and vitamin E, may also reduce the risk of cancer and certain other chronic diseases.

## Keeping food safe to eat

Part of a healthy diet is making sure that the foods that you eat won't make you sick. (Sounds simplistic, but it's something people often take for granted.) You count on producers, packers, and shippers, and supermarkets to comply with sanitation requirements. You expect restaurants to be scrupulously clean. Yet did you know that most food-related illnesses can be traced back to home kitchens?

Eating foods that contain harmful bacteria, toxins, parasites, viruses, and chemical contaminants can cause a host of illnesses. Salmonella and Campylobacter are the most common ones. Plenty of folks can shake off the (sometimes) unpleasant symptoms of food "poisoning" in a matter of hours or days, but for other people, food contamination can be fatal. Pregnant women, young children, older people, and anyone with a weakened immune system are at high risk.

To ensure that the healthy food you bring into the house stays that way, keep these guidelines in mind:

- **Clean.** Wash hands and surfaces often. Use soap and rinse it well.
- **Separate.** Keep raw foods that will be eaten raw, such as salads, from contamination by separating them from raw foods that must be cooked, such as meat, eggs, and poultry.
- **Cook.** Know safe temperatures. Check labels and cookbooks for recommendations. Use a thermometer to make sure the internal temperature reaches a safe level.
- **Keep it cold.** Don't leave food out more than two hours (one hour in 90 degrees Fahrenheit weather).
- **Serve it safely.** Keep hot foods hot, and cold foods cold.
- **When in doubt, throw it out.** Don't take chances.

### Less fat + more calories + less exercise = more weight

Data from 1978 showed that Americans were getting 40 percent of their calories from fat. Ten years later, fat intake dropped to 34 percent. By 1996, that number was down to 33 percent. (Thirty percent is the recommended maximum.) Looks like America is on the lowfat track, right? Wrong.

Although changes in the way consumption data was gathered may be to blame, another reason may be that between 1977 and 1996, the total number of calories that Americans ate rose 7 percent. So although the percentage of calories from fat looks like it decreased from 1977 to 1996, the drop may have been due to an increase in total calories consumed. And considering that 30 percent of men and 45 percent of women say that they rarely or never exercise, it's easy to understand why 64 percent of Americans are considered to be overweight or obese today, compared to only 20 percent in 1977.

# Choosing Sensibly

This last group of guidelines gets specific with advice on choosing foods that have the most significant impact on health. It's no coincidence that the guidance for eating healthfully in general also has a big impact on your weight-loss progress and success.

## Choosing a diet low in saturated fat and cholesterol and moderate in total fat

Yes, you do need *some* fat for good health. Fat supplies essential fatty acids and helps your body absorb the fat-soluble vitamins A, D, E, and K. But eating too much saturated fat and, to a lesser degree, dietary cholesterol is linked to increased risk of heart disease. And because fat has more calories than protein or carbohydrate, cutting down on fat is also the easiest way to cut calories. All kinds of fat, regardless of how saturated or unsaturated they are, have 9 calories per gram and should comprise no more than 30 percent of your total calories. Dietary cholesterol doesn't provide calories, but it too should be limited — to less than 300 milligrams per day.

The number of calories that you consume determines the amount of fat that you can have in your diet. Keep in mind that no more than 30 percent of your daily calories should come from fat.

| *Calorie Level* | *Daily Fat Gram Allowance* |
|---|---|
| 2,000 | Less than 65 grams |
| 1,800 | Less than 60 grams |
| 1,600 | Less than 53 grams |
| 1,400 | Less than 46 grams |
| 1,200 | Less than 40 grams |

To quickly determine your fat gram allowance, drop the last digit of your calorie intake and divide by 3. For example:

1,500 calorie diet = 150 ÷ 3 = less than 50 grams of fat

### Choosing foods low in saturated fats and trans fat

Fats are made up of both saturated and unsaturated fatty acids and are categorized by the predominate kind of fatty acid that they contain. Research shows that a diet high in saturated fatty acids causes blood cholesterol levels to rise even more than eating large amounts of dietary cholesterol does. The fats from meat, milk products, and tropical oils are the main sources of saturated fats in most American diets. Lesser amounts of saturated fat come from vegetable oils.

As a guideline, remember that any fat that's solid or semisolid at room temperature (think of butter and the fat on beef and other meats) is predominantly saturated fat. Your diet should provide less than 10 percent of calories from saturated fat. On the Nutrition Facts panel, 20 grams of saturated fat is the Daily Value for a 2,000-calorie level. That translates into a 13-gram maximum of saturated fat in a 1,200-calorie diet.

*Trans fatty acids* are similar to saturated fats but aren't listed on Nutrition Facts Panels. Trans fats, as they're often called, are a type of fatty acid that forms during *hydrogenation.* A fatty acid becomes more saturated when hydrogen is added to it. It's done to make a fat stable and solid at room temperature and extend shelf life. For example, hydrogenating vegetable oil makes stick margarine. So the softer the margarine, the less saturated it is. Crackers are made with partially hydrogenated oils so that they don't get stale quickly. Those conveniences come at a price. Trans fats are believed to be as much of a threat to heart health as saturated fats — maybe more. Evidence is mounting about how damaging trans fat can be.

In response, the Food and Drug Administration reviewed data to determine how the trans fatty acids content of food should be labeled. Beginning in January of 2006 all food labels that are required to carry Nutrition Fact panel must also include the trans fat content. Until then, look at ingredient lists. Whenever you see the words *hydrogenated* or *partially hydrogenated,* know that trans fatty acids are contained in that food. Avoid them as much as possible.

### *When you eat fat, choose unsaturated*

All fat has the same number of calories, but eating foods that contain unsaturated fat instead of foods that contain saturated fats can help reduce your blood cholesterol level. Unsaturated fat is classified as either *monounsaturated* or *polyunsaturated.* Monounsaturated fats reduce the harmful low-density lipoproteins (LDLs) and leave the protective high-density lipoproteins (HDLs) in place. Research shows that polyunsaturated fats reduce both LDLs and HDLs.

Confused about what foods contain significant amounts of saturated, polyunsaturated, or monounsaturated fat? Table 10-1 gives you a quick look at what foods contain which types of fat.

**Table 10-1 Figuring Out the Fats**

| *Saturated* | *Polyunsaturated* | *Monounsaturated* | *Trans fats* |
|---|---|---|---|
| Butter, lard | Corn oil | Canola oil | Stick margarine |
| Dairy products (except nonfat) shortening | Fish oils | Olive oil | Solid vegetable |
| Meat and poultry | Cottonseed oil | Peanut oil | |
| Palm oil, palm kernel oil | Safflower oil | Other nut oils | |
| Coconut oil | Sesame oil | | |
| | Soybean oil | | |
| | Sunflower oil | | |

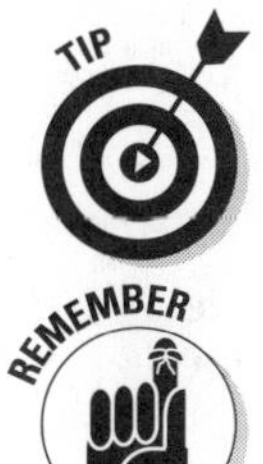


Most varieties of fish contain omega-3, a type of polyunsaturated fatty acid that's associated with a decreased risk of heart disease in certain people.

Here's the bottom line when it comes to fat. Choose

- Mostly monounsaturated fats
- A little less polyunsaturated fat
- Very few saturated fats
- As little as possible trans fats

### Selecting a low-cholesterol diet

Your body (specifically, the liver) can make all the cholesterol it needs. This type of cholesterol is referred to as *blood cholesterol*. But cholesterol also comes from foods that you eat; it's known as *dietary cholesterol*. You can get dietary cholesterol *only* from animal sources, such as egg yolks, meat (especially organ meats like liver), poultry, fish, and higher-fat dairy products. Plant foods don't contain cholesterol.

Often, foods that are high in cholesterol are also high in saturated fats. Although it was believed that dietary cholesterol was mainly responsible for raising blood cholesterol levels, researchers now know that saturated fat is the main culprit that causes your body's cholesterol factory to work overtime. For more information about saturated fat, refer to the "Choosing foods low in saturated fats and trans fat" section, earlier in this chapter. The Nutrition Facts panel lists the Daily Value for cholesterol as 300 milligrams, no matter what your calorie intake is.

## Picking beverages and foods to moderate your intake of sugars

Sugars, which are simple carbohydrates, are found naturally in many foods, including milk, fruits, some vegetables, breads, cereals, and grains. And sugars are sometimes used as preservatives and thickeners; they're also added to foods during preparation, during processing, and at the table.

In the process of digestion, the body breaks down carbohydrates (with the exception of fiber) into sugars. Interestingly, no matter whether the sugar is added or found naturally in a food, your body can't tell the difference because, from a chemical standpoint, all sugar is the same. For example, whether you eat canned fruit packed in natural juices or canned fruit packed in heavy syrup, your body digests it in exactly the same way. The difference is that fruit packed in its own juices is much lower in calories than fruit packed in syrup, because natural juice contains less sugar than syrup does.

Contrary to popular belief, sugar doesn't cause hyperactivity or diabetes. But it can cause dental cavities and supply unnecessary calories. Sugary foods are usually low in nutrients, too, so eat foods with added sugar sparingly if you want to lose weight.

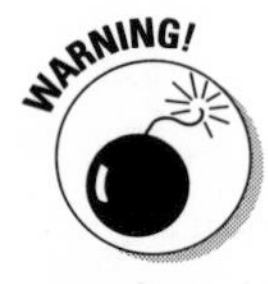


Sugar shows up on food labels in many forms. If one of the terms in the following list (from the USDA Dietary Guidelines) appears as the first or second ingredient on a food label, or several are used in a single product, it's an indication that the food is probably high in sugar. It also means that the food has sugar added to it, because the sugars that are naturally present in foods aren't listed in the ingredients.

- Brown sugar
- Corn sweetener or corn syrup
- Dextrose
- Fructose
- Fruit juice concentrate
- Glucose (dextrose)
- High-fructose corn syrup
- Honey
- Invert sugar
- Lactose
- Maltose
- Malt syrup
- Molasses
- Raw sugar
- [Table] sugar (sucrose)
- Syrup

Keep in mind that many reduced-fat and fat-free products are high in sugar, which also keeps their calorie contents high; so check labels before you decide to splurge. Finally, unlike the ingredient list, the Nutrition Facts panel on most food products includes sugars, which include both naturally occurring and added sugars, so it's easy to see at a glance how much sugar a food provides.

## Preparing foods with less salt

Many foods naturally contain sodium, albeit usually in tiny amounts. Although some people add salt to their food at the table, most dietary sodium in the U.S. diet comes from foods to which salt has been added during preparation or processing. Many foods that are high in sodium don't taste salty, so beware.

Salt is chemically known as sodium chloride. Although sodium accounts for only part of table salt, most people use the words *salt* and *sodium* interchangeably.

Sodium plays an important role in the body, helping to regulate fluids and blood pressure. But if you consume too much salt, you may need more calcium, because the excess salt may cause your body to excrete calcium in your urine.

## The skinny on sugar substitutes

Sugar substitutes, such as sorbitol, saccharin, and aspartame, are ingredients in many foods. Most sugar substitutes don't provide significant calories, and therefore, may be useful in the diets of people who are concerned about calorie intake. Foods containing sugar substitutes, however, may not always be lower in calories than similar products containing sugars, so check labels. Unless you reduce the total number of calories you eat, the use of sugar substitutes will not help you lose weight. For more information on sugar substitutes, see Chapter 11.

Keep the following tips in mind when trying to consume less sodium in your diet:

- Limit the amount of salt you add to foods during cooking and at the table. Measure the amount you use so that you don't overdo. A sprinkle here and a sprinkle there can add up quickly. Remember: Taste before you shake.
- Season with spices, herbs, fruit juices, and vinegars rather than salt to heighten the flavor of your food.
- Gradually cut back on the amount of sodium that you consume. It takes about two weeks for your palate to get accustomed to the reduced amount — but your taste for salty foods will change.
- Use fresh and plain frozen vegetables. Not only are they lower in sodium than vegetables in sauce, but they're generally lower in calories, too.
- When selecting canned foods, select those labeled without salt, low-sodium, or reduced-sodium. Or with regular canned beans or vegetables, rinse before preparing.
- Many frozen dinners, packaged mixes, canned soups, and salad dressings also contain considerable amounts of sodium. Again, choose low- or reduced-sodium versions when possible.
- Use condiments, such as soy and other sauces, pickles, olives, ketchup, and mustard in moderation. They're high in sodium.
- Fresh fruits and vegetables are a lower-sodium (and lower-calorie) alternative to salted snack foods, and they still provide the "crunch" factor.
- If you eat out frequently, be sodium-conscious. Request that foods be prepared without added salt; ask for sauces and dressings on the side; and pay attention to the terms that signal a high-sodium content: *smoked, pickled, au jus, soy sauce,* or *in broth.*

The Nutrition Facts Label lists a Daily Value of 2,400 milligrams per day for sodium. Just 1 teaspoon of salt contains 2,300 milligrams of sodium — almost your entire day's allowance!

### Sodium and weight gain

Eating too much sodium may make the number on the scale jump, but that's probably water weight, not fat. In time, your body will adjust and rid itself of the extra sodium.

### Sodium and high blood pressure

Many studies have shown that eating plenty of sodium is associated with high blood pressure. Sodium doesn't cause high blood pressure any more than sugar causes diabetes, but research indicates that people at risk for high blood pressure — because it runs in their families — may reduce their chances of developing this condition by consuming less sodium. Other ways to help decrease high blood pressure include losing excess weight if you're overweight, eating enough fruits and vegetables for adequate potassium, getting sufficient calcium through lowfat and fat-free dairy products, and keeping alcohol consumption moderate to low.

## Drinking alcoholic beverages in moderation

Beer, wine, and spirits may enhance your enjoyment of meals, but they supply calories and few or no nutrients. Dieters who eliminate alcoholic beverages save about 150 calories per 12-ounce bottle or can of beer or 8-ounce mixed drink, and 100 calories per 5-ounce glass of wine. In addition, the alcohol in these beverages has physiological effects and is harmful when consumed in excess. If you're an adult and you choose to drink alcoholic beverages, consume them only in *moderation,* defined as no more than one drink per day for women and no more than two drinks per day for men. (One drink equals 12 ounces of regular beer, 5 ounces of wine, or 1.5 ounces of 80-proof distilled spirits.)

Naturally, if you're trying to cut calories, alcohol is the ideal place to start. Any healthy benefits that you would get from a glass of wine with dinner will be surpassed by the health payoff of losing weight.

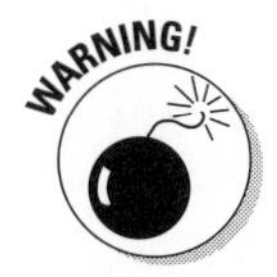


If you're on this list, which was compiled by the USDA and can be found in their Dietary Guidelines, you shouldn't drink, even in moderation. The health risks for you outweigh any benefits:

- **Children and adolescents.**
- **Women who may become pregnant or who are pregnant.** A safe level of alcohol intake has not been established for women at any time during pregnancy, including the first few weeks. A pregnant woman who drinks heavily can bring on major birth defects in the fetus she is carrying. This is commonly known as *fetal alcohol syndrome.* Other fetal alcohol effects may also harm the fetus in ways that are not as obvious.
- **Individuals who plan to drive, operate machinery, or take part in other activities that require attention, skill, or coordination.** Most people retain some alcohol in the blood up to two to three hours after a single drink.
- **Individuals taking prescription or over-the-counter medications that can interact with alcohol.** Alcohol alters the effectiveness or toxicity of many medications, and some medications may increase blood alcohol levels. If you take medications, ask your healthcare provider for advice about alcohol intake, especially if you're an older adult.
- **Individuals of any age who can't restrict their drinking to moderate levels.** This is a special concern for recovering alcoholics, problem drinkers, and people whose family members have alcohol problems.

## Chapter 11

# A Matter of Taste: Using Fat Substitutes and Artificial Sweeteners

### *In This Chapter*

- Sticking exclusively to fat-free doesn't work
- Finding out why calories still count
- Understanding fat replacers and the lowfat label
- Changing your food preferences

Trailer loads of food made with artificial sweeteners and fat substitutes are rolling down highways and into supermarkets. Since 1997, more than 3,000 fat-reduced foods have been shipped to supermarkets, and an equally staggering number of foods sweetened with artificial sweeteners are available. Just about every one (nine out of ten people, according to industry estimates) eats something made with a fat or sugar substitute. But just as there are no free lunches; there are no free calories. This chapter tells you why some fat and sugar substitutes may help you lose weight, but also why they aren't the only answer.

## Wising Up to the Fat-Free Fake-Out

A 1998 study conducted by the Calorie Control Council, an industry group that represents manufacturers of lowfat and sugar-free foods, showed that 62 percent of consumers say they always try to check the nutrition label to determine fat content in the products they buy. But only 55 percent check the label for calories. That discrepancy may be one of the reasons that more people are obese today, despite the fact that total fat consumption is down.

On a gram-by-gram basis, fat has more calories than carbohydrates or protein. Therefore, eliminating fat or cutting down on the amount you eat helps you lose weight. However, if fat is replaced with carbohydrates, as it is in many fat-reduced and fat-free products, the total number of calories in a serving may not be reduced. Consequently, no weight loss occurs.

Table 11-1 shows you how reducing fat in a product doesn't always mean that its calories are reduced, too.

**Table 11-1 Lowfat Doesn't Always Mean Low Calorie**

| *Food* | *Portion* | *Calories* |
|---|---|---|
| Refrigerated whipped topping | 2 tablespoons | 25 |
| Lite refrigerated whipped topping | 2 tablespoons | 25 |
| Canned turkey gravy | ¼ cup | 30 |
| Canned fat-free turkey gravy | ¼ cup | 30 |
| Fig bars | 2 | 110 |
| Fat free fig bars | 2 | 100 |
| Canned refried beans | ½ cup | 100 |
| Canned fat-free refried beans | ½ cup | 100 |
| Peanut butter | 2 tablespoons | 191 |
| Reduced-fat peanut butter | 2 tablespoons | 187 |
| Vanilla frozen yogurt | ½ cup | 104 |
| Nonfat vanilla frozen yogurt | ½ cup | 100 |
| Homemade caramel topping | 2 tablespoons | 103 |
| Fat-free caramel topping | 2 tablespoons | 103 |

But in some cases, a lower fat content *does* mean fewer calories, especially when it comes to dairy products. Table 11-2 gives a few examples.

**Table 11-2 Where Lowfat *Does* Mean Lower Calorie**

| *Food* | *Portion* | *Calories* |
|---|---|---|
| Cottage cheese, 4% milk fat | ½ cup | 110 |
| Cottage cheese, 1% milk fat | ½ cup | 82 |

| Food | Portion | Calories |
|---|---|---|
| Whole milk | 8 ounces | 150 |
| Fat-free milk | 8 ounces | 85 |
| Yogurt, lowfat | 8 ounces | 155 |
| Yogurt, nonfat | 8 ounces | 135 |
| Vanilla ice cream | ½ cup | 135 |
| Vanilla ice milk | ½ cup | 90 |

# Investigating the Role of Fat Replacers

Fat in the diet provides calories (or energy) and important vitamins, such as vitamin E. In addition to carrying flavor and giving foods taste appeal, fat also gives foods texture — whether it's crispy or smooth and creamy. The concern about eating fatty foods is not only the number of calories they contain but also, depending on the type of fat, their potential for increasing the risk for disease. A diet high in saturated fat, for example, increases blood cholesterol levels and, therefore, increases the risk of heart disease.

The problem with eating high-fat foods is that fat doesn't immediately satisfy hunger the way that sugary carbohydrates do. Therefore, eating too many fat calories before realizing that you've had enough is easy to do. (Think about how easy it is to eat a whole bag of French fries or chips and still feel hungry.)

## Exploring the different types

Fat is complicated stuff. The kind and amount of fatty acids that make up a particular type of fat determine how the fat feels in your mouth and how it tastes, among other functions. So finding one universal fat replacer is impossible.

Therefore, three basic types of fat replacers are used:

- **Carbohydrate-based fat substitutes** duplicate the taste and function of fat in foods but contain fewer calories than real fat. They work by combining with water to thicken and add bulk, which makes the food *feel* like fat in your mouth.

Foods that use carbohydrate-based fat substitutes include lowfat and nonfat baked goods (such as brownies, cakes, and cookies), lowfat ice creams, and fat-free salad dressings. Pureed fruits, including prunes and applesauce, are also used as fat replacers in some baked goods.

- **Fat mimetics (fat-based replacers)** copy some or all the properties of the fat they replace. Most are made from fat but have fewer calories per gram than fat because the chemical structure of the fat has been altered. The body is unable to fully absorb the fatty acids and the calories they would otherwise provide.

  *Salatrim* (brand name *Benefat*) is one example of a fat-based replacer. It's used in baked goods, dairy products, and candies, providing 5 calories per gram compared to fat's usual 9 calories per gram.

  *Olestra* (brand name *Olean*), known in chemistry labs as a *lipid analog,* is a calorie-free fat replacer made from vegetable oils and sugars, which contributes no calories. Olestra mimics the characteristics of fat when fried. It's currently used in potato chips, tortilla chips, and other snack foods. For more information about olestra, see the sidebar "A food industry case study: Olestra (Olean)" in this chapter.

- **Protein-based fat replacers** are made with egg whites or skim milk. They provide a creamy texture and an appealing appearance when fat is removed. Lowfat cheeses and ice creams made with protein-based substitutes mimic the taste and appearance of their full-fat counterparts.

  Simplesse is an example of a protein-based fat replacer. It's used primarily in frozen desserts, providing 1 to 2 calories per gram. Protein-based fat replacers have great potential for use in many products, especially frozen and refrigerated items.

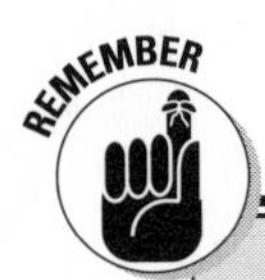


Table 11-3 lists the most commonly used fat replacers in foods.

## Cutting only fat isn't the answer

Research from the University of Vermont [published in *Obesity Research* 6(3), May 1998] proves that there's more to weight loss than counting fat grams. A group of dieters was told to restrict their fat to 22 to 28 grams per day, but nothing was said about counting calories. Another group restricted calories but wasn't given specific instructions to cut back on fat. After six months, the calorie counters lost more than twice as much weight as did those who restricted fat. One reason is the incredible number of fake-fat products on the market that are not low in calories. Many people view these products as a license to overeat. Don't fall into that trap.

**Table 11-3 Fat Replacers That You May See on Labels**

| *Carbohydrate-Based* | *Protein-Based* | *Fat-Based* |
|---|---|---|
| Cellulose (carboxy-methyl cellulose, microcrystalline cellulose) | Modified whey protein concentrate (Dairy-lo) | Caprenin |
| Dextrin | Microparticulated protein (Simplesse) | Olestra (Olean) |
| Fiber | | Salatrim (Benefat) |
| Gum (alginates, carrageenan, guar, locust bean, zanthan) | | |
| Polydextrose | | Emulsifiers |
| Maltodextrin | | |
| Inulin | | |
| Oatrim (hydrolyzed oat flour) | | |
| Polyols | | |
| Starch (modified food starch) | | |

## Determining if they work

Some fat replacers are fat free. Others contribute calories, but fewer than they replace. Fat replacers can reduce the amount of fat you eat *only if* you do not consume additional fat at other meals. Research shows that test subjects who were fed fake-fat foods did not eat additional fat when only fat-reduced and fat-free foods were available. But people don't live in laboratories, and plenty of full-fat foods are always available.

However, consider this fact: Most of the fat in people's diets comes from eating and cooking with fats and oils. Add red meat, poultry, fish, and dairy products to that mix, and you'll discover that all these foods account for about 90 percent of the fat that you eat. Meanwhile, few of these foods contain fat replacers. Other foods, especially snack foods, use fat replacers. Adding fat-reduced snack foods to an eating plan without also reducing the major sources of fat in your diet — from foods such as oils, red meat, poultry, fish, and dairy products — will *add* calories, not reduce them.

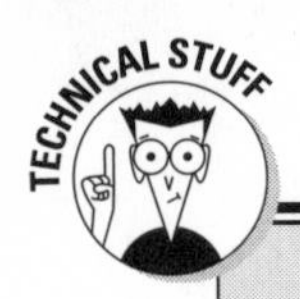


## A food industry case study: Olestra (Olean)

More than 150 scientific studies and 25 years of testing have made *olestra* (brand name *Olean*) the most thoroughly tested new food ingredient ever approved by the Food and Drug Administration (FDA). Yet, a 2003 report in the American Journal of Public Health exposed the fact that 80 percent of the authors who published articles supporting olestra had financial ties to Procter & Gamble (P&G), the company that manufactures the fat substitute. (To prepare their report, the researchers grouped all the journal articles published on olestra and classified them as supportive, critical, or neutral. The researchers also surveyed the authors about their relationships with P&G. All the authors who disclosed an affiliation with P&G wrote supportive articles.)

So, what exactly is olestra? Binding a fatty acid, a fat-building block, to a sugar makes *olestra,* a specific type of fat-based fat replacer known as a *sucrose polyester.* Because the human body doesn't have a way to separate the fatty acid from the sugar, it can't be used, and the body can't absorb the calories in it. So it passes through the body without being digested. The downside of it not being digested is that it also carries away some fat-soluble vitamins, such as vitamin A and vitamin E with it. That's why foods made with olestra have fat-soluble vitamins added to them. Unlike many other fat replacers, olestra is heat stable, so it can be used in fried foods and baked goods. Currently, it's approved for use only in snack foods, however.

The warning label that olestra-containing products were required to carry certainly didn't enhance consumer comfort: "This product contains olestra. Olestra may cause abdominal cramping and loose stools. Olestra inhibits the absorption of some vitamins and other nutrients. Vitamins A, D, E, and K have been added."

The Center for Science in the Public Interest, an industry watchdog group, reports that more complaints about olestra have been filed with the FDA than all other food additives in history — combined. After an explosive launch in the late '90s, sales of olestra have fallen dramatically. Still, be prepared for another marketing blitz for olestra-containing products soon.

On August 1, 2003, the FDA dropped the warning label requirement after reviewing new scientific data of people consuming olestra under real-life conditions. The studies showed only infrequent, mild gastrointestinal effects. Instead of a warning, consumers see only a tiny asterisk after each of the added fat-soluble vitamins listed in the ingredient statement of products containing olestra. The asterisk references the statement, "Dietary insignificant."

# Examining Sweeteners' Place in Your Diet

Two kinds of sweeteners are widely used to replace sugar. Some are classified as *nutritive,* because they provide calories; others are *nonnutritive,* because they don't.

Everyone can relate to the story about the woman who had a huge meal and an even bigger dessert and then insisted that the waiter bring a sugar substitute for her coffee. Maybe you've even done something like this yourself!

Sure, every calorie saved counts, and a sugar substitute saves you about 16 calories for every teaspoon of sugar replaced. Most people's diets include an estimated quarter pound of sugar a day, and theoretically, if that sugar were replaced by nonnutritive sweeteners, this replacement would result in a deficit of 720 calories per day, or about 1 pound of weight loss in 4 to 5 days. But much of the sugar that we eat isn't even visible as sugar; it's buried in our diets as ingredients in other foods.

When artificial sweeteners were introduced, everyone thought that people would eat less sugar. But evidence now suggests that people simply add the sweeteners to their diets. In reality, artificial sweeteners didn't replace anything. Just the opposite is true — consumers are eating three times the amount of sweeteners that they were ten years ago.

## Nutritive sweeteners

Most nutritive sweeteners used as replacements for sugar have just as many calories as sugar. They're simply another way to sweeten foods. Refined sugars, high-fructose corn syrup, crystalline fructose, glucose, dextrose, corn sweetener, honey, lactose, maltose, invert sugar, and concentrated fruit juice are examples of nutritive sweeteners that are just as caloric as plain old sugar.

Sugar alcohols are used in many sugar-free foods and have about half the calories of sugar, because the body absorbs them slowly and incompletely. You may know these sugar alcohols more specifically as *sorbitol, mannitol,* and *xylitol.* Unfortunately, in some people, a side effect of this slow absorption is diarrhea — particularly if large amounts of sugar alcohols are consumed. That's why the labels of some gums and candies that contain these sweeteners carry the statement "Excess consumption may have a laxative effect."

## Nonnutritive sweeteners

*Saccharin, aspartame, acesulfame potassium* (or *acesulfame-K*), *sucralose,* and *cyclamates* are the most commonly used no-calorie sweeteners in North America. They help add sweetness to foods for people who need to limit their intake of sugar, such as those with diabetes, and they also aid in the prevention of dental cavities. They're so intensely sweet that tiny amounts can be used, so the calories that they provide are undetectable. Whether they can help you lose weight depends on the other foods that you eat. Although these no-calorie sweeteners may seem like a dream come true, most come with some warnings. So you can recognize the sweeteners in the low- and sugar-free products that you buy, the sections that follow include the brand name in parentheses next to its chemical name.

### Acesulfame-K (Sunette)

*Acesulfame-K,* which is 200 times sweeter than sugar, is used as a tabletop sweetener. It's also an ingredient in soft drinks, chewing gum, desserts, candies, sauces, and yogurt in more than 15 countries. It's often combined with aspartame or other sweeteners in foods. Like saccharin, *acesulfame-K* is heat stable, so it can be used in cooked and baked goods. However, it may not work well in some recipes due to its finer texture.

*Acesulfame-K* doesn't provide calories, because it's not metabolized by the body and is excreted in the urine.

### Aspartame (Nutrasweet, Equal)

*Aspartame,* which is 160 to 220 times sweeter than sugar, is added to more than 6,000 foods, personal care products, and pharmaceuticals. It has 4 calories per gram, but because it's so intensely sweet and so little is needed to replace sugar, it's considered calorie free.

*Aspartame* is a combination of two amino acids: *phenylalanine* and *aspartic acid.* People who have *phenylketonuria* (PKU), which is only about 1 in 15,000 people, have adverse neurological reactions when they consume phenylalanine, because they can't metabolize it. Therefore, foods that contain aspartame are required to carry a label warning consumers that the product contains phenylalanine. In the United States, all infants are screened for PKU at birth.

Many studies have been conducted on aspartame to evaluate the numerous claims of allergic reactions, respiratory problems, and dermatological problems that consumers have reported. However, challenge studies have failed to reproduce those reactions.

Aspartame isn't heat stable and loses its sweetness in liquids over time, so it is used mostly in foods that don't require cooking or baking. Look for it in puddings, gelatins, frozen desserts, hot cocoa mixes, soft drinks, chewing gum, and tabletop sweeteners. Aspartame is approved for use in a broad variety of products in more than 18 countries, including the United States, Canada, Japan, and the United Kingdom.

### Cyclamate

*Cyclamate* is 30 times sweeter than sucrose and is heat stable. It's approved in Canada and more than 50 other countries around the world. Since 1970, however, it's been banned in the United States based on a study suggesting that cyclamate may be related to the development of bladder tumors in rats. Although more than 75 subsequent studies have failed to show that cyclamate is carcinogenic, the sweetener has yet to be reapproved in the United States.

## Stevia — sugar sub or herb sup?

You won't find *Stevia,* also sold as *sweet leaf* and *sweet herb,* in a soft drink, because the FDA classifies it as an herb supplement. Three hundred times sweeter than sugar, this Native-American herb is sold in health food stores and touted for sweetening without causing dental cavities the way that sugar does.

Stevia has been used for more than 30 years in Japan, but the FDA won't clear it in the United States because of the lack of long-term studies. Why not? The companies who manufacture new products, such as sugar substitutes that must be approved before they can use them, do most of the research studies that are submitted for the FDA's review process. Because Stevia is a natural product and wasn't invented in a laboratory (and therefore doesn't qualify for a patent), there is no industry incentive to study it.

### Saccharin (Sweet 'N Low)

*Saccharin,* which is 300 times sweeter than sugar, was discovered more than 100 years ago and has been back on the market in the United States since 1991, after having been banned in 1977, because it was found to cause cancer in rats. Newer studies cleared saccharin of links to cancer. A little bit of saccharin goes a long way — just 20 milligrams provides the same amount of sweetness found in 1 teaspoon (or 4,000 milligrams) of table sugar. Saccharin is calorie free, because the body can't break it down.

Saccharin is heat stable and, unlike aspartame, can be used in cooked and baked goods. However, because it doesn't have the bulk that sugar has, it may not work well in some recipes as a substitute. Saccharin is currently used in many food and beverages in more than 80 countries.

### Sucralose (Splenda)

*Sucralose,* which is 600 times sweeter than sugar, doesn't contain calories. It's the only low-calorie sweetener that's made from sugar. Sucralose is heat stable in cooking and baking and can be used virtually anywhere sugar can without losing its sugarlike sweetness. Currently, sucralose is approved in more than 25 countries around the world for use in food and beverages. It's mainly a tabletop sweetener, and you can find it in desserts and candy.

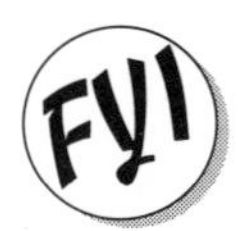


The FDA gave the Nutrasweet Company, developers of aspartame, approval for their new sugar substitute, *Neotame.* It's 7,000 to 13,000 times sweeter than sugar, it's heat stable, and can be used in soft drinks, chewing gums, syrups, and other similar foods. It'll be in a low-cal food soon.

# Seeing the Dangers of Depriving Yourself of Real Foods

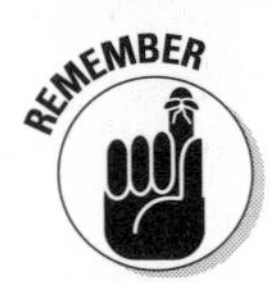


One of the problems with eating fake foods is that you don't learn to like foods that are naturally low in fat or sugar. Continually tricking your palate with foods that taste and feel like fat and sugar may reduce the amount of fat and sugar you eat, but you're not making progress toward a naturally healthier way of eating.

Although people are born with a love of sugar and a predisposition to enjoy fat, those preferences can be replaced over time. If you've already made the switch from whole milk to lowfat or fat-free milk, you know that the full-fat version is almost unpleasantly rich after you're accustomed to the way fat-free milk tastes and feels in your mouth. The change in preferences takes a few weeks to several months, depending on your present diet, but stick with it.

Try these tricks to train your taste buds:

- **Use ingredients that are naturally low in fat or fat free.** Try pureed fruits as a sauce for desserts or meats, lowfat yogurt to thicken shakes or fruit smoothies and dips, and evaporated fat-free milk to add body to cream sauces.
- **Add sweetness without sugar.** Instead of adding a spoonful of sugar, squeeze citrus juice over fresh fruit to enhance flavor. Cut the amount of sugar that you add to coffee or tea by half. Sprinkle fresh fruit over pancakes and waffles instead of syrup. Do the same over cereal. Add dried fruit and sweet spices, such as nutmeg, cinnamon, and ginger to hot cereals to intensify sweetness without adding sugar.
- **Enjoy the real thing.** A small portion of a high-fat or high-sugar food can be super satisfying if you eat it slowly and deliberately. Giving in to a sweet craving from time to time may be healthier than trying to eat around the craving or feeling unsatisfied by artificial concoctions. Instead of gulping big portions of a "fake" food, train yourself to savor a saner sized dessert, cookie, or even candy — on occasion.

You *can* discover a preference for less sweet and less fatty foods — all it takes is a little time and effort.

# Chapter 12

# Becoming More Active

***In This Chapter***

- Understanding the importance of exercise
- Calculating your exercise prescription
- Balancing aerobics with muscle building
- Overcoming excuses for not exercising

In this book, we talk about consuming fewer calories and eating less fat to lose weight. And that's exactly what you must do if you're going to shed pounds. But adding exercise increases the number of calories you burn so that you speed up your weight-loss efforts. Plus, you build muscle, which keeps your metabolism in high gear to burn calories more readily. You feel better about yourself, too. This chapter tells you how to work exercise into your lifestyle and keep at it.

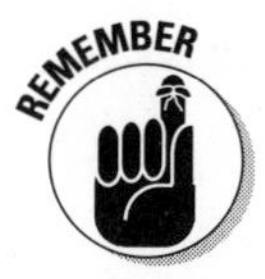


Naturally, if you have any medical conditions that would make exercising difficult or dangerous for you, see your doctor. This caution is especially important if you're over 40 years old. Your physician can perform an exertion test, evaluate your overall health, and suggest forms of exercise that are safe for you.

## Knowing Why Exercise Is Key to Weight Loss

Exercise is important for everyone. The fitter you are, the less your risk of having a heart attack or stroke or developing diabetes or some other crippling and deadly disease. Exercise also offers true, tangible benefits that are a real plus to dieters. The following sections describe those benefits.

### Curbing your appetite

Many people eat out of boredom or habit. True hunger has little to do with why or how much people eat. Think of the mindless nibbling that you do while watching TV, for example. When you're busy and out of the house, on the other hand — or at least diverted from the call of the kitchen — you eat less.

Some people say that exercise increases their hunger. But that's one of the greatest exercise-avoidance excuses of all time. The reason? Exercise pulls stored calories — or energy — in the forms of glucose and fat out of tissues so that blood glucose levels stay even and you don't feel hungry.

When you first start becoming more active, after a long stretch without any exercise, you may feel hungry initially. It's only temporary. After a day or so into your exercise commitment, any sensations of hunger will be replaced with feelings of well-being. In fact, it's a well-known phenomenon that people who exercise regularly automatically eat better and more healthfully.

## Increasing calorie burn

The math is simple: The more calories that you burn over the amount that your body needs to maintain its current weight, the greater your weight loss. That's why adding exercise to your reduced calorie plan speeds up your weight-loss efforts. Another way that exercise burns calories is by increasing your *metabolic rate* — the pace at which your body uses calories. And exercise helps you to lose fat but not muscle, which determines how fast or slow your body burns calories. Fat is relatively inert, but muscle is active and needs energy to maintain itself. So the more muscle you have, the more calories your body needs.

## Protecting against muscle loss

Many studies demonstrate that when a person diets, the weight that's lost is 75 percent fat and 25 percent muscle. And that ratio isn't good. As muscle is lost, your body's ability to burn and use calories efficiently is decreased, too.

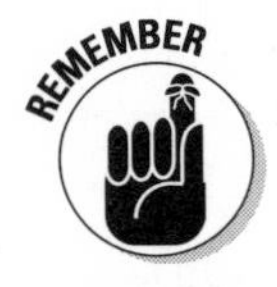


To build muscle, you need to add resistance training, such as lifting weights, to your exercise program. See the section called "Strength Training," later in this chapter, for details.

## Improving self-esteem

Exercise pays off physically, but its psychological benefits are dramatic as well. And we're not just talking about a runner's high or an endorphin buzz. Each time that you exercise, you're doing something positive for yourself. Some psychologists even prescribe daily exercise for depressed patients and see mood improvements equal to those of prescription antidepressant drug therapy.

So much of the weight-loss process involves giving up, limiting, and cutting out. But exercise is a positive addition, not a take-away negative, and that's a powerful incentive to stick with. When you feel good about yourself, staying with your weight-loss commitment is easy.

### Losing weight more easily and keeping it off

The National Weight Control Registry maintained at the University of Colorado includes more than 3,000 individuals who have lost more than 30 pounds and have kept it off for more than a year. But amazingly, the *average* loss is 60 pounds, and the average maintenance is six years. So many people actually lost more weight as time went on and have kept it off for a long period of time.

Researchers looked carefully at these success stories and found that one common thread, besides reducing the number of calories they ate, is that these successful losers expended about 2,800 calories in physical activity per week. That translates into about 60 minutes of activity a day. Typically, they combined walking with medium-to-heavy exercise, such as cycling, running, stair climbing, aerobic exercising, and weight lifting. This activity level, researchers say, may be the most important factor in maintaining their success.

## Determining How Much Exercise Is Enough

The current guidelines from the Centers for Disease Control and Prevention and the American College of Sports Medicine recommend 30 minutes or more of moderate-intensity physical activity on most — and preferably all — days of the week. That amount is enough for most people, and it's a good starting point. But for weight loss, you need to expend a minimum of about 200 to 300 calories a day on a *minimum* of three to five days a week. See the section "Going for the (Calorie) Burn" for a list of common exercises and the number of calories each activity burns.

How do you define moderately intense? You can count your heartbeats to determine how intensely you're working, but we think the American Heart Association's *conversational pace* rule is the easiest way to determine whether you're setting the right pace.

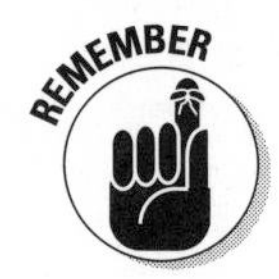


If you can talk and walk at the same time, you're probably walking at the right pace. If you can sing and maintain your level of effort, you're probably not working hard enough. And if you get out of breath quickly, you're probably working too hard — especially if you actually have to stop and catch your breath.

Researchers in Italy who wanted to know why some people stay with their exercise commitments and some don't suspect that success may have something to do with intensity. Their 2003 report in the *Journal of Endocrinology Investigations* explained that people who did short bouts of moderately intense activity lost an equal amount of weight as folks who spent more time doing lower intensity exercise. But here's the kicker: The people who increased their energy output by upping how hard they exercised stayed committed longer.

How frequently and intensely you exercise, as well as how long you work out, determines how much fat you burn. But don't overdo it. To burn fat, you need oxygen — get your heart and lungs pumping with aerobic activities. However, if you exercise so vigorously that you can't breathe, your workout is actually *anaerobic* (not using oxygen), which means that you're using carbohydrate and possibly protein (from your lean muscle) for energy, not fat. And that's not the point. If you want to lose weight, you want to lose fat.

# Getting Started on Exercising

Expending 2,800 calories a week in exercise or committing to one hour every day, as the folks in the weight-loss registry did, may sound like a tall order if you're among the 78 percent of American adults who are totally sedentary or not active enough. So how do you go from doing little or no exercise to developing a daily routine? Make it a habit. The easiest way to do that is to *commit to exercise every day.* That's seven days a week! Start with 20 minutes of walking every day. You can do two 10-minute walks if you like. Just commit to 20 minutes a day.

You may think you're already walking at least 20 minutes a day between all the things you do — and you may be. One way to find out is to attach a step counter (pedometer) to your belt. Pedometers don't calculate time; they log the number of steps you take. Twenty minutes equals 2,000 steps or about 1 mile. (See the sidebar, "10,000 steps" in this chapter for more information.)

After about 2 weeks, lengthen your walks to 40 minutes. In another 2 weeks, lengthen them to 60 minutes. Table 12-1 outlines the exercise program.

**Table 12-1 Your Exercise Prescription**

| *Time Period* | *Activity* | *Comments* |
|---|---|---|
| Weeks 1 and 2 | Walk 20 minutes a day | Intensity isn't important |
| Weeks 3 and 4 | Walk 40 minutes a day | Gradually increase the intensity |
| Week 5 | Walk 60 minutes a day | Walk briskly |
| Lifelong | Add recreational sports or aerobics for cardio respiratory conditioning | Supplement with walking on off days |

If you're new to exercise, keep in mind that you don't have to do exercise in one lump sum. Finding a continuous 30 to 60 minutes in which to work out is difficult for almost everyone. Focus initially on the day's total amount of activity — it doesn't matter how or if you break it up. For example, find three 20-minute periods in your day for exercising. Exercising at least 10 minutes at a time, several times a day, adds up to sufficient exercise quickly.

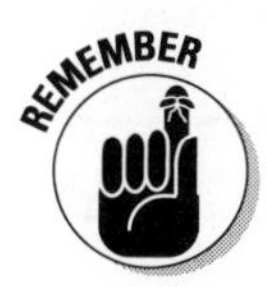


Don't try to make up for a slow day with an overly active one. But if you do go overboard with an activity that's too strenuous, still try to do something the next day, even if it means a slow walk. The important thing is to do some kind of exercise every day. That's how you make it a habit.

# Keeping an Exercise Log

In Chapter 9, we ask you to keep a pyramid score sheet. Table 12-2 has another chart to put up on your fridge, or you can tape it to the bathroom mirror, your computer monitor, or wherever you're sure to see it every day.

Make a grid on a piece of paper with space to record the date along the side and 10-minute time slots along the top, as in Table 12-2. As you complete your exercise sessions, make an X in the box that corresponds to the amount of time that you exercised.

**Table 12-2 Sample Minutes of Walking Log**

| *Date* | *10* | *20* | *30* | *40* | *50* | *60* | *Total* |
|---|---|---|---|---|---|---|---|
| Sunday | XX | XX | | | | | 60 |
| Monday | | | | X | | | 40 |

*(continued)*

**Table 12-2 (continued)**

| Date | 10 | 20 | 30 | 40 | 50 | 60 | Total |
|---|---|---|---|---|---|---|---|
| Tuesday | | X | | X | | | 60 |
| Wednesday | XX | | X | | | | 50 |
| Thursday | X | XX | X | | | | 80 |
| Friday | | | | | | X | 60 |
| Saturday | XX | X | X | | | | 70 |

Focus first on increasing the length of time that you exercise and then shift your efforts to increasing the intensity. For example, after you're comfortable with walking, you can add a variety of activities to total your 60 minutes — for example, jogging, hiking, or working out with weights. After you reach your goal of 60 minutes of daily exercise, begin jotting down the kind of exercise that you do in the column that corresponds to the amount of time you're active. (Your goal, even after you've moved past the walking-only stage, is still 60 minutes a day.) Your exercise log may look like Table 12-3.

**Table 12-3 Sample Exercise Log**

| Day | 10 | 20 | 30 | 40 | 50 | 60 | Total |
|---|---|---|---|---|---|---|---|
| Sunday | jog | swim | walk | | | | 60 |
| Monday | walk | | walk | | | | 40 |
| Tuesday | | | jog | walk | | | 70 |
| Wednesday | | | cycle | | walk | | 80 |
| Thursday | walk | | jog | | | hike | 100 |
| Friday | | | | | | walk | 60 |
| Saturday | | | walk | | | cycle | 90 |

# Going for the (Calorie) Burn

The more you weigh, the more calories you burn. It's a simple matter of physics: Moving a heavier mass takes more energy than moving a lighter one. In people terms, a 250-pound person burns twice as many calories while walking the same distance as someone who weighs only 125 pounds.

## 10,000 steps

Rather than time your walks, you can count your steps. The goal is 10,000 steps, which translates closely to the recommendations made by the Surgeon General to engage in at least 30 minutes of exercise most days of the week. A simple $20 to $30 pedometer attached to your belt can do the counting for you.

Wear a pedometer for a few days to get a sense of how many steps your normal routine takes. (Most inactive people take only 2,000 to 4,000 steps a day.) When you know how many steps you normally take, add about 500 extra steps for a few days, then add 500 more, and so on. Moderately active people take 5,000 to 7,000 and active people reach the 10,000-step mark, or about 5 miles. To help with your weight-loss plan, you'll need to move up to a minimum of 12,000 to 15,000 steps a day (or 45 minutes) — and ideally 20,000 steps or about 1 hour.

As you step up your count, you'll find that you'll need to add walking to your day in order to make your target. Check out the following ways to work more walking into your day:

- Take the stairs instead of the elevator
- Park in the farthest spot in the lot
- Walk with the dog
- Walk to the bus stop with the children
- Dance
- Park the golf cart and walk the course
- Cruise around the shopping mall three times before starting to shop
- Pace the long corridors of the airport while waiting for a flight, and stay off the moving sidewalks
- Give up e-mail or phone calls and walk to your coworkers' desks

Table 12-4 shows how engaging in various aerobic activities burns calories.

**Table 12-4 Calories Burned in 20 Minutes of Continuous Exercise**

| *Activity* | *Body Weight of 134 Pounds* | *Body Weight of 183 Pounds* |
|---|---|---|
| Aerobic dance | 128 | 170 |
| Ballroom dance | 64 | 84 |
| Basketball | 172 | 220 |
| Canoeing | 54 | 74 |
| Cleaning | 76 | 102 |
| Cross-country skiing | 148 | 198 |

*(continued)*

**Table 12-4 *(continued)***

| *Activity* | *Body Weight of 134 Pounds* | *Body Weight of 183 Pounds* |
|---|---|---|
| Cycling | 80 | 106 |
| Football | 164 | 220 |
| Jumping rope | 204 | 272 |
| Mopping floors | 76 | 102 |
| Mowing (push mower) | 138 | 186 |
| Racquetball | 220 | 296 |
| Raking | 66 | 90 |
| Running (9 minutes/mile) | 240 | 320 |
| Scrubbing floors | 134 | 180 |
| Snowshoeing | 206 | 276 |
| Squash | 262 | 352 |
| Stacking wood | 110 | 146 |
| Swimming, breaststroke | 200 | 268 |
| Tennis | 136 | 180 |
| Volleyball | 62 | 84 |
| Walking | 100 | 134 |

# Strength Training

Strength or resistance training, such as lifting weights or working out on exercise equipment, builds muscle. This type of exercise isn't just for body builders. Building muscle offers several benefits:

- Your body develops definition and firmness.
- You burn more calories.
- Bones strengthen, which helps protect against osteoporosis.
- Balance improves significantly.
- The pain from arthritis decreases, and your range of motion improves.
- Your spirits are boosted.

## Activities that don't burn calories

Unfortunately, some activities just don't burn as many calories as others. If the types of activities listed comprise the extent of your exercise habits, it's time to get into gear and get moving!

- Jumping to conclusions
- Running off at the mouth
- Catching your breath
- Standing on ceremony
- Toeing the line
- Jogging your memory
- Hitting the books
- Raking in the bucks
- Sweeping it under the rug
- Playing the field
- Marching to the beat of a different drummer
- Skipping a beat
- Exercising caution
- Swinging on a star
- Social climbing
- Running scared
- Jumping for joy

If you're new to exercise, you don't have to run to the gym; simply walking may be enough for you to increase your muscle mass. When you can walk easily for 60 minutes at a brisk pace, having followed the plan outlined in Table 12-1, you may need and want to push for more of a workout. Adding resistance training is a good way to go.

Table 12-5 outlines a suggested program for weight training. Get the help of a personal trainer or gym instructor to build a routine for you that you can do at home with hand-held weights or do at the gym on the machines. Or pick up an exercise video or a copy of Liz Neporent and Suzanne Schlosberg's *Weight Training For Dummies,* 2nd Edition (Wiley).

**Table 12-5 Recommended Program for Weight Training**

| *Training Factor* | *Comments* |
|---|---|
| Frequency | 3 days a week |
| Resistance | Use a weight that you can lift comfortably |
| Repetitions | 12 to 15 in 30 seconds (The last lift should be difficult.) |
| Stations | Work 8 to 12 muscle groups |
| Total time | 20 to 30 minutes |

# Ten Inexcusable Excuses for Not Exercising (And How to Cope with Them)

We've all heard them. Most of you have used them: so-called justifiable excuses for not being more active. Some ways to get around every good reason not to exercise are as follows:

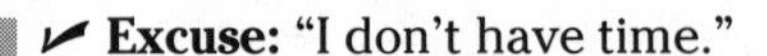

- **Excuse:** "I don't have time."

  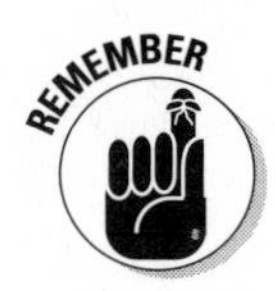
  

  This is the number-one reason most people give for not exercising. But you must make exercise a priority. That's one reason to make your daily activity a habit — because then it becomes a priority. Remember, you don't have to commit to a full hour all at once. Three 20-minute walks count.

  *Coping strategies:* Turn off the TV. Americans watch about 30 hours a week. Trade one hour of TV watching each day for one hour of exercise.

  Get somebody else to watch the children, get up a half-hour early, or walk during your lunch hour. Or take the children with you. You can be a good role model for them and have some quality one-on-one time, too. Make it part of the day's routine as some moms do: When the kids get off the bus in the afternoon, they have a quick snack, grab the dog, get on their bikes, and bike away for an hour of action.

- **Excuse:** "I don't feel like it."

  *Coping strategies:* Grab a buddy or several friends and make a commitment to them. Chances are that one of you will want to keep moving even when the others don't. And don't forget to give yourself credit for every bit of exercise you do, even if you don't make your 60-minute goal on some days. Remember, some physical activity is better than none.

- **Excuse:** "I can't do exercises well."

  *Coping strategies:* We're talking about walking, not jogging, running, or race walking. You can saunter, meander, or stroll. Just move. After a few weeks, you'll feel more comfortable. When you do, you can increase your speed and improve your technique.

- **Excuse:** "I can't get to my workout place easily."

  *Coping strategies:* You don't have to go to a special place, although you may find it motivating to go to a school track, a mall, the woods, or some other walker-friendly environment. You can take the stairs, get off the bus a little earlier and walk the rest of the way, park at the far end of the lot, or pace instead of sitting while waiting for the train.

- **Excuse:** "Exercise didn't work for me in the past."

  *Coping strategies:* Maybe you tried to do too much. Maybe you were forced to be on a sports team as a child. Or you were always the last person to be chosen for a team in the schoolyard. Try to figure out why past attempts to stick with exercise failed, or why you believe that your past gets in your way. Work out your own way around the problem. It's worth repeating: We're talking about going for a walk, not training for a marathon.

- **Excuse:** "I'm too fat to move."

  *Coping strategies:* Have you tried "chair dancing"? You can get tapes to guide you through a seated exercise routine. (Call 1-800-551-4386 or visit www.chairdancing.com.)

  *Active at Any Size*, a publication from the National Institutes of Health's Weight-Control Information Network, has many ideas and resources. You can download it from www.niddk.nih.gov/health/nutrit/activeatanysize/active.html or call its toll-free number 1-877-946-4627 to order one.

  Eventually, as your weight comes down and your fitness level improves, your ability and enjoyment will improve, too. Watch for little signs of encouragement, such as walking up the stairs without huffing and puffing. Or notice that your thighs don't rub together as much as they did a few weeks earlier. The more active that you become, the more progress you'll see.

- **Excuse:** "I have poor balance."

  *Coping strategies:* Balance is a problem for very large people who have been sedentary. You may want to start with strength training because one of the key health benefits of building muscle is improved balance. When you're ready to add walking, make sure that you have comfortable footwear that has a wide sole and good support. Choose flat, paved surfaces for walking.

- **Excuse:** "I'm afraid."

  *Coping strategies:* Fear stops people from doing all kinds of things, but the best antidote for fear is action. Grab a buddy to encourage you. Keep your sense of humor primed. Make exercise fun!

- **Excuse:** "Exercising hurts."

  *Coping strategies:* If an activity doesn't feel good, don't do it. Never exercise to the point of exhaustion. You don't want to wake up stiff. If you feel any pain at all, slow down or cut back on the exercise you do and slowly work your way back up. Listen to your body. If you're new to exercise and have been sedentary, it's possible to translate any discomfort you feel while exercising as pain. Chances are you're experiencing the sensation of physical effort. Effort is important to work to the next level; pain is not. If the distress you feel continues after you stop moving, that's pain. If you feel better when you stop, you're putting in effort and that's good. Keep going.

- **Excuse:** "I'm too embarrassed."

  *Coping strategies:* Don't worry about looking foolish. When you walk for exercise, you don't have to join a gym filled with perky, spandex-clad instructors. You can be as private or as public as you like, depending on where you walk. You can wear whatever you want, too.

# Eating Smart for Your Workout

Eating a small meal two to three hours before a workout is ideal. Two to three hours is how long it takes for a meal to reach your muscles, but it's not always practical. Not substituting exercise for eating is important; you can accommodate both. Keep reading to get some ideas for scheduling your meals to boost your workout productivity. And be sure to read through Chapter 23 for more specifics on when and what to eat before you exercise.

## Early birds

If the only time that you can sneak in a workout is first thing in the morning, try to eat something before you start. Your body needs fuel constantly, and your carbohydrate stores have most likely been tapped out in the six to seven hours since your last meal. Without eating, you'll feel sluggish and weak. Exercise should make you feel good. It takes only 20 minutes for a piece of fruit to give you the energy that you need to make your workout work for you.

## Lunch-hour or after-work crunchers

Split your lunch: eat half a few hours before the workout and finish the rest when you get back to your desk. If you exercise after work, say about 5:30 p.m. or 6:00 p.m., plan a minimeal — perhaps a small bowl of cereal, a piece of whole-grain bread with just a dab of PB&J, or a cup of lowfat yogurt at 3:00 or 3:30 p.m. in the afternoon.

## Drink, drink, drink

Regardless of how you define "workout," you need to replace fluid losses, which tend to be great after aerobic activities. Don't wait for thirst as an indicator; by that time, you're already down half a quart of fluids.

Water is fine if your workout lasts less than an hour. But sports drinks are helpful if you're exercising longer. They're better than soda and fruit juices, which can cause stomach upset during exercise and interfere with fluid absorption because they have *too much* carbohydrate — about 12 to 15 percent by weight. Sports drinks contain 6 to 9 percent carbohydrate.

So why not water down fruit juice? Research shows that fluid and energy are better absorbed when the drink contains several carbohydrates (sports drinks contain maltodextrins, sucrose, and fructose) that use different absorption mechanisms than when the sweetener comes from a single source. In addition, the small amount of electrolytes, including sodium, that sports drinks provide can replenish those lost through sweat. And as an added bonus, the sodium helps make you thirsty, encouraging you to drink more even after you think that you've had enough. Few people drink enough fluids to replenish lost stores.

## Weekend warriors

When you're doing extra exercise — a charity bike ride or a minimarathon fun run, or a long hike, for example — and stay at it for more than an hour, you need to refuel during the event. The human body can store only about an hour's worth of carbohydrate; it's in the muscles in the form of glycogen. (See Chapter 8 for further explanation of metabolism.) So if you want to finish the race without dragging yourself over the finish line, you need to eat or drink some form of carbohydrate. A sports drink is one option. A small energy bar works, too.

After an especially long workout, you need to refuel to restore your energy. A small high-carbohydrate, moderate-protein, and lowfat meal is best. Reach for fruit, lowfat yogurt, whole-wheat crackers, or bread.

Energy bars come in all kinds of formulations from the calorie, and sugar-packed cereal bars to the protein-dense energy bars. For a meal replacement, be sure that the bar contains at least 10 grams of protein. If you exercise for more than an hour and need a bar to refuel, carbohydrate-heavy ones are best.

# Part IV
# Shopping, Cooking, and Dining Out

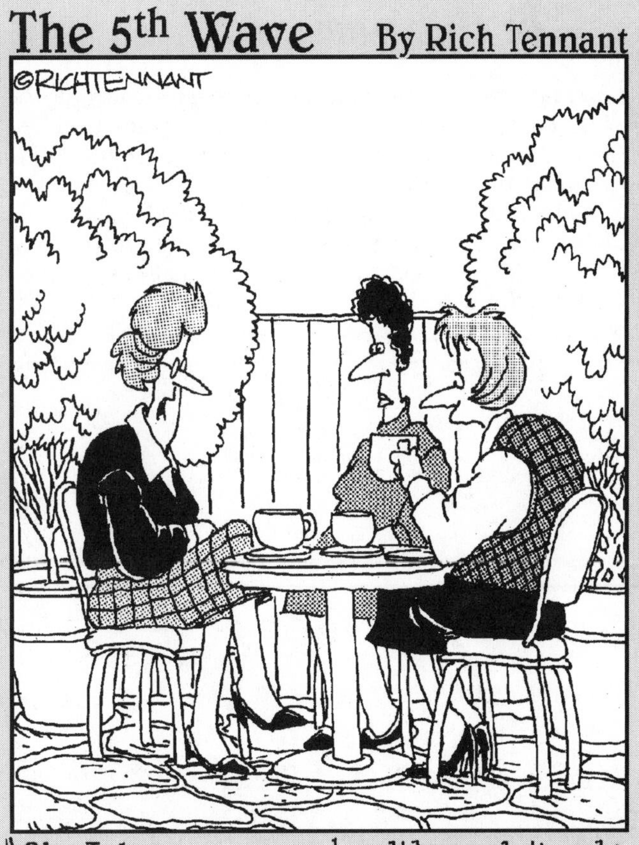


"Oh, I have a very healthy relationship with food. It's the relationship I have with my scale that's not so good."

## In this part . . .

You may have the best intentions to eat healthfully, but if diet-friendly foods aren't within your reach, you'll have trouble shedding pounds. This part shows you how to make the best choices at the grocery store and cook in nutritious, low-calorie ways. It also helps you navigate your way through restaurants and their often-deceptive menus, making smart choices that keep you on the right track.

# Chapter 13

# Healthy Grocery Shopping

***In This Chapter***

- Taking inventory of your edibles
- Choosing what's wholesome
- Checking out the details before you buy
- Figuring out how much is in a serving

More places sell food today than at any other time in history. Just five years ago, people bought gas at a gas station. Today, they can buy all kinds and sizes of snacks and sodas — and plenty of calories. If you don't plan ahead and do a weekly or twice-weekly grocery run, you may be forced to shop at the quick stop. That means being faced with aisles of foods that shout, "Buy me! Eat me!" It's a jungle of temptation out there. To stay on the weight-loss track, arm yourself with the tips in this chapter.

## Making a Healthy Grocery List

Shoppers who use lists spend slightly more money per trip to the grocery store than nonlist users, but they don't have to run back to the market as frequently to pick up forgotten items. The benefit to dieters: Temptation has fewer chances.

Some tips for making sure that your grocery list is diet friendly and that your trip to the store is as quick and painless as possible are as follows:

- Plan your menus when you're hungry. They'll be more interesting. But shop when you're not hungry, so you'll have more control.
- Forget using coupons, unless they're for food items that you usually buy. The savings can be tempting, but the purchase can add up to a diet disaster.

- Check your cupboards, freezer, and refrigerator in advance to avoid duplicating purchases.
- Find out the store's layout and write your list according to it. You'll be less likely to forget items. Or write your list according to categories: frozen foods, produce, meat, and dairy, for example.

# Filling Your Grocery Cart the Right Way

Your menus, shopping list, and filled grocery cart should be in the same proportion as the Food Guide Pyramid: whole grain bread, cereal, rice, and pasta should occupy the largest space and be the foundation on which the rest is built. Fruits and vegetables come next in order of predominance and then meat and dairy. Fats, oils, and sugar should take up the least amount of space. Keep reading for some specifics about the Food Guide Pyramid's recommendations.

## Breads, cereals, rice, and pasta

Thick-sliced, thin-sliced, with sugar or without, whole-grain or white, this category has grown to one of the most confusing and calorie dense in the store. Shop carefully and heed these hints.

- When you buy breads, make sure that the first grain on the ingredient list is a whole grain, such as whole wheat, oats, or millet. Note that rye and pumpernickel breads aren't whole grain, even though their color may make you think that they are. Their fiber content is similar to that of white bread, but the calorie content is often slightly higher, because molasses is added for color.
- Baked goods should have 3 grams of fat or less per serving. And cereal should have at least 3 grams of fiber per serving.
- Pizza dough or crusts should be whole wheat. Search them out or ask your grocer to stock them.
- Frozen waffles and pancakes should be lowfat.
- Baked goods from the in-store bakery don't usually have nutrient labeling. Look at the ingredient list to see what kinds of flour are used. Go for the ones that list whole-grain flours first.

- Avoid giant muffins, biscuits, and scones. One has several servings' worth of fat and calories.

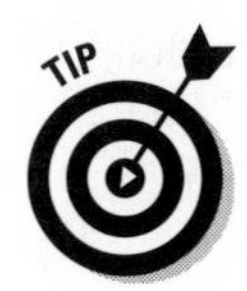


One store-bought brand name bran muffin has 160 calories and 7 grams of fat. Depending on the recipe, a homemade bran muffin may have much less. One muffin made per the recipe in the 1964 edition of *The Joy of Cooking,* for example, has 135 calories and 4 grams of fat.

- When you read labels on packaged mixes, be sure to look at the *As Prepared* column. Many mixes call for fats or eggs to be added in preparation.

- Brown rice has almost three times the fiber of white rice.
- Ramen noodle soups are flash-cooked in oil before packaging, which means that they're high in fat.
- A sugar-sweetened cereal that has 8 grams of carbohydrate per serving has the same amount of sugar as an unsweetened cereal to which one rounded teaspoon of sugar has been added.
- Seeded crackers have slightly more calories than plain ones, but they have more fiber, too.

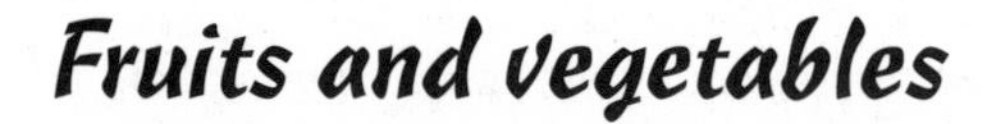

## Fruits and vegetables

No question about it: Fruits and vegetables are almost *free* foods for dieters. But eating healthfully means more than counting calories. Vitamins and minerals are important, too. Want to get more nutrition out of your fruits and vegetables? Follow these tips:

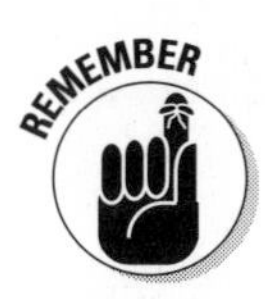


- In general, the darker the color, the higher the nutrient content. Dark salad greens, such as spinach, watercress, and arugula contain more nutrients than pale ones, such as iceberg lettuce. Deep orange- or red-fleshed fruit, such as mangoes, melon, papaya, and oranges, are richer in vitamins C and A than pears and bananas, but pears and bananas are especially good sources of potassium and fiber.
- For the best buy and best flavor, get fresh fruits and vegetables while they're in season. Otherwise, canned or frozen forms processed without added sugar, fats, or sauces are a good choice.
- Fresh produce doesn't carry nutrient labels; look for nutrition fliers or posters in the produce department for specifics. If prepared without sauces, butter, or added sugar, most fruits weigh in at less than 60 calories per ½ cup serving. Most vegetables contain a mere 25 calories per ½ cup cooked serving or per 1 cup raw.
- Most fresh produce is virtually fat free, with the exception of avocado and coconut.

- Shop the salad bar when you need ingredients for a recipe but don't purchase more than you can use at one time. Cut ingredients will lose nutrients faster than whole. Cut produce in bags is packaged in special material that cuts down on moisture loss and, therefore, nutrient loss, too.
- Prebagged salad is a staple in every supermarket. Buy the salad that's packaged without dressing packets or garnishes. (These items are high in fat and calories.) And for a longer shelf life at home, buy bags of single variety lettuces and create your own mix. Fragile leaves in salad blends can spoil quickly, ruining the whole bag.
- Dried fruits are a healthy, high-fiber snack food, but because most of the water has been removed from them, the nutrients are concentrated and the calories are higher. Keep an eye on serving size.
- Many dried fruits, especially bananas, cranberries, and dates, have sugar added to them.

## Dairy

One of the first foods to be cut from many dieters' shopping lists and menus is dairy. What a shame! Most people, women in particular, need to *increase* their dairy consumption, because they don't get enough precious bone-building calcium. Plus, incorporating more dairy products can actually enhance weight loss according to accumulating research. In the February 2002 issue of *Lipids,* a medical journal, research at the University of Tennessee concluded that increasing dietary sources of calcium, especially from dairy products, reduces body fat, even without calorie restriction and accelerates weight loss when calories are reduced.

Lowfat dairy products are among the best-tasting fat-reduced items in the supermarket, and they have all the calcium of the full-fat varieties. Don't cut out dairy products altogether — just cut down on the high-fat (and high-calorie) dairy foods. Look for the following when you shop:

- Buy only lowfat (1 percent) or fat-free (skim) milk. Two-percent milk isn't lowfat. Lowfat or fat-free milk is often fortified with nonfat milk protein to improve its texture. An added bonus is that it has a bit more calcium than whole milk.
- Buy only lowfat or nonfat yogurt and cottage cheese. Creamed cottage cheese (4 percent milk fat) doesn't have cream added to it; it's made with whole milk. The name refers to the way it's processed.
- Search out and buy lowfat cheeses. They're labeled *part skim, reduced fat,* or *fat free.* However, strongly flavored full-fat cheeses are fine if used sparingly.

- Buttermilk contains no butter and is available in lowfat and fat-free varieties. Some dieters find that its thicker texture is more satisfying than that of fat-free milk.

## Meat, poultry, fish, dry beans, eggs, and nuts

Many dieters make the mistake of thinking that if they cut out meat, they cut out calories. Unfortunately, they often substitute high-fat cheese, nuts, and nut butters for protein. Without meat, getting enough zinc and iron — two nutrients that help maintain your energy and performance — is tough. Don't shortchange yourself nutritionally by making sacrifices that don't help. Shop smart instead. See the suggestions that follow:

- Some of the leanest cuts of beef are flank, sirloin, and tenderloin. The leanest pork is fresh, whole canned hams, cured, and boiled ham. Canadian bacon, pork tenderloin, rib chops, and roast are also on the lean side. Lean lamb includes roasts, chops, and legs; white-meat poultry is lower in fat than dark.
- Meat labeled *select* is leaner than meat graded *choice.*
- Turkey or chicken skin is high in fat and calories. When you shop, look for a label that reads ground turkey or chicken *meat* for the lowest fat. Or better yet, look for a label that reads *ground turkey breast,* which is lower still.

- Self-basting turkeys have fat injected into the meat. Dieters should avoid them.
- Buy water-packed tuna and sardines rather than those packed in oil.
- Buy only fresh seafood or seafood that's frozen without added breading or frying.
- Cold cuts should be lowfat. Turkey and chicken franks don't always have fewer calories than beef or pork; check the labels.
- A half-cup of beans or 3 ounces of tofu equals a serving of protein. Check the ingredient list for calcium sulfate. Tofu processed with it is a good source of calcium.
- Two tablespoons of peanut butter counts nutritionally as an ounce of meat, but at 190 calories and 16 grams of fat, it's hardly a dieter's best bet. Even reduced-fat peanut butter has 12 grams of fat, and because it has added sugar, the reduced-fat and regular versions have the same number of calories.

## Better beef for your burger

When well done, the nutritional difference between a burger made with regular ground beef and one made with extra lean doesn't amount to much. When broiled on a rack or grilled, about 2 ounces of fat drips out of the regular meat. Lean meat loses a similar amount of weight, but it's fat plus water. A well-done burger made with 4 ounces of regular ground beef or chuck has only 12 calories more than a same-size, extra-lean burger, and has almost the same number of calories as one made with lean ground beef. The big difference is in price and flavor — regular ground beef or chuck wins on both counts.

| | ***Raw*** | | ***Cooked (Well Done)*** | |
|---|---|---|---|---|
| ***Ground Beef*** | ***Calories*** | ***Fat (Grams)*** | ***Calories*** | ***Fat (Grams)*** |
| Extra lean (17% fat) | 264 | 19 | 186 | 11 |
| Lean (21% fat) | 298 | 23 | 196 | 12 |
| Regular (chuck) (27% fat) | 350 | 30 | 198 | 13 |

### Fats, oils, and sweets

At the very top of the Food Guide Pyramid is the tiny triangle of fats and sweets. These foods add calories without contributing much in the way of other nutrients to your diet. Use them sparingly. But do remember that when you plan carefully, you can make room for these fun foods, too. Consider these tips:

- With the exception of whipped or diet spreads, all butter, margarine, and oils have about 100 calories per tablespoon. Whipped has about 70, and light varieties have 50 to 60.
- Sugar, syrups (such as pancake and maple), and jelly beans don't add fat, but that doesn't mean that they're free foods. They still have calories. One *level* teaspoon of sugar has 16 calories — surely not enough to ruin your diet, but if you have 3 cups of coffee and a bowl of cereal a day and use 2 teaspoons of sugar in each, that's a quick 128 calories. If you substituted no-calorie sweeteners for this amount of sugar and made no other changes in the way you ate, you'd lose 1 pound in a month.
- Keep nuts on your shopping list, because they contain heart-healthy antioxidants and make great snack foods. But buy them in the shell. Opening the shells as you eat will slow you down, so you don't wolf them by the fistful.

# Navigating the Supermarket Maze

Supermarkets are sophisticated marketing systems. Everything you see and smell in a grocery store is specifically crafted to entice you to buy more. Where items are placed in the store, whether a package meets you at eye level or your child's eye level, the amount of time the aroma of chickens roasting in the deli wafts under your nose, the brightness of the lights, the tempo of the music — everything is carefully chosen. To effectively navigate the supermarket maze, remember to

- Double-check the end-of-aisle displays against the usual in-aisle stock. The items featured at the ends of the aisles aren't always on special.
- Eat before shopping and feed the children, too. Hunger makes controlled shopping difficult for adults and nearly impossible for children.
- Refuse to be tempted by free samples. (If you're not hungry, you're better able to pass them by.)
- Realize that the most frequently purchased foods are placed farthest from the door. That setup forces you to pass many other tempting items.
- Look up and down. The more expensive items are generally placed at eye level. Bargains can often be found on less convenient shelves.
- Become a label reader and use the nutrition information. A label shows the size of a serving (it may be smaller than you think), the number of servings in the package, and the ingredients, as well as the food's nutrient profile. (See the following section "Label Reading 101 for Dieters," for more information.)

# Label Reading 101 for Dieters

Since 1990, when the Food and Drug Administration's Nutrition Labeling and Education Act (NLEA), went into effect, all packaged food products (with a few exceptions) carry labeling, which states the nutrition content in the package. The law also allows manufacturers to use certain food-and-health claims on the labels of their products too.

But such labeling can be overwhelming. When you understand how to read and use the information on a food label, you'll discover that the label can help you choose foods that fit into your diet. This section explains everything you'll see on a typical label and how to use the information to your advantage.

## Nutrition Facts label

Choosing foods wisely based on the information that you can glean from Nutrition Facts labels is key to successful dieting. At first, the label may seem awfully confusing, but if you know what to look for, interpreting a label is really pretty simple. See the list that follows for the skinny on the most important information featured on the Nutrition Facts label:

- **Calories:** The calorie total is based on the stated serving size — so if you eat more or less than what the label lists as one portion, you need to do the math.
- **Dietary fiber:** Choose the foods with the most fiber. Research shows that people who eat plenty of fiber also eat fewer calories. You get the most fiber in foods made from whole grains, such as cereals and breads. Fruits and vegetables have fiber, too. A food is considered to be high in fiber if it has at least 5 grams of fiber per serving.
- **Serving size:** Notice how the food manufacturer's serving size compares to the size you usually eat. For example, does your normal serving of ice cream measure more than the standard ½ cup? And remember that serving amounts are given in *level* measuring cups or spoons. Servings per container can help you estimate sizes if a measuring cup or spoon isn't handy.
- **Total fat:** For dieting, keep total fat to less than about 20 to 30 percent of calories. For someone who eats 1,500 calories a day, that's no more than 33 to 50 grams. Remember, the Percentage Daily Value numbers on Nutrition Facts labels are based on 65 grams of fat a day (30 percent of total calories) and calculated on a 2,000-calorie-per-day diet.

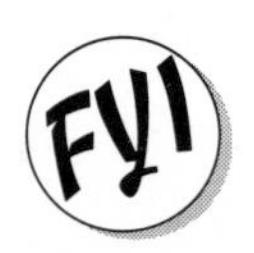


*Trans fatty acid* is the newest item to be added to the Nutrition Fact label. By January 2006, all foods required to carry nutrition labeling will have to state the amount of trans fatty acids in their product. Like saturated fat, trans fat is a type of fat. The grams of these fats, and their calories, are already accounted for in the total fat.

To quickly figure the number of grams of fat that 30 percent represents, start with your total number of daily calories. Drop the last digit and then divide the remaining number by 3. So if you allow yourself 1,800 calories for the day, divide 180 by 3 to get 60 grams of fat as your daily limit.

## More labeling lingo

In addition to the information on the nutrition panel, food packagers can also use descriptive terms, which are very specific and legally defined. Table 13-1 lists some of the terms that are particularly important when on a weight-loss plan.

**Table 13-1 Label Lingo**

| *What the Food Label Says* | *What It Means* |
|---|---|
| Fat-free | Less than ½ (0.5) gram of fat in a serving. |
| Calorie-free | Less than 5 calories per serving. |
| Lowfat | 3 grams of fat (or less) per serving. |
| Lean (on meat labels) | Less than 10 grams of fat per serving, with 4.5 grams or less of saturated fat and 95 milligrams of cholesterol per serving. |
| Extra lean (on meat labels) | Less than 5 grams of fat per serving, with less than 2 grams of saturated fat and 95 milligrams of cholesterol. |
| Less | Contains 25 percent less of a nutrient or calories than another food. |
| Reduced | A nutritionally altered product that contains at least 25 percent fewer calories, sodium, or sugar than the regular one. |
| Lite (Light) | Contains ⅓ fewer calories or no more than ½ the fat of the higher-calorie, higher-fat version; or no more than ½ the sodium of the higher-sodium version. |
| Cholesterol-free | Less than 2 milligrams of cholesterol and 2 grams (or less) of saturated fat per serving. |
| Healthy | The food must be low in fat and saturated fat and contain limited amounts of cholesterol and sodium. |
| Percent fat free | The food must be low in fat or fat free. Plus, it must reflect the amount of fat present in a serving. In other words, if a food contains 5 grams of fat in a serving, it can be labeled "95 percent fat free." |
| Low-calorie | Fewer than 40 calories per serving. |

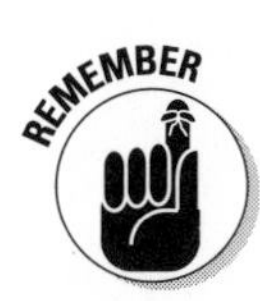


Don't confuse total fat and calories with cholesterol, saturated fat, and sodium. All the nutrients that a food contains are important; however, to achieve weight loss, the total fat and calories are the most important to track. Cholesterol and sodium (salt) don't add calories but eating too much sodium can contribute to water retention and therefore water weight. The calories from saturated fat are included in the *calories from fat* total.

## Sneaky Servings and Other Portion Tricks

Many dieters find that portion control is real tricky. Manufacturers certainly don't help in this regard. Some containers look as though they should contain one serving, because that's probably how most people consume them. However, consider that

- A 16-ounce container of iced tea is 2 servings.
- A 6½- to 7-ounce can of tuna is 2½ servings.
- A 4-, 6-, or 8-ounce container of yogurt is considered one serving.
- A 20-ounce bottle of soda is 2 servings.

See Chapter 9 for tips on estimating portion sizes with your hand.

# Chapter 14

# Outfitting and Using Your Kitchen

### In This Chapter

- Using appliances and gadgets for healthy cooking
- Adopting good-for-you cooking techniques
- Stocking your cupboard, refrigerator, and freezer

If you read Chapter 8, you know how many calories you need to lose weight. And if you read Chapter 13, you know what foods make the healthiest choices in the supermarket. If you look ahead to Chapter 15, you can find out how to eat low-cal when dining out. But eventually, you'll have to brave going into the kitchen and actually prepare the foods that you eat. Take courage! You can do it. And this chapter shows you how. Cooking and eating low-cal and lowfat needn't be mysterious. Armed with the information in this chapter, cooking and eating low-cal and lowfat can become second nature.

## Amassing Your Cooking Arsenal

You don't need to reoutfit your kitchen to make the switch to lowfat, low-calorie cooking techniques. In fact, you probably already own many of the most useful fat-fighting gadgets:

- **Nonstick skillet:** Using a skillet with a nonstick surface eliminates the need for oil, butter, or some other fat to prevent sautéed foods from sticking. If you've tried nonstick pans but gave up on them because they required special cooking spoons and spatulas and gentle washing, take another look: Nonstick coatings have come a long way since the early days of scratch-and-peel Teflon. Today, it's chip resistant and durable.

  Invest in top quality. Look for a heavy skillet with a tough, textured coating. Heavy pans deliver even, high heat without hot spots, because they don't warp. A ringed, circular pattern or a grid of squares on the cooking surface is a good investment because it makes deglazing easy — after you sauté meat or fish in the pan and remove the fat, you can add water, wine, or broth and make a sauce from the browned bits that cling to the bottom of the skillet.

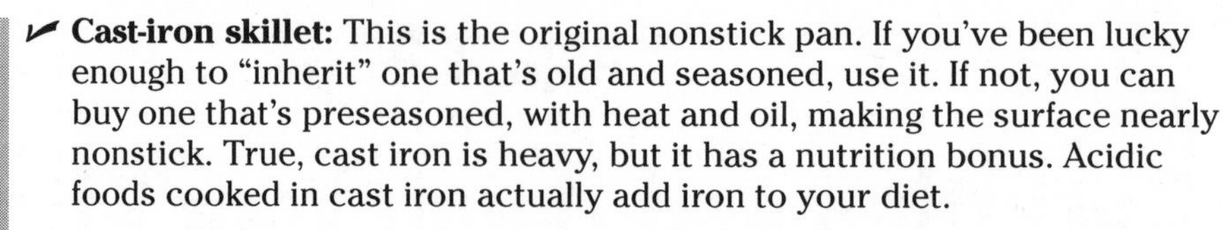

- **Cast-iron skillet:** This is the original nonstick pan. If you've been lucky enough to "inherit" one that's old and seasoned, use it. If not, you can buy one that's preseasoned, with heat and oil, making the surface nearly nonstick. True, cast iron is heavy, but it has a nutrition bonus. Acidic foods cooked in cast iron actually add iron to your diet.

  To clean a cast-iron skillet, scrape it with a spatula and then wipe it with a damp paper towel. To remove the occasional stubborn bit stuck to the pan, scrub it with coarse salt using a paper towel dipped in vegetable oil. Don't use soap. It will ruin the seasoning, and you'll have to give it a new coat of vegetable oil and set it in a 325-degree Fahrenheit oven for about an hour.

- **Instant-read thermometer:** Lean meats and egg whites have very little fat, so they can be a dieter's best friends. But because they don't have fat, which also tenderizes them, cooking times must be brief. Cook pork, beef, or chicken too long, and it becomes tough and chewy; overcook an egg white and it bounces. However, food poisoning from undercooked foods is really scary and, unfortunately, a fact of life. To avoid this situation, take your food's temperature periodically with an instant-read thermometer. This kind of thermometer isn't meant to stay in a food as it cooks. Chefs keep these pencil-size thermometers in their chest pockets for quick access.

  Minimum safe food temperatures include

  - **Eggs:** 140 degrees F
  - **Beef and lamb:** 145 degrees F for medium rare; 160 degrees F for medium
  - **Poultry:** 170 degrees F for breast meat; 180 degrees F for the whole bird
  - **Pork:** 160 degrees F

- **Measuring cups, measuring spoons, and a kitchen scale:** No, you don't need to portion out every ingredient or serving of food before it passes your lips, but watching portions is the easiest way to cut calories. So when you start out, keep track of how much you eat by measuring your portion sizes. Doing so will make a difference in your weight-loss efforts. For example, a measuring spoon that's been leveled, rather than a heaping soupspoon full of mayonnaise or creamy salad dressing can mean up to 100 calories saved. Likewise, you can save 75 calories by using a scale to measure your 3-ounce steak serving versus estimating and serving yourself 4 ounces instead.

- **Plastic bottles:** A refillable pump bottle beats cans of fluorocarbon-fortified vegetable oil cooking spray. Fill a bottle with olive oil and use it to lightly coat baking dishes and pans or spray a shimmer of oil over vegetables before roasting. Or fill one with salad dressing to make calorie-wise serving sizes a blast.

Squeeze bottles (such as the ones used for ketchup at diners) can shave calories, too, because you can put just a bit of sauce or gravy only where you need it. You just can't do that with a spoon, pitcher, or ladle. Even high-fat sauces, when dotted judiciously, are condoned in a lowfat kitchen.

- **Food processor:** A processor speeds up chopping, grating, and/or blending of vegetables and low-cal, lowfat sauces and marinades — jobs that seem daunting if done by hand are a snap with one of these. Mini-processors are particularly helpful for small jobs, such as chopping a cup's worth of vegetables. They're more affordable than the large-size processors, too.
- **Gravy strainer:** A gravy strainer is a measuring cup with a pour spout that starts at the base. It makes skimming fat from sauces, broths, and meat drippings a snap. Instead of spooning away the fat that floats to the surface, a strainer lets you pour out the nonfat portion from the bottom, leaving the fat behind. Buy a large one and use it for soups as well as pan drippings.
- **Sharp knives:** One of the greatest detriments to cooking low-cal or otherwise is not being able to quickly and safely cut and chop. The basics: a serrated-edge bread knife (which is great for tomatoes, too), a paring knife (about 3 inches in length), and a chef's knife (8 to 10 inches in length) for chopping.
- **Microwave oven:** If you use it for nothing else than zapping leftovers or "steaming" vegetables and fish without the added fat, a microwave is worth having.

- **Popcorn popper:** Invest in an air popper or a popper that you can use in the microwave without added oil. After it's popped, spray the popcorn with a light mist of water before adding salt or herbs — the seasonings will stick better.
- **Plastic bags:** Store washed, trimmed vegetables and fruits in plastic bags, so they're ready to go when you need a snack or when meal prep time is short. Plastic bags made specifically for storing vegetables and lettuce have tiny holes in them and help ready-to-eat and perishable vegetables keep for up to a week.

# Becoming a Calorie-Conscious Cook

Standard cooking methods need some reworking to make them lowfat and low calorie, and some foods can be used as substitutes, making them great, healthy stand-ins for others. Every calorie-conscious cook should use the following tricks:

- **Sauté onion and garlic the lowfat way:** When a recipe calls for onion and garlic to be cooked in oil, use a nonstick pan and 2 tablespoons of water in place of the oil. Use low heat and cover the pan to coax the natural juices out of the onion and garlic while they tenderize.
- **Make and use yogurt cheese:** Spoon a 16-ounce container of plain, low-fat yogurt (made without gelatin) into a colander lined with cheesecloth or into a paper filter-lined coffee cone. Place it over a bowl in the refrigerator and allow the yogurt to drain for 8 to 24 hours, depending on how firm you want the "cheese" to be. Use well-drained yogurt as a cream cheese substitute; when softer, you can use it in place of sour cream or heavy cream.
- **Make your own vinaigrette salad dressing:** The standard vinaigrette dressing (3 parts oil to 1 part vinegar) weighs in at about 90 calories a tablespoon. If you used more vinegar than oil, the calorie count would be great, but your salad would be unbearably pungent. Instead, use 1 part oil; 1 part flavorful yet mellow vinegar, such as balsamic; and 1 part strong black tea or citrus juice, such as orange or grapefruit.
- **Roast garlic:** When roasted, garlic is transformed into a rich, buttery, nonbiting, nonodorous spread that you can substitute for mayonnaise in potato, pasta, and chicken salads. It's also delicious when spread on bread in place of butter or oil. Bake a head of garlic, trimmed to expose the cloves and sealed in foil with a scant tablespoon of water, for 45 minutes in a 400 degree F oven. Unwrap and cool it until it's easy to handle and then simply squeeze the garlic from its skin.
- **Use aged cheese:** The stronger the flavor, the less you need. When a recipe calls for a mild cheese, such as mozzarella or Monterey Jack, whose flavor often disappears when cooked, substitute aged cheddar, Asiago, imported Parmesan, or an aged and smoked cheese, such as smoked Gouda. For the greatest bang for the bite, use these cheeses only where you see them, like on top of a dish, or when the recipe would suffer without the taste of cheese.
- **Roast vegetables:** You know that you need to eat more vegetables, but you may be bored by plain steamed ones. Roast them instead in a hot oven, and you'll caramelize the natural sugars that they contain and add a depth of flavor that naked veggies lack. Set the oven to 450 degrees F. Slice large vegetables in half or cut them into ½-inch thick slices and arrange in a single layer. Lightly spritz them using a pump bottle filled with olive oil to prevent them from drying. Cook them according to the following suggested guidelines:
  - **Beet halves:** Roast for 1 to 1½ hours.
  - **Winter squash slices:** Roast for 8 to 12 minutes.
  - **Carrots:** Roast for 15 to 20 minutes.
  - **Green beans and red pepper strips:** Roast for about 12 minutes.
  - **Onion halves:** Roast for about 30 minutes.

- **Sweet potato slices:** Roast for 15 minutes.
- **Summer squash or zucchini slices:** Roast for 5 to 8 minutes.
- **Eggplant slices:** Roast for 10 to 15 minutes.

To lightly and evenly coat vegetables before roasting or to lightly dress a salad, drizzle a bit of oil or vinaigrette in an empty bowl. Then add the ingredients and toss.

- **Use sun-dried tomatoes in place of bacon:** You can easily duplicate the mellow richness and smokiness that fatty pork adds to soups, stews, and pizzas with chopped sun-dried tomatoes. Don't use the oil-packed ones unless you drain them well and blot them dry. You can soften up the dried ones in a bit of hot water.
- **Swap fruit for most of the fat in baked goods:** You can't remove all the oil or butter from baked goods and still have something worth eating. But you can reduce the fat to about one-quarter of the original amount and replace the rest with prune pie filling (*lekvar*), apple butter, or applesauce.
- **Brown butter to use less:** Heat a bit of butter in a skillet until it becomes fragrant and begins to turn nutty brown. You'll punch up its flavor, so you can use less. A tiny bit drizzled over corn on the cob, eggs, or vegetables tastes like you're using much more.
- **Toast nuts for greater flavor bang:** Heat the oven to 350 degrees F and toast nuts — on a cookie sheet in a single layer — for five minutes or until fragrant. Stir them to prevent scorching. Treat toasted nuts in a recipe as you would cheese: Use them only where the flavor really counts or where they'll be seen, such as on the top of a bread.
- **Switch from chocolate to cocoa powder:** You can replace one ounce of chocolate (135 calories) with 3 tablespoons of cocoa (35 calories). Dutch-processed cocoa is richer and more intense than the American varieties; dutching neutralizes the natural acidity in cocoa powder, making the flavor mellower and the color darker.

Table 14-1 lists a few more diet-friendly switches to consider.

**Table 14-1 Calorie-Shaving Switches**

| *Instead Of* | *Use* | *Calories Saved* |
|---|---|---|
| 1 medium white potato | 1 medium sweet potato | 100 |
| 3 ounces ground beef | 3 ounces ground turkey meat* | 100 |
| 1 tablespoon mayonnaise | 1 tablespoon lowfat mayonnaise | 65 |
| 10 fried tortilla chips | 10 baked tortilla chips | 20 |

*(continued)*

**Table 14-1 (continued)**

| *Instead Of* | *Use* | *Calories Saved* |
|---|---|---|
| 1 cup whole milk cottage cheese | 1 cup fat-free or 1% milk | 64 (fat-free) or 48 (1%) |
| 1 flour tortilla | 1 corn tortilla | 50 |
| 1 cup whole milk | 1 cup 1% cottage cheese or ricotta cheese whirled in a blender | 268 |
| 1 whole egg | 2 egg whites | 46 |
| ½ cup cream | ½ cup evaporated fat-free milk | 145 |
| ½ cup premium ice cream | ½ cup regular ice cream | 100 |
| 3½ ounces tuna in oil | 3½ ounces tuna in water | 80 |
| ½ cup canned fruit in syrup | ½ cup canned fruit in juice | 25 |

**Make sure that you select ground turkey breast meat. When the label says simply "ground turkey," skin may be included, and that means added fat.*

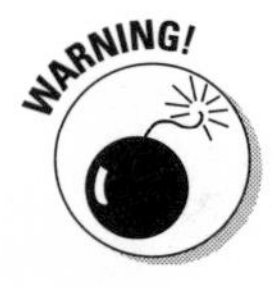


Not all reduced-fat products are reduced calorie. See Chapter 11 for more information about this danger.

# Stocking Your Cupboard, Refrigerator, and Freezer

To cook low calorie, you don't need to keep many bottled salad dressings, canned cream soups, and oils in your kitchen. Instead, stock your pantry with canned tomatoes, a flavorful olive oil, vinegars, and herbs and spices. Keep reading to find out about some good foods to keep on hand, by category.

## On the shelf

You may have to dig a bit deeper into your pockets for these basics, but after you taste them, you'll agree that paying more is worth the extra flavor they deliver.

- **A good stock:** Use stock (or broth) in salad dressings in place of some of the oil, to cook vegetables for more flavor, to start a homemade soup, or in place of butter or oil when a recipe says to sauté in oil.

  Store extra stocks (or broths) frozen in an ice cube tray to punch out 2 tablespoons whenever needed. You also can buy canned broth. We think low-sodium chicken broth has the best flavor. For beef or fish, try stock base. They're superconcentrated, and you must add water to them before use. Look for them in gourmet shops. They're pricey but worth it.
- **A selection of vinegars:** Sherry, rice, raspberry, wine, and balsamic vinegar are all milder than acidic white or cider vinegar. To make a lowfat vinaigrette, you must cut back on oil as you do when you cook low-cal. But oil helps tame the punch of vinegar's acid, making the dressing taste mellower. Therefore, you need a milder vinegar. Also consider using vinegar to sauté chicken breasts, or add a splash instead of fattening butter or cream sauces.
- **Hills of beans:** You can keep beans dry and cook them or stock many different kinds in cans. Either way, beans can be pureed into sandwich spreads and dips, added to soups, and sprinkled on salads as a nearly fat-free yet protein-packed alternative to meats and cheeses.
- **Tomatoes galore:** Take advantage of the variety of canned tomato products sprouting in the supermarket. Many of them are already seasoned, which is a time-cutting, but not calorie-building, bonus for you. Thicken them with a little cornstarch (about 1 teaspoon to an 8-ounce can) or reduce them simply by boiling, and you have the start of a sauce for pasta, vegetables, grilled fish, or chicken.

## Condiments with more flavor than fat

Tired of the same old broiled chicken breast or plain potato? Reach for one of these flavor-makers to spice up your palate:

- Mustard
- Hot sauce
- Chili powder
- Aged balsamic vinegar
- Salsa
- Grated horseradish
- Wasabi
- Harisa (Moroccan pepper paste)
- Pickles

*Tip:* Add 2 tablespoons prepared mustard to ½ cup pan drippings (that you have skimmed of their fat) and heat to boiling. You get a velvety sauce without needing to add cream, butter, or flour.

## In the refrigerator and freezer

Of course, your fridge will be stocked with many fresh fruits and vegetables and plain frozen ones, which are a lot lower in calories than the frozen ones packaged in sauce or butter. But leave room for these diet helpers, too:

- **Good extra-virgin olive oil:** You should use less oil on a reduced-calorie diet, so flavor counts. The earlier the press, the more flavor the olive delivers. Extra-virgin oil is made from the first press and has much more flavor than oil made from olives pressed several times.

  Olive oil spoils quickly. In a hot kitchen, it can turn rancid in as little as six months, so keep it in the fridge. It thickens and turns cloudy when chilled, but a few minutes at room temperature returns it to a golden liquid without damaging the flavor.

- **Lowfat and reduced-fat cheeses:** These can help you save fat and calories. Lowfat American, Monterey Jack, cheddar, and Havarti are good bets.
- **Aged cheese:** Compared to soft cheese, aged ones are typically high in fat, but because their flavor is so pungent, you can use less — a cooking bonus. (See the section "Becoming a Calorie-Conscious Cook," earlier in this chapter.)
- **Whole grains:** Whole grains don't have fewer calories than white, but they do have extra fiber, which helps fill you up. Studies show that people who eat an abundance of fiber have diets that are low in fat.

  Because whole grains go rancid quickly, store them in the fridge. Whole-wheat flour, corn meal, cracked wheat, brown rice, and wheat germ lasts longer when kept in cold storage.

- **Fresh herbs:** Use fresh herbs for garnish and flavor. Piney herbs, such as rosemary, sage, and thyme last longer than basil, oregano, cilantro, and mint. When using fresh herbs in recipes, add them at the end of cooking so that their flavors don't dissipate. (Dried herbs, on the other hand, are generally added early in the cooking process to coax as much flavor as possible from them.) Treat bunches of fresh basil like flowers; keep their stems in a vase of water outside of the refrigerator. Cold temperatures blacken and wilt the leaves.

## Chapter 15

# Eating Healthfully While Eating Out

### In This Chapter

- Understanding how dining out can add calories
- Spotting the high-fat cues on menus
- Knowing your best ethnic food choices
- Eating before you take off and during your flight

Eating out can pose special problems for dieters. New menu choices are tempting, portion sizes are large, and many professional kitchens don't normally use lowfat or low-calorie cooking methods as standard practice. In fact, as a rule, the less expensive the restaurant, the more likely it is that the kitchen uses generous amounts of fat and high-fat cooking techniques — inexpensive and easy ways to add flavor to food. A fish fillet, for example, must be high quality and cooked skillfully if it's going to taste delicious simply broiled or baked without a coating of oil or buttery sauce.

But don't fear. This chapter can help you navigate menus and still enjoy going out to eat. Armed with the information we give, you can be a dining detective, avoiding the high-fat items and zeroing in on the lower-calorie and lower-fat meals with ease.

## Knowing Your Enemy

The whole dining-out experience can cost you plenty of calories. How many times have you had to wait in the bar until your table was ready? Cocktails add calories and lessen your diet resolve — you get to the table famished and not exactly steeled against temptation. And then the impulse to clean your plate overtakes you because, after all, you're paying big bucks for the meal. But take heart: You can maneuver around these predicaments.

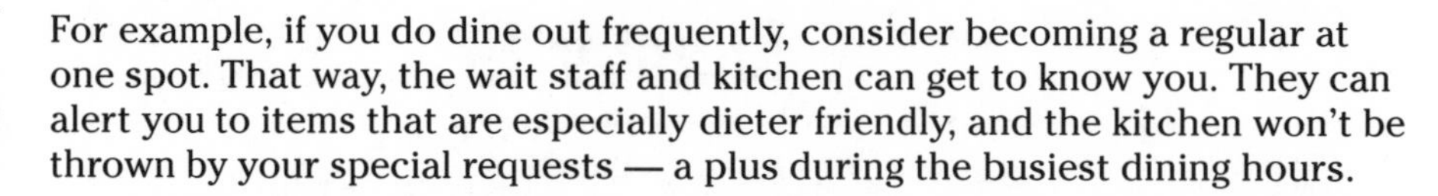

For example, if you do dine out frequently, consider becoming a regular at one spot. That way, the wait staff and kitchen can get to know you. They can alert you to items that are especially dieter friendly, and the kitchen won't be thrown by your special requests — a plus during the busiest dining hours.

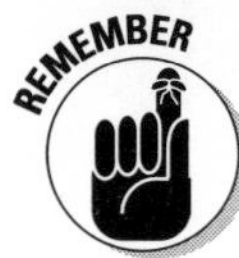

Whether dining out is more special or a routine part of your day, keep this advice in mind:

- **Restaurant meals are often considered special occasions.** More frequently, though they're last-minute solutions when you're too tired or stressed to make dinner. Both scenarios set you up for overindulging. Remember to look at the meal in context of the entire day's eating or what you'll eat over several days.
- **Restaurant meals are often loaded with fat.** Fat is an easy way to make foods taste good. Fat is also cheap compared to lean meat, so restaurants use it liberally because it makes their bottom line healthy — although it doesn't do much for the shape of *your* bottom. Be a fat detective. Ask questions about preparation and request substitutions.
- **Portions may be huge.** You often get twice the amount that you really need to eat. Share an entree with a friend or order two appetizers instead of one entree. Don't be embarrassed to ask for a doggie bag.
- **Menus are organized with the focus on protein, and the servings of protein are much too large.** Meat, chicken, and fish often get the most "ink," with little attention paid to side dishes. So cast your eye over to the side dishes section and choose from the plainer ones. (That is, those without sauces.) Another way to create a better balance may be to order your entree from the appetizer section.
- **Most meals eaten out include alcohol.** Not only is alcohol calorie heavy and nutrient poor, but it also lowers your resolve to eat healthfully. If you enjoy a cocktail or a glass of wine when eating out, plan to limit your intake to one, and drink it with, not before, the meal.

These are important tactics to keep in mind wherever you dine. They're a start. But menus are always going to be written to entice and seduce you into ordering more than you intend. If you can discover how to read between the lines and spot the red flags for dieters, you'll rarely be duped into ordering and eating more than you want. And when you eat ethnic, try to find out a little about the cuisine, the ingredients, and the typical methods of cooking so that foreign phrases don't throw you.

# Menu Sleuthing

If you know how to translate the code, menu descriptions can yield clues to the fat and calorie contents of a dish. For example, "Grande taco salad served in a crispy tortilla shell, topped with lean sautéed ground beef" may sound like a good choice at first. But the words *grande, crispy,* and *sautéed* tell you that this is no low-cal salad. In fact, it contains about 700 calories! If you're restricting your intake to 1,200 calories a day, do you really want to get more than half your calories from a single dish?

Following are the most commonly used menu words that speak volumes — calorically, that is.

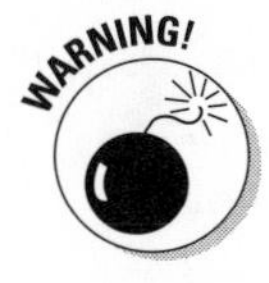


**Lots of fat:**

- Alfredo
- Basted
- Batter-dipped
- Breaded
- Buttery
- Creamy
- Crispy and crunchy (except when describing raw vegetables)
- Deep-fried
- Marinated
- Pan-fried
- Rich
- Sautéed
- Coated
- Dressed
- Dipped
- Bathed

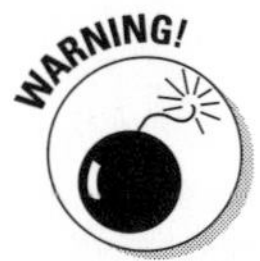


**Huge portion sizes:**

- Combo
- Feast
- Grande
- Jumbo
- King-size
- Supreme

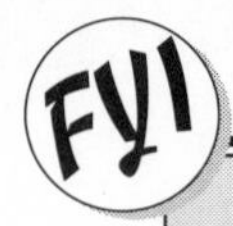

## A portion to a restaurant may not be a portion to you!

Restaurant portion sizes have more to do with controlling operation expenses than with balancing nutrients. Most restaurants use standardized ladles, spoons, cups, and scoops, and their capacity is generally larger than what you would use at home. Some typical institutional measures are:

- Salad dressing ladle = ¼ cup
- Pat of butter = 2 teaspoons
- Scoop of ice cream = 1½ to 2 cups
- Burger = 6 to 8 ounces
- Meat, poultry, or fish = 8 to 12 ounces
- Beverages: small = 2 cups, medium = 4 cups, large = 6 cups
- Theater popcorn: small = 4 cups, large = 10 cups, jumbo = 15 to 20 cups
- Wine = 6 to 8 ounces

**Saner sizes:**

- Appetizer
- Kiddie
- Luncheon
- Petite
- Regular
- Salad-size

# Taking a Dieter's Tour of Restaurants

You may think that you must avoid certain types of restaurants or cuisines while you're dieting. Not true. Keep reading if you want to be guided through various cuisines and food scenarios and find out what's "safe" and what's not.

## Chinese

Depending on your order, you can get a healthy low-cal meal or a calorie nightmare in a Chinese restaurant; foods are either lean or fatty. Generally, the protein foods in Chinese cuisine — duck, spareribs, and pork — are extremely fatty, although you can also find chicken, shrimp, and lean beef.

Much of the food is deep fried — even items that may surprise you, such as vegetables in a simple stir-fry are sometimes blanched in hot oil instead of water. And the amount of oil in stir-fries can be staggeringly large.

Family-style dining (large dishes are placed on the table for guests to help themselves) offers another temptation to eat too much simply because the food is there. So start with small portions and have seconds only if you're *really* hungry.

**Dieter's aid:** Eat the way the Chinese do. Rice is the centerpiece of the meal, and diners eat from their small rice bowls, not from big dinner plates. Meat and vegetables are selected from the serving dishes, almost one bite at a time, added to the bowl, and eaten with rice. Also, if you can't pass up an especially fatty dish, be sure to balance it with lean ones. Ask for brown rice, which has more fill-you-up fiber.

**Choose more of these:**

- Bean curd (unless fried)
- Fish, shrimp, and scallops
- Hot and spicy, as opposed to deep fried
- Served on a sizzling platter (which means the entrée is broiled or roasted)
- Vegetables
- Velvet sauce

**Eat less of these:**

- Anything served in a bird's nest
- Batter-fried foods
- Breaded and fried foods
- Crispy noodles on the table
- Sweet-and-sour dishes
- Sweet duck sauce
- Twice-cooked dishes

## Delis and sandwich shops

True delicatessens are overly generous on servings, piling sandwiches so high with meat that you need a knife and fork to eat them. What delis do vertically, sub shops (those that sell grinders and hoagies) do horizontally. Therefore, portion control is a must. Menus are usually flexible, so this is one type of restaurant where you can exercise your calorie-smart creativity.

**Dieter's aid:** Go to lunch with a friend, split a sandwich, and order an extra roll or bread to make two sandwiches out of the meat in one. Or if you're by yourself, order half a sandwich and extra bread and create two sandwiches for the price of one — taking one home for later, of course. Most restaurants that serve sandwiches also have soup. Order a bowl of a soup made without cream and eat it with an unbuttered roll, and you have a lower-calorie meal.

**Choose more of these:**

- Baked or boiled ham
- Beet salad
- Whole-grain bread
- Carrot and raisin salad
- Extra tomato, lettuce, and veggies for sandwiches
- Mustard (not mayo)
- Pickles
- Roast or smoked turkey
- Sliced chicken (not chicken salad with lots of mayo)
- Tuna
- Sauerkraut

**Eat less of these:**

- Bagels (They're huge!)
- Bologna
- Corned beef
- Eggplant or chicken Parmigiana
- Extra cheese
- Hot pastrami
- Knockwurst
- Liverwurst
- Meatballs
- Mortadella
- Reuben sandwiches (grilled corned beef, sauerkraut, and Swiss cheese with Thousand Island dressing)
- Salami
- Sausage and peppers
- Tongue

## Fast food

You can swear never to eat another burger, fry, or shake again, but get real. Often, the one and only option on America's interstates is fast food. And certainly, a trip to the mall usually means passing the food court, with its aromas seducing you to stop for just a little something.

Ever noticed where they put the restrooms in shopping malls? Other than the ones located within department stores, the men's and women's rooms are stacked near the food court. It's no accident — mall designers plan it that way.

**Dieter's aid:** To balance all the grim news about fast foods, consider the following few happy thoughts:

- You get no surprises. You know what will be on the menu. With few exceptions, the menus are the same from coast to coast, so you can choose a restaurant that you know offers items that fit into your diet.
- Except for beverages, portions are generally small, especially if you stick to the regular or kids' sizes.
- Most restaurants post nutrition information or will provide it when asked, so you can make informed choices.

Even a small soda is a generous portion, so be sure to order a diet one or a seltzer and drink it all before going back for more food — it *will* fill you up.

**Choose more of these:**

- Baked potato
- Grilled chicken
- Fat-free or lowfat milk
- Fat-free salad dressing
- Salad with the dressing on the side
- Single burger (regular or kid-size)
- Small fries

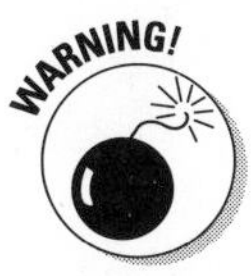


**Eat less of these:**

- Cheese sauce
- Chicken nuggets (they often include the skin)
- Croissants

- Fish sandwich (it's fried)
- Fried chicken
- Large and jumbo-size fries
- Onion rings
- Salad dressing (unless it's fat-free)
- Sauces and high-fat add-ons such as cheese, chili, and tartar sauce
- Specialty burgers

## French

Fat is the pitfall when it comes to French cuisine, from the butter on the table to the cream sauces, rich salad dressings, and desserts. Even lean meats and fish have added fat. Unless the restaurant specializes in *nouvelle cuisine* (the updated style of cooking that relies more on fresh ingredients and less on classic butter-enhanced sauces), you'll be hard-pressed to find diet-friendly foods.

**Dieter's aid:** Start with an appetite-taming green salad (easy on the dressing) or a clear soup.

**Choose more of these:**

- *Au vapour* (steamed)
- *En brochette* (skewered and broiled)
- *Grillé* (grilled)

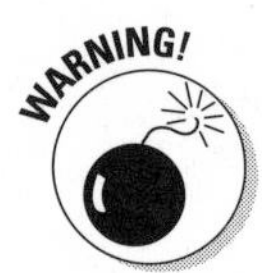


**Eat less of these:**

- *A la crème* (in cream sauce)
- *A la mode* (with ice cream)
- *Au gratin* or *gratinée* (baked with cheese and cream)
- *Crème fraîche* (similar to sour cream)
- Drawn butter
- *En croûte* (in a pastry crust)
- Hollandaise
- Puff pastry
- *Remoulade* (a mayonnaise-based sauce)
- Stuffed

# Indian

Some styles of Indian cooking are vegetarian, but don't let that lull you into thinking that these foods are low-cal. Plenty of fat is used in Indian cooking — usually clarified butter called *ghee.* Roasting tandoori style (in a clay oven called a *tandoor*) is a good lowfat cooking method, but other dishes are often stewed and fried. Indian breads are many and varied, ranging from *chapatti* to high-fat, deep-fried *poori.* Often, the chef gives the breads a shimmer of butter before serving them.

**Dieter's aid:** Indian cuisine doesn't focus on meat; rather, it uses carbohydrates, such as basmati rice (an aromatic long-grain variety) and lentils as its foundation. Vegetables are a part of almost every dish, and the sauces are enriched with yogurt, not cream.

**Choose more of these:**

- Chutney
- *Dahl* (lentils)
- *Masala* (curry)
- *Matta* (peas)
- *Paneer* (a fresh milk cheese)
- *Pullao* or *pilau* (rice)
- *Raita* (a yogurt and cucumber condiment)

**Eat less of these:**

- Chickpea batter used to deep-fry
- *Ghee* (clarified butter)
- *Korma* (cream sauce)
- *Molee* (coconut)
- *Poori* (a deep-fried bread)
- *Samosas* (fried turnover appetizers)

# Italian

Most Americans think of heavy southern Italian food when they think of high-cal items: meatballs, eggplant Parmigiana, veal Parmigiana, and lasagna. However, the food of northern Italy, while it may appear less caloric, also has its detractors: butter, olive oil, and cream.

**Dieter's aid:** Portions are overly generous in most Italian restaurants, so this may be a good place for sharing — particularly important when you consider that an antipasto of cheese, marinated vegetables, salami, and garlic bread can use up a day's calorie budget before the main course arrives. Bread on the table served with butter or olive oil can be a diet buster. Ask for tomato sauce for dipping if you must fill up on bread and have the fats removed. Or better yet, out of sight, out of mouth; have the bread removed, too. Order vegetables à la carte as long as they're not cooked with plenty of fat or deep-fried. And instead of a creamy dessert, order a lowfat cappuccino with fruit.

**Choose more of these:**

- Light red sauce
- Marinara sauce
- Pasta (other than those stuffed with cheese)
- *Piccata* (lemon-wine sauce)
- White or red clam sauce (but ask the wait staff; some clam sauces are made with cream)
- Wine sauce

**Eat less of these:**

- Alfredo
- *Alla panna* (with cream)
- Butter
- *Carbonara* (butter, eggs, bacon, and sometimes cream sauce)
- Fried eggplant or zucchini
- *Frito misto* (fried mixed vegetables or seafood)
- Olive oil
- *Parmigiana* (baked in sauce with cheese)
- Prosciutto
- Salami

## Japanese

Japanese can be one of the healthiest cuisines, with only a few fattening dishes, such as tempura, teriyaki, katso, and sukiyaki. If eaten in the balance that the Japanese apply — heavy on the vegetables and light on the fats and meats — Japanese food can be a dieter's dream.

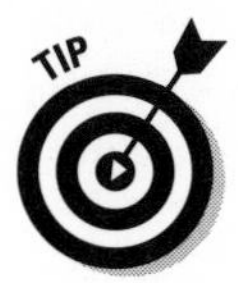


**Dieter's aid:** Portions are small, and rice and noodles are the foundation. Cooking techniques are most often broiling, steaming, braising, or simmering — all of which generally produce low-cal and lowfat dishes.

**Choose more of these:**

- Clear broth
- *Miso* (fermented soy)
- *Miso* dressing
- *Mushimono* (steamed)
- *Nabemono* (a one-pot dish)
- *Nimono* (simmered)
- Sashimi
- Sushi
- *Udon* (noodles)
- *Yaki* (broiled)
- *Yakimono* (grilled)

**Eat less of these:**

- *Agemono* (deep-fried)
- *Katsu* (fried pork cutlet)
- *Sukiyaki* (a one-dish meal made with fatty beef)
- *Tempura* (batter-fried)

## Mexican

The good news is that Mexican cuisine places minimal emphasis on meat protein. The bad news is that most Mexican food is fried or cooked in abundant amounts of fat.

For example, a flour tortilla is fine on its own, but roll it around a filling and deep-fry it, and you have mucho calorica. Many of the national Mexican food chains don't use lard or animal fat drippings, which is typical in many independent restaurants, but they do use plenty of vegetable oil. As far as calories are concerned, there's no difference between animal fat and vegetable fat.

**Dieter's aid:** Use salsa instead of salad dressing, guacamole, or sour cream on entrees. Ask for cheese toppings to be omitted or ask if lowfat sour cream and cheese are available.

**Choose more of these:**

- Black bean soup
- *Ceviche* (fish or scallops marinated in lime juice)
- Chili
- Enchiladas, burritos, or soft tacos (skip the sour cream, guacamole, and most of the cheese)
- Fajitas
- Gazpacho
- Mexican salad minus the fried taco shell

**Eat less of these:**

- Chimichangas
- Extra cheese
- Refried beans
- Sour cream
- Tortilla shells

## Pizza

The trend toward newfangled pizza is a real plus for dieters. You can add or subtract ingredients to fit your particular tastes. Meat choices have moved from extra pepperoni, sausage, and bacon to grilled chicken and shrimp. You can specify the kind of cheese you like and replace high-fat, low-flavor mozzarella with a smaller amount of full-flavored goat cheese or feta. Even a traditional pizzeria can be diet friendly if you order selectively.

**Dieter's aid:** If you can, start with a small salad to take the edge off your appetite. Order it with the dressing on the side or extra vinegar to thin it.

**Choose more of these:**

- Canadian bacon
- Grilled chicken
- Part-skim cheeses, or strongly flavored ones
- Shrimp
- Tuna
- Vegetable toppings, especially broccoli and spinach

**Eat less of these:**

- Bacon
- Extra cheese
- Extra olive oil
- Meatballs
- Olives
- Pepperoni
- Sausage

# Thai

Light on fats, most Thai dishes are stir-fried, steamed, braised, or marinated. The one exception is Thai curry, which is made with coconut milk. It's loaded with calories — 1 cup of the milk contains 445 calories.

**Dieter's aid:** Rice and noodles are staples. Ask the chef to substitute leaner scallops, shrimp, or skinless chicken for fatty duck. The ingredients in many Thai dishes are interchangeable, so asking for substitutions shouldn't pose a problem.

**Choose more of these:**

- Basil sauce
- Bean thread noodles
- Fish sauce
- Lime sauce
- *Sâté* (skewered and grilled meats)
- Sizzling
- Thai salad

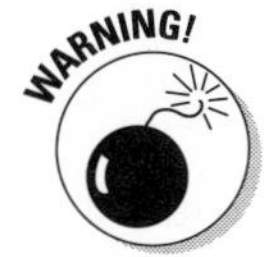

**Eat less of these:**

- Coconut milk soup
- *Mee-krob* (crispy noodles)
- Peanut sauce
- Red, green, and yellow mussman curries (They contain coconut milk.)

## Low calorie by law

You can be sure that you're getting a low-calorie meal when you order one. The Food and Drug Administration (FDA) has ruled that all restaurants (including airlines) must demonstrate that special menus comply with the same federal regulations as those used on the labels of packaged foods. The only difference is that restaurateurs aren't held to the same grueling standards applied to food manufacturers. They're not required to do laboratory nutrition analysis — they can use computer programs to do their calculations and show that the menu items are prepared from recipes that comply with the standards. They don't have to post the nutrient contents of their food, but they must have it available if you ask.

If you see these terms on a menu, they must comply with FDA standards.

- **Low calorie:** It contains 120 calories or less per 100 grams (about 3½ ounces).
- **Lowfat:** It has less than 3 grams of fat per 100 grams.
- **Low-cholesterol:** These items must contain less than 20 milligrams of cholesterol per 100 grams and no more than 2 grams of saturated fat.
- **Low sodium:** It has 140 milligrams or less of sodium per 100 grams.
- **Light:** This means that the item is low in fat or calories. (Restaurants may continue to use the term *light* as in "Lighter Fare" to mean smaller portions, as long as they make it clear how they're using the word.)
- **Healthy:** It's low in fat and saturated fat, has limited amounts of cholesterol and sodium, and provides significant amounts of one or more key nutrients: vitamin A, vitamin C, iron, calcium, protein, and fiber.

# Eating on the Fly: Airline and Airport Food

Airline food must meet a few standards. First-class servings are larger than those offered in coach; international flights are catered differently than domestic ones; meal service varies with the time of day. One thing is sure, though: If you fly coach, portions are tightly controlled, and that may be the best thing about eating on board.

Your larger challenge is probably the wait between connecting flights. Making sane, low-calorie choices from all the fast food available in terminals is tough, but it is getting easier because the variety of restaurants is enormous. A word of caution: Don't use food and eating as a way to kill time. Visit the magazine stand. The long corridors make great walking space if you stay off the moving sidewalks. Walk the corridors.

## Rules for the road

Whenever you're traveling, you're at the mercy of the food service industry. Their job is to get you to buy, and eat, more than you planned. Your responsibility is to your health. Advertising is seductive, and your resolve may be weak. But you can win the battle for your dinner dollars if you follow these suggestions.

- **Control your portions.** Go for the children's menus at fast food chains, such as McDonald's and Burger King. The portions are small but as filling if you eat slowly. One caveat: Don't drink even the kid's-size regular soda: It's too much — 15 oz. milk or diet soda or juice is better and all are allowed with the kid's meal. Add a salad if available.
- **Stick to your regular meal schedule.** If you normally have lunch at 1:00 p.m., then pull over at that time and get something to eat. This is particularly important when you're traveling with kids. Hungry children quickly become cranky children. Also, by not letting yourself get completely famished, you'll be better able to make smart food choices.
- **Get out of the car to eat.** You will pay more attention to what you're eating and have more healthy foods to choose from if you skip the drive-through and sit down at a table for lunch. If you eat too quickly, overeating is easy to do.
- **Eat with a fork and spoon.** Order foods that force you to slow you down. You can't eat salad or chunky soup easily with your hands.
- **Travel with plenty of water.** The air conditioning in cars and plane cabins is really dehydrating. Bring plenty of water for you (and your kids) to drink along the way.
- **Pack plenty of fruits and vegetables.** Eating in the car can easily become a bad habit if food is a way to occupy bored children. If you must pack snacks because you're traveling at snack or mealtime and can't stop, make them fruit and vegetables. It's much better to keep your hands and mouth busy with apples and baby carrots than crackers and potato chips.

# Part V
# Enlisting Outside Help

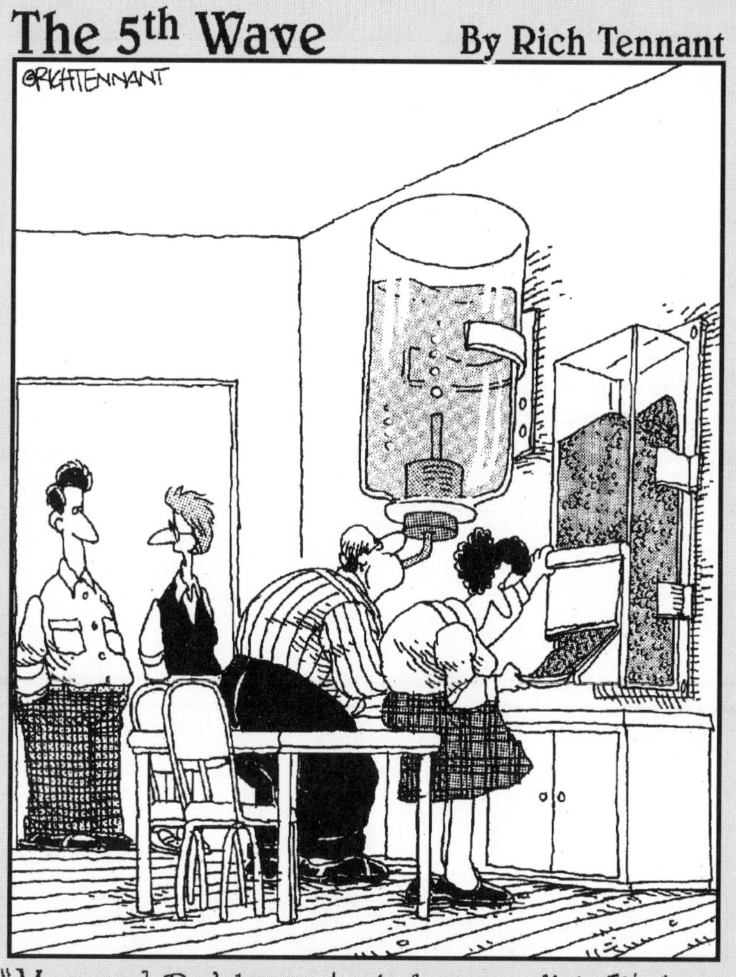


"Mom and Dad have started a new diet. It's been proven quite effective when used on hamsters."

## In this part . . .

Some dieters have more success when they enlist outside help, whether it comes from a weight-loss program, a doctor-prescribed medication, or a dietitian. People who are at least 100 pounds overweight may even need surgery to get their weight down to a healthy range. This part explains the many options that can help you to achieve success and spot questionable resources that may be best avoided. It also talks about some of the most popular diets out there today. In particular, Chapter 20 supports the ones that work and exposes the ones that don't.

## Chapter 16

# Getting Help from a Weight-Loss Professional

### *In This Chapter*

- Finding a bona fide weight-loss expert
- Knowing what to expect from pro counseling
- Hunting through the right organizations for help

Reading this book is a good way to get started toward your weight-loss goal. But sometimes going it alone isn't the best route. That's especially true if you

- Are involved in competitive sports and would like to enhance your performance.
- Have tried to lose and maintain your weight many times and have regained it (and more).
- Have health problems and need to modify your eating habits both to lose weight and to control your condition.
- Are worried about your child's weight or suspect she has an eating disorder.

If you look up *nutritionist* in the Yellow Pages, you're apt to find a hodgepodge of qualifications. How do you know whether the person that you find is qualified to help you? This chapter helps you sort the pros from the charlatans. Knowing the difference is important — your health depends on it. (For information about weight-loss centers, which also may be listed in the phone book under *nutrition* or *diet,* turn to Chapter 19.)

## Weeding Out the Pros from the Hoi Polloi

No nationwide law mandates what qualifications people must have before they call themselves a "nutritionist," "diet counselor," or "health advisor." However, the majority of states license or certify qualified nutritionists and dietitians. (In Canada, dietitians must be registered in the province in which they practice.) Unfortunately, a few states have no requirements or standards of practice yet. So being fooled into thinking that the advisor you meet is qualified to dispense accurate weight-loss information is an easy trap to fall into.

Just because someone *says* that she went through such-and-such a program or hangs a shingle outside her backdoor that has a title after her name on it doesn't mean that the so-called pro actually went through any training whatsoever or that she has any title, either. So before you spend your hard-earned cash on potions, pills, and quackery that some wannabe has sold you on, check out her credentials with the proper authority.

Table 16-1 lists some abbreviations that you're likely to encounter in your search for a nutrition specialist. But be sure to ask the counselor to explain his degree.

**Table 16-1 Abbreviations for Nutrition-Related Degrees and Other Related Designations**

| *Abbreviation* | *Degree or Designation* |
|---|---|
| CCP | Certified Culinary Professional |
| CD or CN | Certified Dietitian or Certified Nutritionist (granted by some states) |
| CDE | Certified Diabetes Educator |
| CDN | Certified Dietitian/Nutritionist (granted by some states) |
| CSP | Board Certified Specialist in Pediatric Nutrition |
| DTR | Dietetic Technician, Registered |
| EPC | Exercise Physiologist Certified |
| LD | Licensed Dietitian (granted by some states) |
| MD | Doctor of Medicine |
| MEd | Master of Education |
| MA | Master of Arts |
| MS | Master of Science |

| Abbreviation | Degree or Designation |
|---|---|
| MPH | Master of Public Health |
| ND | Naturopathic Doctor |
| PhD | Doctor of Philosophy |
| RD | Registered Dietitian |
| ScD | Doctor of Science |

## Registered dietitian

One way to ensure that you receive accurate nutrition and diet information is to search out a *registered dietitian* (RD) — a professionally trained authority on the role that food and nutrition play in health. RDs are a reliable source of information about nutrition and can provide sound advice on eating and health.

To earn an RD, an individual must have a bachelor's degree in nutrition or a related field from a regionally accredited college or university. The Commission on Accreditation and Approval of Dietetics Education of the American Dietetic Association must accredit the program of study. Courses include food science, nutrition, biochemistry, anatomy, physiology, biology, organic chemistry, and management. The individual must also complete a 6- to 12-month supervised practice experience at a healthcare facility, community agency, or foodservice corporation and pass an extensive examination to become registered.

All RDs are required to stay current by completing a minimum of 75 hours of continuing education every 5 years. Only dietitians who have passed the exam and maintain their continuing education are considered registered. Many RDs go on to earn additional degrees, such as master's (MS or MPH or MEd) or doctorates (PhD or ScD) in nutrition or a nutrition-related specialty.

Registered dietitians can also hold additional certifications in specialized areas of practice, such as pediatrics (CSP) and renal nutrition (CSR). These individuals must not only pass an extensive exam in their specialty but also accumulate a specific number of practice hours in their specialty.

Forty-six states certify or license dietitians and/or nutritionists who meet specific criteria established by the state agency that regulates health professionals. Certification entitles professionals to use "dietitian" or "nutritionist," depending on how the law is written within an individual state. The initials CD or CN appear after the name of a dietitian who is also state certified as a dietitian or nutritionist. Licensure protects the title "dietitian" or "nutritionist" and defines how they practice. The initials LD appear after the name of a licensed dietitian or nutritionist. In some states, dispensing nutrition advice without a license is against the law.

Individual state regulations determine which one of the following terms can be used:

- **Licensing** statutes include an explicitly defined scope of practice, and performance of the profession is illegal without first obtaining a license from the state.
- **Statutory certification** limits use of particular titles to persons meeting predetermined requirements, while persons not certified can still practice the occupation or profession.
- **Registration** is the least restrictive form of state regulation. As with certification, unregistered persons are permitted to practice the profession. Typically, exams aren't given and enforcement of the registration requirement is minimal.

## Dietetic technician, registered

The initials DTR stand for *dietetic technician, registered.* A person who is a DTR is qualified to be part of the nutrition care team, which may include teaching nutrition classes, diet counseling, and nutritional assessment. To become a DTR, an individual must earn an associate degree from a regionally accredited U.S. college or university, complete a dietetics practice program accredited by the Commission on Accreditation and Approval of Dietetics Education of the American Dietetic Association, pass a registration exam, and maintain at least 50 hours of continuing professional education every 5 years.

## Exercise physiologist

Exercise physiologists can help you plan an exercise program to aid in your weight-loss efforts, but they should not dispense diet advice. An exercise physiologist holds a bachelor's degree with an emphasis in exercise physiology. In addition to basic science courses, exercise physiologists study human anatomy and physiology, biomechanics, cardiopulmonary rehabilitation, exercise physiology, sports nutrition, electrocardiography, stress tests, and research and statistics. They also take a variety of specialized courses.

The American Society of Exercise Physiologists Board of Certification offers a national certification test for all graduates of an approved exercise physiology curriculum. A certified exercise physiologist is allowed to use the initials EPC, which stands for *Exercise Physiologist Certified,* after his name.

The American College of Sports Medicine (ACSM) also offers certification. Three levels of certification are offered to any professional within the preventive and rehabilitative exercise field who meets established prerequisites:

- **ACSM Registered Clinical Exercise Physiologists** have met education and clinical requirements. These individuals are competent in cardiovascular, metabolic, immunological, inflammatory, and neuromuscular ailments.
- **ACSM Exercise Specialists** can do exercise testing, exercise prescriptions, emergency procedures and health education for patients with cardiovascular, breathing, or metabolic diseases.
- **ACSM Health/Fitness instructors** conduct fitness testing and design and implement exercise programs for low-to-moderate-risk clients or with individuals who have any complicating diseases under control.

Each level of certification requires a written exam to test knowledge and a practical exam to measure hands-on skills. After earning ACSM certification, an exercise physiologist must participate in continuing education and maintain a current CPR certification.

## Physician

Medical doctors (MDs) offer medical weight-loss programs, which may include the use of prescription drugs and low-calorie diets (VLCD). Although any licensed physician can offer this kind of treatment, a *bariatrician* (from the Greek word *barros,* meaning heavy or large) specializes in treating obesity and has received special training and extensive continuing medical education. Often, a physician refers a patient to a registered dietitian for help with working out specific food issues.

VLCD, which stands for *very low calorie diet,* describes a plan — usually liquid — of 800 or fewer calories per day. These diets are generally considered safe when supervised by a healthcare team. Optifast and Health Management Resources are examples of a medically supervised VLCD. (See Chapter 19 for more information about these programs.)

# Understanding What the Pros Can Do

A nutritionist, dietitian, exercise physiologist, or physician can tailor an exercise and weight-loss program to meet your needs. The program should include personal, ongoing care. You attend an evaluation session, during which the healthcare professional assesses your history, preferences, and needs. He then gives you a personalized plan to follow and schedules follow-up appointments to check your progress and make adjustments to your program as needed.

Medical nutrition therapy, which is what insurance companies call *nutrition counseling,* may be covered by your health plan if a registered dietitian provides it. Be sure to ask your physician or insurance provider for information. Often insurance companies refuse to cover "diet," "weight," and "obesity" counseling. Yet they cover nutrition counseling if you also have been diagnosed with diabetes, high cholesterol, high blood pressure, or other complications of being overweight. Be sure to ask your health insurance carrier what the regulations are especially if you use an HMO — their coverage varies greatly.

If your insurance company doesn't cover nutrition therapy and you feel like you need counseling but can't afford the one-on-one that a Registered Dietitian provides, check out Chapter 19. You may find support from other like-minded and action-oriented individuals by joining a program that provides support but requires only member contributions in return.

The Internal Revenue Service (IRS) can help you recover some of the expenses that insurance companies refuse to cover. A 2002 change to the tax law allows you to add the cost of weight-loss programs to your unreimbursed medical expenses. Not surprisingly, there are restrictions: You can include amounts you pay to lose weight only if your doctor has referred you because you have a specific disease diagnosis (such as obesity, hypertension, or heart disease). You can include fees you pay to join a weight-reduction group and attend periodic meetings. But you cannot include membership dues in a gym, health club, or spa. You cannot include the cost of diet food or beverages in medical expenses because that substitutes for what you normally consume to satisfy your nutritional needs.

## Assessing your situation

A dietitian or other medical professional will want to know your health status before making dietary recommendations. He assesses your blood pressure, plus information from a blood test, including your cholesterol, glucose, hemoglobin, and hematocrit levels. These measurements are helpful for determining the best diet recommendations for you.

An exercise physiologist also needs to know whether any health concerns would limit your ability to exercise. Therefore, before you discuss your diet and exercise habits with the physiologist, it may be necessary to have a medical checkup.

Your dietitian may ask you to fill out a food diary for several days before your first visit so that no details are missed. Bring this diary, along with any vitamin and mineral or herbal supplements that you're taking, too. These supplements figure into your daily nutrient needs. In some cases, taking large doses of one nutrient or a combination of large doses can throw an otherwise healthy eating plan out of balance. Your dietitian may want to make adjustments or recommendations.

Expect to spend at least an hour at your first visit with a dietitian. Be prepared to answer questions — many of them. The dietitian will want to know whether you have food sensitivities or allergies, what foods you like and dislike, what you usually eat, how much you eat at one time, when you eat, and where you eat — the whole ball of wax. Your weight history is also important.

You will be asked about your family as well. Who does the cooking? Who does the food shopping? What is your normal routine? Do you work out of your home? What kind of employment do you have? Do you exercise? How often do you eat out and what kind of restaurants do you usually go to? Do you eat plenty of take-out food? Do you use supplements or herbal preparations? Be honest in your answers; trying to paint a rosy picture of your habits serves neither you nor the dietitian.

The dietitian records your starting weight and helps you set realistic weight-loss goals. He may do skin-fold measurements (see Chapter 3) as well to determine what percentage of your weight is fat and what percentage is muscle. (You can expect the same from an exercise physiologist.) All these factors help you and the dietitian build a diet that meets your individual needs.

From the information that the dietitian gathers from your interview, he determines your normal calorie intake and expenditures and, with your input, designs a weight-loss plan.

You may want to bring your spouse, parent, or child with you to your first meeting, especially if one of them does the food shopping and cooking. Support is important throughout your weight-loss program, so consider starting out by taking your "team" along.

## Creating a plan

A dietitian focuses on lifestyle and food choices, not quick results, so don't expect miracle cures. Nor should your weight-loss success depend on your buying and taking expensive weight-loss supplements or aides. (See the sidebar "Ten red flags that signal bad nutrition advice" in this chapter.) A qualified exercise physiologist should not expect you to purchase special equipment or a health club membership.

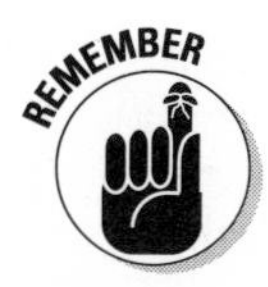


If you don't understand something about a plan that a dietitian or exercise physiologist creates for you, then ask questions until you do. You may hear nutrition or sports lingo that throws you, understanding exactly what's being said is important. Remember, the only dumb question is the one you *don't* ask. You can comply with the diet and exercise recommendations only if you understand what's expected.

## Ten red flags that signal bad nutrition advice

How do you know whether the nutrition advice you receive or the weight loss materials provided to you are reliable? Consider any combination of these ten red flags as a signal of questionable nutrition advice:

1. Recommendations that promise a quick fix
2. Dire warnings of dangers from a single product or regimen
3. Claims that sound too good to be true
4. Simplistic conclusions drawn from a complex study
5. Recommendations based on a single study
6. Dramatic statements that are refuted by reputable scientific organizations
7. Lists of "good" and "bad" foods
8. Recommendations made to sell a product
9. Recommendations based on studies published without peer review
10. Recommendations from studies that ignore differences among individuals or groups

*Source:* Food and Nutrition Science Alliance (FANSA) of which the ADA is a member.

### Following up

The dietitian will ask you to commit to follow-up visits while you work toward your goal weight. Not only will you get moral support, but also the dietitian can adjust your plan, answer questions, and record progress. Positive changes take time, encouragement, and most likely some tweaking. Plan your schedule to allow time for follow-up appointments.

## Finding a Weight-Loss Specialist

Keep reading to find a healthcare professional who can help you with weight loss. You can contact the organizations that we include or consult your local Yellow Pages to locate healthcare professionals in your area.

### American Dietetic Association (ADA)

The American Dietetic Association (ADA) is the world's largest organization of food and nutrition professionals. For recorded food and nutrition information and a referral to a registered dietitian in your area, call the American

Dietetic Association/National Center for Nutrition and Dietetics Consumer Nutrition Hotline at 800-366-1655. For more information, including a referral to an RD, visit the ADA's Web site at www.eatright.org.

## American Society of Exercise Physiologists (ASEP)

The American Society of Exercise Physiologists (ASEP) is a national nonprofit professional organization committed to the advancement of exercise physiologists. The society sets standards for exercise physiologists through ASEP-approved curricula in universities and colleges in the United States.

To locate an exercise physiologist in your area, contact the

ASEP National Office
The College of St. Scholastica
1200 Kenwood Avenue
Duluth, MN 55811
(218) 723-6046 or 1-800-249-6412
Fax: 218-723-6472
www.css.edu/asep/

## American College of Sports Medicine (ACSM)

The American College of Sports Medicine (ACSM) is the largest sports medicine and exercise science organization in the world with more than 16,500 members in more than 70 countries. The ACSM is dedicated to promoting and integrating scientific research, education, and practical applications of sports science and exercise science to maintain and enhance physical performance, fitness, health, and quality of life.

To locate a certified exercise specialist in your area or for more information, contact

ACSM National Center for Certification Department
P. O. Box 1440
Indianapolis, IN 46206-1440
317-637-9200
www.ACSM.org

## American Society of Bariatric Physicians (ASBP)

The American Society of Bariatric Physicians (ASBP) is a national professional medical society of licensed physicians who offer specialized programs in the medical treatment of obesity. ASBP members receive additional training in the field of obesity.

To locate a physician who specializes in treating overweight and obese patients, call 303-779-4833. By following the instructions of the ASBP automated system, you can get a list of all physician members in your state. Enter the state's two-letter postal abbreviation (for example, *NY* for *New York*) and your fax number. Within seconds, a list of names starts printing from your fax machine.

For more information, contact the

American Society of Bariatric Physicians
5453 East Evans Place
Denver, CO 80222-5234
303-770-2526
`www.asbp.org/`

## Tracking down a dietitian

To find a registered dietitian in your area who can provide scientifically based nutrition guidance on weight loss, contact

- Your doctor or health maintenance organization (HMO) for a referral
- The American Dietetic Association/National Center for Nutrition and Dietetics. (Ask for a referral to a registered dietitian in your area by calling 800-366-1655 or by visiting the ADA's Web site at `www.eatright.org`.)
- Your local dietetic association, the nutrition department of an area college or university, or the extension service at the nearest state university
- The chief clinical dietitian at your local hospital

# Chapter 17

# When Surgery Is the Only Solution

### *In This Chapter*

- Going under the knife can help
- Finding out what surgeries are out there
- Deciding whether surgery is right for you
- Getting a grip on what's in store

The previous chapters of this book talk about diet and exercise as the healthiest and safest way to lose weight. But what if you have plenty of weight to lose, say, more than 100 pounds? And what if your blood pressure is soaring and your cholesterol levels are flashing "Warning, Warning, Warning!?" And what if you've tried many times to lose weight with all the methods described elsewhere in this book, yet despite your earnest attempts, your weight has your doctor and family worried, and you have resigned yourself to a life dictated and restricted by your size? Medically necessary weight-loss surgery may offer hope.

In this chapter, we look at the kinds of surgical options that are available, how surgery alters your internal anatomy, who is eligible for it, and the risks associated with such a drastic measure.

## Offering New Options for Severe Obesity

Weight-loss surgery (also known as *bariatric surgery*) has been getting plenty of ink lately. High-profile celebrities who have shrunk before our eyes visibly demonstrated how effective and rapid this kind of weight loss can be. You may even know someone who's had the procedure. When the National Institutes of Health (NIH) established criteria for surgical treatment in 1991, insurance companies began to cover the operations, and the number of procedures being done soared.

An estimated 97,000 people underwent weight-loss surgery in 2003, up from about 63,000 one year earlier. In fact, more surgeons are training in weight-reduction procedures in order to treat the growing numbers of people willing to have the surgery. And the new techniques don't require much of an incision. Although the risks of the operations are considered acceptable, it's worth noting that 10 to 25 out of 1,000 patients can die after surgery. Therefore, lifelong medical follow-up and monitoring is required.

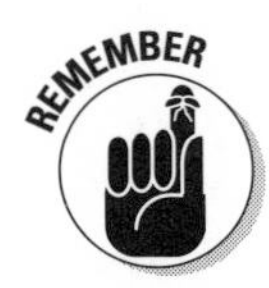


Still, the most encouraging aspect of the procedure is its permanence. People who undergo the procedure do keep their weight off, which is more than most diet plans can claim. All this good news has created long waiting lists for the procedure — often a year or more. But surgery of any kind shouldn't be considered lightly, and it's not for everyone.

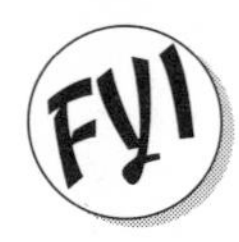


*Liposuction* (the removal of fat under the skin with suction) is a cosmetic surgical procedure and isn't used for weight reduction. Liposuction is used to contour specific areas where fat tends to accumulate. Plastic surgery may be done following the rapid weight loss from gastric surgery to remove excess skin.

## What the surgery involves

For a long time, gastric surgery to remove a portion of the stomach has been used for treating ulcers or cancer. One notable side effect of the procedure was that patients often lost weight or failed to gain weight following their surgeries. Doctors speculated that removing parts of a healthy stomach would help overweight patients lose weight, too. The premise is a no-brainer: If a normal stomach holds about six cups of food, and it's made to hold say, a few tablespoons, fewer calories can be eaten at a time. Fewer calories means weight is lost. No, it's not brain surgery; it's gastric surgery, and it's complicated.

In essence, the plumbing that makes up the stomach, small intestines, and large intestines is rebuilt and retrofitted. Assuming that your memory of high-school anatomy class is as dusty as your yearbook probably is, the following is a quick review.

### Normal digestion

Normal digestion starts in the mouth when you chew. That's where carbohydrates begin to break down with the aid of an enzyme in the saliva. (See Figure 17-1, which is adapted from material from the National Institutes of Health as are the other figures in this chapter.) After chewing, the food travels down the esophagus into the stomach where stomach acids are mixed in to break the food into smaller particles. After it's broken up in this way, the food can be pushed into the small intestines where enzymes are secreted, which break the food particles into nutrients that can be absorbed.

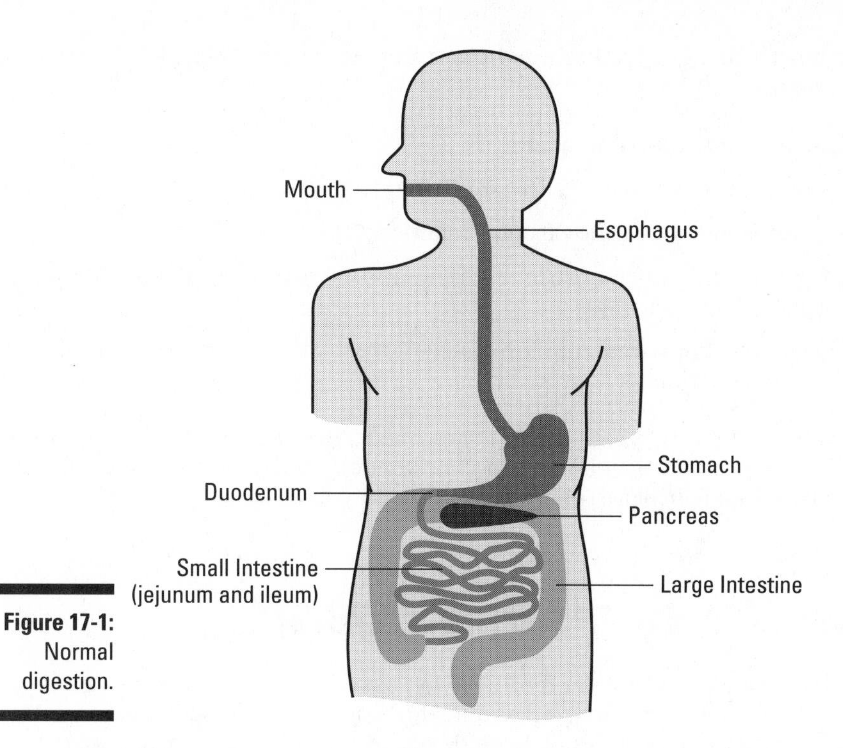


**Figure 17-1:** Normal digestion.

There are three parts of the small intestine: The *duodenum* (attached to the stomach where calcium, iron, and some vitamins are absorbed), the *jejunum* (the midsection), and the *ileum* (connected to the large intestine). The bulk of nutrient absorption takes place in the last two sections. The large intestine is where unabsorbed food particles, mostly fiber, are stored until elimination.

### Digestion after surgery

When parts of the normal digestive tract are removed, reconfigured, and reconnected, the path the food takes is altered, and the amount of nutrients absorbed is decreased. When it comes to calories, that's a good thing. But decreased absorption of key minerals and vitamins causes deficiencies and their resulting complications. See the section, "Understanding What to Expect before, during, and after Surgery" later in this chapter for more details.

## Benefits of weight-loss surgery

The obvious and perceptible payoff of the surgery is rapid, and mostly permanent, weight loss, which continues for one and one-half to two years. Most patients lose between 30 to 40 percent of their preoperative weight. Less visible are the health improvements that result from losing weight. These are the same health advantages that weight loss from less extreme means delivers. For example:

- Reduction in blood pressure
- Normalization of blood cholesterol and triglycerides
- Improvement of cardiovascular function
- Normalization of glucose levels and improvement in or disappearance of type 2 diabetes symptoms
- In women, improvement of menstrual irregularities, fertility, and urinary-stress incontinence

Like any weight loss, what you don't see makes this surgery worthwhile. You may not be aware of the changes in your lab data, but you feel the results. And mirrors and airplane seats won't threaten you anymore.

# Detailing the Types of Surgery

The first procedures done in the 1960s bypassed the small intestines altogether. The results were unpredictable and, unfortunately, sometimes fatal. New, safer methods have since been developed and fall into one of two categories: *Gastric restriction* and gastric restriction with malabsorption, also known as *gastric bypass.*

## Gastric restriction

Only the stomach is involved in this procedure. Staples and bands are used to reduce the amount of food the stomach can hold. An adult stomach normally holds about six cups of food. Gastric restriction creates a pouch that initially holds only an ounce. If the patient follows the postsurgical eating restrictions, the pouch stretches to hold two to three ounces. The intestines continue to function normally to absorb nutrients — just a lot less of them. Two techniques are used:

- **Adjustable Gastric Banding (AGB).** The mechanics for this method work much the same way as the belt that holds up your slacks. After eating a big meal (remember last Thanksgiving? Or last Saturday's binge?), you may have loosened your belt to feel more comfortable and most likely make room for dessert.

  As the name of this technique implies, an inflatable band is wrapped around the top part of the stomach much like a belt (see Figure 17-2).

The band is inflated with a saline (salt) solution to tighten it and regulate how quickly food leaves the new stomach pouch to go into what remains of the old stomach, and then into the intestines. The band can be tightened or loosened as needed to maintain weight loss or improve a patient's comfort level.

- **Vertical Banded Gastroplasty (VBG).** This type of gastric restriction is more common and successful than AGB. The top part of the stomach, nearest the esophagus, is sectioned off with gastric staples to create a small pouch, as shown in Figure 17-3, limiting the amount of food that can be eaten at one time. A band is also used in this procedure to create a small opening from the pouch, about the size of a dime, to slow the rate at which the food leaves the pouch. This makes the patient feel fuller longer.

  Success rates vary for VBG. About 30 percent of patients achieve normal weight, and 80 percent lose some amount of weight. Unfortunately, after about three to five years, many patients regain their lost weight. Because the stomach is quite elastic, eating larger and larger meals stretches the pouch.

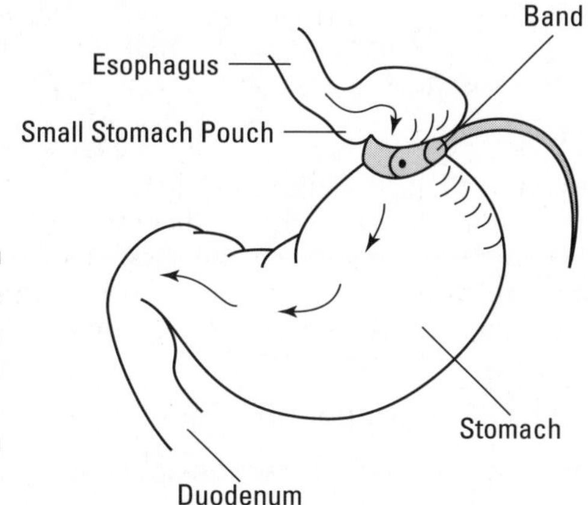


**Figure 17-2:** Adjustable gastric banding.

Risk of death or infection from complications from either gastric restriction surgery is less than 1 percent. Immediately after either surgery, however, vomiting is common, especially if food hasn't been well chewed. Heartburn and abdominal pain are common in both, too. In addition, the staples used in VBG to seal off a portion of the stomach can break, and in a small number of cases, stomach acids may seep into the abdomen and require emergency surgery to fix the leak. Over time, the band used in ABG can let go or wear out and lose its elasticity with repeated inflations, so it will not stay inflated and tight. These are some of the reasons that these procedures are not used as frequently as gastric bypass.

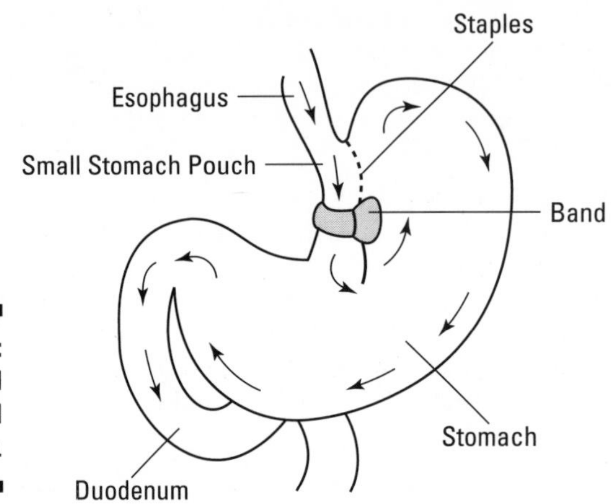


**Figure 17-3:** Vertical banded gastroplasty.

## Gastric bypass

An improvement over the gastric restriction is one that, as the name implies, bypasses the stomach and a portion of the small intestine. With gastric bypass, weight loss is better and more patients are more likely to keep most of their lost weight off. *Biliopancreatic diversion* and *roux-en-Y* are the two types of gastric bypass.

- **Biliopancreatic diversion (BPD):** "If you can't absorb calories, you lose weight," is the thinking behind this technique. The stomach size is reduced as it is in gastric restriction surgery and is connected directly to the last part of the small intestine, the ileum. Because this surgery is so aggressive, weight loss is impressive with patients losing 75 to 80 percent of their excess weight.

  Figure 17-4 illustrates what the operation involves.

- **Roux-en-Y:** This is the most commonly used procedure in the United States for weight loss. The upper portion of the stomach is restricted and all the first part of the intestines is taken out of the digestive loop. Therefore some, but not all, of the nutrients from a meal — the volume of which is also reduced — are absorbed.

  You can see what a Roux-en-Y bypass looks like in Figure 17-5.

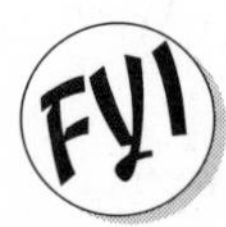


Many surgeons routinely remove the gallbladder during gastric bypass surgery. It's done to prevent having to perform another surgery if the patient develops gallstones — which are common. This is much like removing the appendix when doing any abdominal surgery.

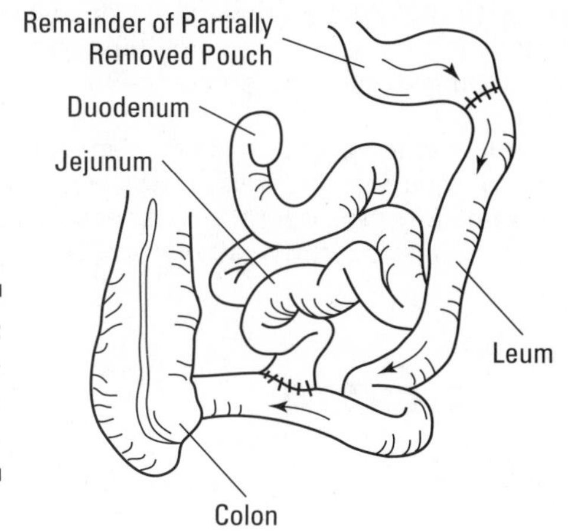


**Figure 17-4:** Biliopancreatic diversion.

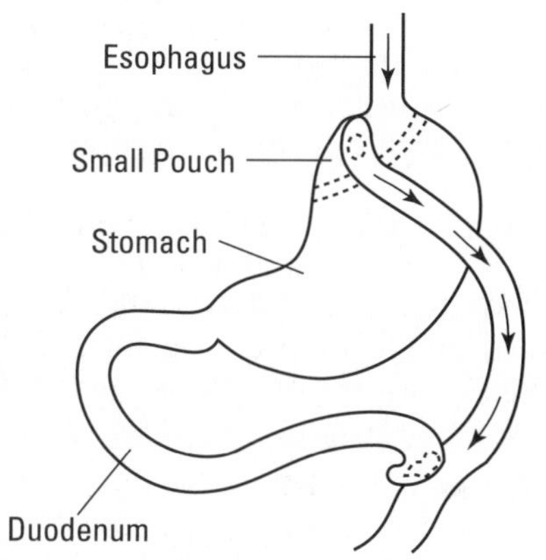


**Figure 17-5:** Roux-en-Y gastric bypass.

Both types of gastric bypass surgeries come with risks and complications. Stomach acids may seep into the abdomen and require emergency surgery to fix the leak. Additional surgery can be required if scar tissue forms and restricts or blocks the narrow opening between the stomach pouch and the intestines. Gallstones can form following rapid weight loss. Iron and vitamin B12 deficiency anemia occurs in more than 30 percent of patients. Patients who have BPD face additional risks: Thirty to 50 percent become deficient in fat soluble vitamins, which are usually absorbed in the middle section of the intestines, and 3 to 5 percent get a form of malnutrition from lack of protein and total calories that requires hospitalization. Less common, but still problematic after either surgical method is *dumping.* Because the *pyloric valve* (which regulates the rate at which food enters the intestines) is bypassed, food sometimes leaves the stomach too rapidly and "dumps" into the last part of the digestive track. This results in adrenalin being released, and it causes lightheadedness, palpitations, and sweating up to one and one-half to two hours after eating especially if the patient has eaten high-sugar or high-fat foods. Diarrhea and foul-smelling stools are also common.

Despite all those drawbacks, success for gastric bypass is impressive. Most patients lose about 60 percent of their starting weight. However, some weight can be regained three to five years after the operation, especially if the patient doesn't follow the doctor's postoperative advice strictly.

# Recognizing Who Is a Good Candidate for Surgery

Although surgery almost seems routine and may appear to be an easier way to lose weight than counting calories, that doesn't mean that surgery is risk free or simple. Nor does it mean that you don't have to actively work at maintaining your new weight. The National Institutes of Health's (NIH) criteria regarding who is a good candidate are specific and clear. If you can't answer *yes* to all the following questions, you aren't yet ready to commit to surgery:

- **Is your BMI more than 40?** That translates to being about 100 pounds or more overweight. (See Chapter 3 for information about calculating your BMI.) You may be a good candidate if your BMI is 35 to 40, *and* you have other health problems, such as high blood pressure, high cholesterol and triglycerides, sleep apnea, type 2 diabetes or other serious cardiopulmonary disorders. (Chapter 2 goes into detail about these health risks.)
- **Have you tried other weight-loss methods?** You've changed your eating habits, increased your physical activity, and tried medication. And you have repeatedly lost and regained large amounts of weight but your BMI is still in the "danger" range.
- **Is your weight affecting your quality of life?** Is it getting in the way of performing your job or engaging in routine daily activities? Is your weight keeping you from enjoying your family?
- **Is your obesity not the result of an endocrine disorder?** Meaning that you don't have a thyroid condition that causes you to gain weight.
- **Do you use alcohol and drugs responsibly?** Abusers are considered to be high risk, because they're mentally unstable.
- **Are you willing to wait at least a year after the surgery to become pregnant?** While you're losing the greatest amount of weight, there won't be enough nutrition to support a developing fetus.
- **Are you ready to make a lifelong commitment to maintain the results?** Regular physical exercise and a new eating plan are required after the surgery. (See the following section.)

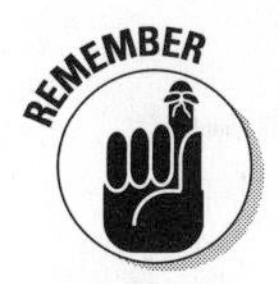


Each person's medical risk is different and only you and your healthcare team can determine if the benefits of weight-loss surgery outweigh the risk.

# Understanding What to Expect before, during, and after Surgery

After you and your doctor decide that surgery should be considered, you've only just started down the long road to the actual procedure. At this point, there are tests to be done, specialists to see, and plenty of questions both to ask your doctor and to answer.

Patients weighing more than 500 pounds may be required to lose some weight before an operation is possible. In fact, your pre and postoperative eating plans will be discussed in detail before the procedure. Likewise, psychological evaluation and support may be needed. Of course, you'll want to be sure that your loved ones are supportive of this enormous step you're considering.

To help you understand the process better, this section takes a quick look at what happens before, during, and after surgery.

## Before surgery

You'll be carefully evaluated. Tests will be done to check on your cardiovascular and endocrine health and how well your lungs and digestive systems work. A psychological evaluation will determine how well you will respond to the changes in your appearance and body image after surgery. And a dietitian will determine your dieting history and instruct you in your post-operative eating plan. You'll probably have several appointments with a dietitian who will help you understand the major changes you'll need to make in how you eat. The success of your surgery depends on how willing you are to follow the dietary advice.

We recommend talking with other people who've had the surgery that you're considering. In addition, be sure to talk with the important people in your life to see what they think of your decision to have the procedure. Finally, check out some Internet sites related to bariatric surgery. The National Institutes of Health has a good explanation of the surgery at `www.niddk.nih.gov/health/nutrit/pubs/gastric/gastricsurgery.htm`. Other sites that offer good basic information are `www.webmd.com` and `www.mayoclinic.com`.

Many insurance companies can cover the cost of bariatric surgery. However, finding that out for sure is important, because the tab can run between $15,000 and $20,000 or more depending on complications and individual health status. Most insurance companies use the NIH criteria that I list in the previous section to determine eligibility. Yet, coverage varies among companies so be sure to talk with your plan provider.

## During surgery

You'll undergo general anesthesia, and the surgery can be performed in either of two ways:

- **Traditional open surgery** needs an incision 6 to 8 inches long and requires about four weeks of "down" time for recuperation.
- **Laparoscopic bariatric surgery** is more common and less invasive. Small incisions, less than an inch long, are made in the abdomen for instruments to be passed through. This technique is less painful, the scarring is lessened, and recovery time is faster. Recuperation for laparoscopic gastric restriction is about one week and two weeks for gastric bypass — though your actual recovery depends on the other health conditions that you have. Laparoscopic surgery is not for everyone. Certain medical conditions and the presence of scar tissue from prior surgery may preclude the laparoscopic option for some patients. Your doctor will decide which type of operation should be performed.

## After surgery

So many things will be different after your surgery. You'll encounter both physical and emotional changes. This section takes a look at both.

### Physical changes

Your first few weeks at home will require a specific diet and vitamin supplements. The foods will need to be soft or semiliquid, such as cottage cheese, mashed potatoes, and scrambled eggs. You may be prescribed a high-protein shake because healing the surgical incision is crucial. After about two weeks, your dietitian will help you transition to solid food. If meat and milk products cause you discomfort (they do for many people just after surgery), another protein source will be found for you, probably a supplement. When adding new foods, try a spoonful at a time.

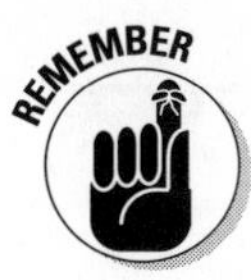


Typically, for at least the first one to two months after surgery, it's recommended that the following foods and beverages be eliminated from your diet, because they can cause stomach irritation and discomfort:

- Alcohol
- Caffeine-containing beverages such as coffee and tea
- Carbonated beverages
- Citrus foods and juices
- Fruits and vegetables that are raw, except bananas
- Fruit and vegetable skins
- Sugar and other sweeteners like molasses, jams, and preserves

Because the surgery drastically reduces the size of your stomach, your meals will have to be smaller than 1 cup. Therefore, you'll have to eat small meals throughout the day. Also, you'll have to slow down the pace at which you eat, because you must chew slowly and thoroughly.

Instead of having a beverage with your meal, you'll need to take small sips at least a half-hour after you eat. Your stomach will be too small to hold both liquids and solids at one time and spacing fluids around meals reduces the chance of vomiting. You'll also need to restrict fried foods and sugary foods to avoid dumping, which I explain in the "Gastric bypass" section, earlier in this chapter.

If you have bypass surgery, you'll be prescribed a vitamin and mineral supplement because you will no longer be able to absorb all the nutrients in the foods you eat. Your dietitian will help to ensure that the food choices you're making provide adequate protein.

### Emotional changes

After the operation, you'll need new clothes and maybe a new hairstyle. But those things are external. The emotional adjustments will be less visible but equally significant. This is one of the reasons that you will be required to have a psychological evaluation before the surgery, and why you may need counseling afterward as well.

You'll have to change what you eat and how much you can handle at one time. That can create stress at restaurants and in front of coworkers or business associates. Your new shape may cause anxiety and tension in social situations that had been easy when you were a large person.

## Other unpleasant (but nonlife-threatening) side effects of gastric surgery

You should be aware of a few other unappealing side effects of this type of surgery:

- **Carbohydrate intolerance:** Rice, pasta, and bread are not well tolerated right after surgery. Crackers and cereal are good substitutes until tolerance improves.
- **Constipation:** Because you'll be eating smaller portions of foods with very little fiber, bowel movements will be smaller and harder. A stool softener may be recommended.
- **Dehydration:** Because vomiting is common, and the size of your stomach is so small, drinking large amounts of water is difficult. Small sips of water between meals will help.
- **Hair loss:** This can occur two to three months after surgery. As your weight stabilizes and you're able to eat more protein foods, the hair loss should resolve. Avoid hair treatments like perms and coloring.
- **Muscle loss:** When weight loss is rapid, protein, not fat is the preferred for of energy. You can slow muscle loss by exercising routinely.
- **Protein intolerance:** Red meats and milk are often not well tolerated. Eating them at the beginning of a meal sometimes helps.

Likewise, your friends and family — even your spouse — may treat you differently. Perhaps you will see yourself differently in response to their reaction to you. You may be faced with greater expectations as a thin person. You'll be able to be more physical with your children (and spouse) and they may demand more attention from you.

You'll be faced with so many changes — most of them positive. However, any change, no matter how good, is still stressful. Be sure to enlist the help you'll need from medical professionals and/or your own personal support system. Finally, be aware that you'll need regular follow-up visits for the first year. Many patients also need plastic surgery to remove excess skin that has lost elasticity.

# Chapter 18

# Using Medications for Weight Control

## *In This Chapter*

- Determining whether medication can help
- Evaluating prescription drug choices
- Considering over-the-counter medications
- Knowing the risks and limits of drug use

Using drugs to lose weight is nothing new. In the 1950s and 1960s, people swallowed many diet pills, mostly amphetamine derivatives (speed). Addiction and abuse were common, so physicians gradually stopped prescribing drugs for weight loss.

For a long time after that, diet and exercise, not drug therapy, were the preferred forms of treatment. But in 1973, the Food and Drug Administration (FDA) approved a new drug for weight loss. Its name was *fenfluramine (Pondimin)*. Next came *dexfenfluramine (Redux)* in 1996. Some physicians prescribed *phentermine* (a different kind of weight-loss medication in use since 1959) in combination with *fenfluramine,* and the medication became known as *fen-phen.* Phentermine has also been used in combination with *dexfenfluramine* (also known as *dexfen-phen*). But in September 1997, after reports of serious heart valve disease, the manufacturers of fenfluramine and dexfenfluramine withdrew the drugs from the market. Prescriptions were no longer written for Redux, Pondimin, or fen-phen.

It's been several years since any new diet drugs have been approved. *Sibutramine* (trade name *Meridia*) and *Orlistat* (trade name *Xenical*) are the newest weight-loss drugs being prescribed. A conga line of others is in development or waiting for FDA approval, and a handful of drugs currently used for other conditions are showing promise for weight loss as well. But you don't need a prescription to find medications that claim to help weight loss — plenty of over-the-counter medications are available. Can they help you lose weight? This chapter gives you the scoop.

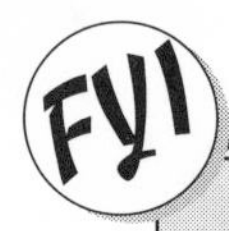


## Redux, redux

During the year and a half that *fenfluramine (Pondimin)* and *dexfenfluramine (Redux)* were being used as weight-loss drugs, 14 million prescriptions were written. The drugs increased the levels of *serotonin* — a brain chemical, a neurotransmitter that's associated with improved mood and has a role in the feedback system of appetite and satiety.

People did lose weight on these medications, but in September 1997, the FDA requested that they be removed from the market, because it was becoming clear that taking the drugs, either alone or in combination, was associated with fatal heart valve problems. In fact, patients who took the drug had a 30 percent chance of developing heart valve abnormalities, often without symptoms.

The FDA advises that anyone who took Pondimin or Redux or fen-phen should have an echocardiogram (ECG) — even if the individual showed no symptoms of heart or lung disease, such as a heart murmur or shortness of breath. Undergoing an ECG is particularly important before undergoing any invasive procedure. Even dental work may release bacteria into the bloodstream. ECG results can help to determine whether antibiotic treatment is necessary to prevent *bacterial endocarditis,* a potentially fatal infection of the heart's lining.

# Understanding How Current Weight-Loss Drugs Work

Most of the drugs that the FDA approves for weight loss work by decreasing appetite. But the mechanism of action of today's available medications is far more complex than that of the old pep pills and diet pills of the 1950s and 1960s, most of which were *amphetamines* (central nervous system stimulants, commonly know as *speed*). They're still prescribed, but because of the potential for abuse and addiction, they're rarely used for weight loss anymore.

The new generation of appetite-regulation drugs works on brain chemicals (called *neurotransmitters*) to partially suppress appetite and thereby reduce how much you eat. Another class of obesity drugs, known as *lipase inhibitors,* exerts an effect on fat directly in the gastrointestinal tract. Lipase inhibitors work by blocking the absorption of fat. And then over-the-counter diet preparations act as stimulants to decrease your appetite or as bulking agents to make you feel full.

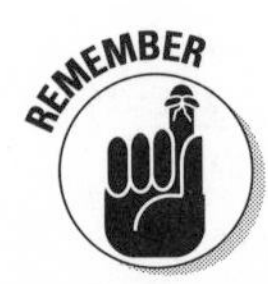


Weight-loss drugs don't work without lifestyle changes. Appetite-suppressant medications must be combined with physical activity and a calorie-reduced diet. Think of these medications as aids — not substitutes — for your weight-loss program.

# Deciding Whether Prescription Weight-Loss Drugs Are for You

Before prescribing a medication to aid weight loss, your physician takes a careful medical history and performs a physical exam. She asks whether any of your relatives have heart disease or diabetes. Your physician also calculates your Body Mass Index (BMI). (For an explanation of BMI and to find out how to calculate your own, see Chapter 3.) The result of this calculation is the primary guideline to determine whether you're a candidate for prescription drugs. If you have a BMI of 30 or greater (or 27 or greater if you have heart disease, diabetes, or other factors that would make your weight a health risk), you're a potential candidate for weight-loss drugs.

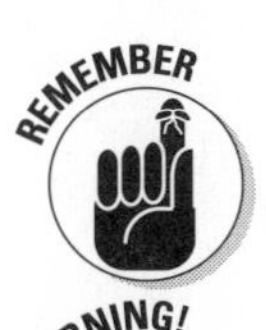


Diet counseling from a registered dietitian should always be provided along with weight-loss medication.

To determine which — if any — weight-loss medication may work for you, your doctor needs to know if you

- Are pregnant or breast-feeding
- Have a history of drug or alcohol abuse
- Have a history of an eating disorder
- Have a history of severe depression or manic-depressive disorder
- Take a *monoamine oxidase* (MAO) inhibitor or any other type of antidepressant medication
- Get migraine headaches and take medication for them
- Have an unstable medical condition such as glaucoma, diabetes, high blood pressure, or heart disease or a heart condition, such as an irregular heartbeat
- Are having surgery that requires general anesthesia

After you've been on your medication for about four weeks, your doctor schedules another visit to see whether the prescription is working and evaluate its effects on your overall health. A weight loss of 1 pound a week is considered "working." If the medication doesn't work in the first three to six weeks of treatment despite adjustments in dosage, chances are good that the diet drug will never work for you. Your physician will tell you to stop taking the drug you're on and may suggest that you try another.

Few severely obese people reach their ideal body weights by using the currently available medications alone. But for these individuals, even a modest weight loss of 5 to 10 percent of their starting body weights can improve health and reduce risk factors for disease. The current weight-loss medications are *not* recommended for people who are only mildly overweight unless they have health problems that their extra weight aggravates. These drugs shouldn't be taken solely for cosmetic reasons. You and your physician must weigh the risk of the potential side effects of the medication against the benefits of weight loss resulting from treatment.

# Using Prescription Medications

Keep reading to find some information about specific prescription medications for weight loss.

## Orlistat (trade name Xenical)

*Orlistat,* the newest of the new drugs, works in the intestinal tract. It doesn't suppress appetite, but it reduces the amount of fat that can be absorbed during digestion. Studies show that people who use Orlistat can lose about 9 percent of their initial weight over the course of a year.

The drug works by preventing the full digestion of fat; about one-third of the fat in a meal is excreted. Also lost are the fat-soluble vitamins in that meal; therefore, a multivitamin is recommended.

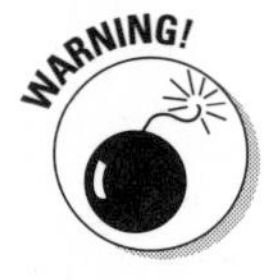


The side effects are not pleasant if you eat a meal containing high amounts of fat: changes in bowel habits, oily discharge, gas with discharge, urgent need to go to the bathroom, and oily stools. These side effects tend to occur after consuming a meal containing higher amounts of fat and tend to lessen with continued treatment.

Before prescribing Xenical, your doctor will want to know if you are

- Under 16 years of age
- Allergic to any medicines, foods, or dyes
- Taking any other weight-loss medication
- Taking cyclosporine, which decreases the effects of your body's immune system or coumadin, an anticoagulant
- Taking any other medicines (including those not prescribed by your doctor)
- Have a *chronic malabsorption disorder* that prevents you from absorbing nutrients from food

- Taking any dietary supplements, including herbal products
- Pregnant, planning to become pregnant, or breast-feeding
- Anorexic or bulimic

## Sibutramine (trade name Meridia)

*Sibutramine* is FDA-approved for both weight loss and weight maintenance. It works on brain chemicals to reduce appetite and give a sense of fullness. Studies have shown that sibutramine can help people lose weight and maintain the loss, but the weight loss tends to plateau after about a year, with a loss of about 10 percent of starting weight. That's enough to produce measurable health benefits but probably not a sufficient loss to satisfy an "ideal" body image.

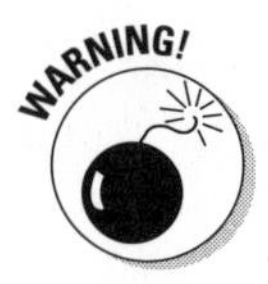


The drug may elevate both blood pressure and heart rate. In fact, the watchdog group, Public Citizen Health Research Group, has petitioned the Food and Drug Administration (FDA) to take Sibutramine off the market. About 30 deaths have been attributed to the drug and about 400 serious adverse reactions. The FDA's ruling is pending.

Before prescribing *Meridia,* your doctor will want to know if you are

- Under 16 years of age
- Taking prescription medicines called *monoamine oxidase inhibitors* (MAOIs) for depression or Parkinson's Disease
- Taking other weight-loss medications that act on the brain (for example, phentermine), including prescription and over-the-counter medications, as well as herbal products
- Being treated for high blood pressure, heart, liver, or kidney disease
- Pregnant, planning to become pregnant, or breast-feeding
- Anorexic or bulimic
- Taking any dietary supplements, including herbal products
- Have an eye disorder called *narrow angle glaucoma* because the drug can cause prolonged pupil dilation

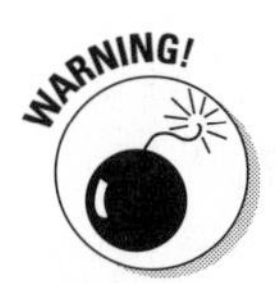


The major drawback to using Xenical or Meridia is that the weight loss achieved is very modest, about 2 to 4 pounds per month. Plus, these drugs are very expensive (about $200 for a one-month prescription) and are generally not covered by insurance companies.

## Other appetite suppressants

The following appetite suppressants are currently available by prescription:

- **Diethylpropion** (trade names *Tenuate* and Tenuate *Dospan*)
- **Benzphetamine** *(Didrex)*
- **Phendimetrazine** (trade names *Bontirl, Plegine, Prelu-2,* and *X-Trozine*)
- **Phentermine** (trade names *Apidex-P, Fastin, Ionamin,* and *Oby-trim*)

In studies that combine these drugs with diet and exercise in long-term tests (longer than six months), about three quarters of the participants lost about 5 percent of their starting weight, about half lost about 10 percent, and about a third lost 15 percent. But because all medications come with side effects, the FDA has approved these appetite suppressants only for short-term use — generally, only a few weeks to a few months. However, some physicians do prescribe them for *off-label use.* (Keep reading for an explanation of this term.)

The FDA regulates how a manufacturer can advertise or promote a medication. These regulations restrict a doctor's ability to prescribe the medication for different conditions, in larger doses, or for different lengths of time. The practice of prescribing medication for unapproved periods of time or for unapproved conditions is known as *off-label use.* Using more than one appetite-suppressant medication at a time (combined drug treatment) or using a currently approved appetite-suppressant medication for more than a few weeks is also considered off-label use. (Meridia and Xenical are approved for long-term use, however.)

## Antidepressants

Some antidepressants (particularly *fluoxetine* — trade name *Prozac* and *Sertraline* — trade name *Zoloft*) have been studied as appetite-suppressant medications. In studies, patients taking antidepressants to suppress appetite lost modest amounts of weight for up to six months. But most reached a plateau after about four months and tended to regain weight while they were still on the drugs. Prozac therapy *has* been effective in the treatment of eating disorders, however. (See Chapter 21 for more information about eating disorders.)

*Bupropion* (trade name *Wellbutrin*) is looking promising for weight loss. It's also an antidepressant but doesn't work the way *Prozac* and *Zoloft* do. Clinical trials are now underway.

## Using nondiet drugs as diet drugs

Drugs that are used to control seizures such as *topiramate* (trade name *Topamax*) and *Zonisamide* (trade name *Zonegran*) also reduce how much patients eat. Patients who take the drugs lose their appetite and therefore lose weight. Both drugs are being tested on obese patients who don't have seizures.

*Glucophage* (trade name *Metformin*) is a drug used to treat type 2 diabetes. The drug helps diabetics by inhibiting how much glucose their livers produce and making their cells more efficient at using glucose. The drug is being studied on children and adults who are obese, but not diabetic, to determine how effective it may be in weight loss.

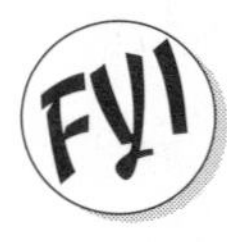


*Axokine* is a brand new drug that has a unique mode of action. It was being developed to treat Lou Gehrig's disease (ALS), but a side effect was weight loss. The drug seems to work on the *leptin pathway,* a system that signals the brain to tell you when to stop eating. Obese people have leptin resistance. Axokine may make their lepin pathway more efficient. Trials are now underway and the manufacturer hopes for FDA approval in late 2004.

# Taking Over-the-Counter Drugs

Most over-the-counter medications have one or more of the ingredients that I describe in the following sections. The front label may not tell you much about the ingredients that they contain so be sure to read the fine print.

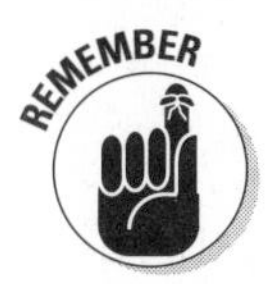


Few long-term studies have been conducted on the safety or effectiveness of over-the-counter drugs. Herbs packaged for weight loss are crowding the shelves. Herbal preparations aren't labeled with amounts of active ingredients, so knowing how much of a drug you're getting is nearly impossible. Remember that just because a product is herbal doesn't mean that taking much of it is safe. Many preparations combine several of the ingredients that we describe in the following sections. Be sure to tell your physician and pharmacist exactly what you're taking so that drug interactions or invalid lab tests can be avoided.

## 5-hydroxytryptophan (5-HTP)

5-HTP is a compound formed during serotonin synthesis from tryptophan. Serotonin is associated with feelings of calm and fullness. Studies using this metabolite in humans are inconclusive, but some experts are concerned that any drug that elevates serotonin levels may be associated with the same kind of risks seen with prescription appetite suppressants.

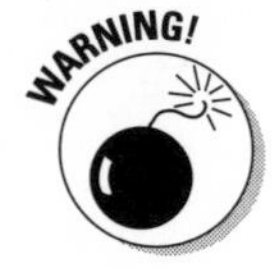


The FDA has found impurities in supplements of 5-HTP. One of those impurities is similar to one found in L-tryptophan supplements that was linked to *eosinophilia-myalgia syndrome* (EMS), a serious illness that can result in death. L-tryptophan was removed from the market because of the contamination.

**The bottom line:** Not recommended.

## Chromium picolinate

*Chromium* is needed for insulin metabolism and plays a small role in energy production. It's found in mushrooms, broccoli, and potatoes. But *chromium picolinate* is a synthetic compound. There's no recommended dietary allowance for chromium, and deficiencies are extremely rare. Supplements increase chromium levels significantly, which may lead to chromosomal damage and may be linked to kidney failure.

**The bottom line:** Not recommended.

## Ephedra (ma huang)

*Ephedrine,* which is structurally similar to amphetamines, is the active ingredient in *ephedra,* which is commonly known as *ma huang.* You may see ephedrine, ephedra, or ma huang listed on the labels of some herbal weight-loss drugs and fat burners. Doses of ephedrine that are sufficient to cause weight loss also can cause tremors, induce severe headaches, heart arrhythmias, and make your blood pressure soar — especially when combined with caffeine, as it often is in over-the-counter diet preparations.

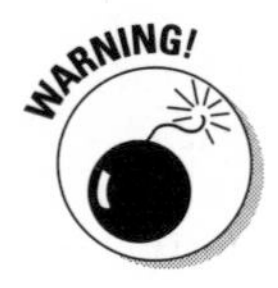


Ephedra has been linked to more than 800 incidents, including high blood pressure, severe headaches, heart-rate abnormalities, seizures, heart attacks, and deaths. The 2003 death of Steve Bechler, a Baltimore Orioles pitcher, was linked to ephedra. Derivatives of ephedra have also been reported to produce acute hepatitis and other unexplained liver injuries. The FDA has little power to regulate the sale or use of ephedra, because it falls under the Dietary Supplement Act, which allows the sale of such preparations as foods.

The FDA has proposed a warning label for products that contain ephedra. The exact wording is still in progress but it's expected to include the following warnings:

- Ephedra is associated with serious adverse reactions.
- Risk of using ephedra increases with the dose you take, how strenuously you exercise, and if you're taking other stimulants such as caffeine.
- People who have heart disease and high blood pressure should avoid ephedra.

Health authorities are worried that extreme political pressure will prevent the approval of the labels as it has in the past.

**The bottom line:** Not recommended.

## Guarana

*Guarana* is sold as a fat burner and a metabolism booster, but its active ingredient is basically caffeine — 100 milligrams of guarana has about the same caffeine content as a cup of black coffee. Taken by itself, guarana is probably not dangerous.

Guarana is often used in herbal preparations in combination with ephedra, making the ephedra even more powerful and dangerous. This combination increases the risk of high blood pressure, stroke, and death.

**The bottom line:** No more effective for weight loss than caffeine.

## Phenylpropanolamine

You won't see many over-the-counter weight-loss drugs on the market with *phenylpropanolamine* (PPA) anymore. Acutrim and Dexatrim voluntarily removed the drug, and the FDA is considering a ban. However, many drugs sold via the Internet still contain PPA, which was used in many cough and cold remedies and for weight loss because it decreases appetite.

The FDA has issued a public health advisory against PPA. A Yale University study linked PPA and *hemorrhagic stroke* (bleeding into the brain or into the tissue surrounding the brain) in women. Men are also at risk.

**The bottom line:** Not recommended.

## Pyruvate

This compound occurs naturally in the body and can be found in foods such as beer, red wine, and cheese. Proponents claim that *pyruvate* can increase metabolism and speed up carbohydrate digestion. Many athletes believe that it can increase their performance and endurance. However, the studies on weight loss and exercise performance have not shown a connection.

**The bottom line:** Probably not harmful but not effective either.

## St. John's Wort

You can find *St. John's Wort* in many herbal diet preparations. It has been used to treat depression in Germany for many years and may increase the brain's serotonin levels, which boosts mood and possibly curbs the depression sufferer's tendency to eat.

Extended use may cause eye and skin sensitivity to sunlight. If you're taking antidepressant medications such as Prozac, Zoloft, Celexa, Lexapro, Effexor, Remeron, Serzone, or Paxil, you should not take St John's Wort.

**The bottom line:** May help relieve overeating due to depression but can be dangerous to people taking prescription antidepressants.

## Senna

*Senna,* one of many herbal laxatives, is an ingredient in herbal "diet teas." It stimulates the colon and can result in extreme diarrhea, nausea, and dehydration. The weight loss is apt to be due to water loss, not fat loss. And drinking tea made with this herb can be as habit forming as regularly using laxatives, making it impossible to have a bowel movement without it.

**The bottom line:** More harmful than helpful.

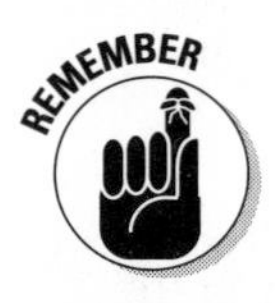


The idea that a pill or potion can make losing weight easy is seductive — that's why dieters spend billions of dollars buying them and drug companies spend billions of dollars developing new ones. But while drug therapy offers hope of thinness to many people, study after study shows that weight-loss medications work only when used in combination with a low-calorie diet and exercise plan.

## Chitosan

*Chitin,* the compound from which *chitosan* is derived, is found in the skeletons of shrimp, crabs, and lobsters. It can bind four to six times its weight in grease, oils, and toxic substances, and has been used in water filtration systems for years. Because it can bind fatty acids, chitosan has been promoted for weight loss. It may be effective in reducing blood cholesterol, but it has not been shown to aid in weight loss.

People who are allergic to shellfish may react negatively to it.

**The bottom line**: No more effective than sugar pills.

## Is the product worth spending your money?

Before you plunk down your hard-earned cash for a product or service that makes weight-loss promises, consider the following points: Your cash is better left in your wallet if the product or service

- Claims or implies a large (more than 1 to 2 pounds a week) or fast weight loss — often promised as easy, effortless, guaranteed, or permanent. (The exception is medically supervised VLCD programs. See Chapter 19 for more info on these programs.)
- Is described as miraculous, a breakthrough, exclusive, secret, ancient, from the Orient, an accidental discovery, or doctor developed.
- Declares that the established medical community is against this discovery and refuses to accept its miraculous benefits.
- Relies heavily on undocumented case histories, before and after photos, and testimonials. By law, weight-loss claims must be typical of all clients or include a disclaimer.
- Implies that weight can be lost and maintained without exercise and other lifestyle changes.
- Professes to be a treatment for a wide range of ailments and nutritional deficiencies as well as for weight loss.
- Includes gadgets, such as body wraps, sauna belts, electronic stimulators, passive motion tables, and cellulite creams.
- Makes a drug claim not allowed by the Food and Drug Administration for any ingredient, food supplement, or nonprescription drug. Claims that ingredients surround calories, starch, carbohydrate, or fat and remove them from the body are illegal drug claims. The only drugs that are allowed to claim that they suppress appetite are phenylpropanolamine (PPA) and benzocaine.
- Is sold door-to-door by a self-proclaimed health advisor or "nutritionist" or by a pyramid sales organization.
- Is distributed through a mail-order advertisement, television infomercial, or ad listing a toll-free number but not an address.

## Spirulina

Enthusiasts claim that *spirulina,* also called *super blue-green algae,* suppresses hunger pangs and is effective in treating diabetes, hepatitis, cirrhosis of the liver, anemia, stress, pancreatitis, cataracts, glaucoma, ulcer, and even hair loss. They also boast that it's protein — and vitamin-packed. The algae does contain protein composed of a good balance of amino acids and offers certain B vitamins, but neither is difficult to find in the American diet.

In theory, because it contains carbohydrate, spirulina can cause an increase in blood sugar and a corresponding reduction in hunger as any carbohydrate food does. However, the recommended doses of the supplement have too little carbohydrate to have such an effect.

**The bottom line:** Not recommended.

## Chapter 19

# Joining a Weight-Loss Program

### In This Chapter

- Determining if you need an organized group
- Sorting out the ragtag from the bobtail programs
- Going online and deciding what's right for you

If you're reading this chapter, chances are you're wondering if the support of an organized group is the kind of commitment that you require. This chapter shows you how these programs compare and gives you the background ammunition that you need to sort through the maze of options.

The programs are grouped in categories based on the kinds of support they offer. Some require more visits than others, some cost an arm and a leg and some are fairly reasonable, and some are more restrictive than others. You can find self-help groups that offer only support, not concrete diet or exercise advice. Others require membership and the purchase of special foods or meal replacements.

The big news in weight-loss support is the growth of online plans. Many programs that may have been geographically off limits in the past can now be accessed through the convenience of your computer — but don't just let your fingers do the walking — move your legs, too! Plus, you can find a crop of new Web-only programs that are worth a look. I give you the lowdown on these in this chapter as well.

Don't think that one of the programs listed in this chapter has all the magic that you're seeking. Two extremely large surveys suggest that weight-loss programs may not hold the key to successful weight loss and maintenance. Consumer Reports conducted a 2002 investigation revealing that of the 8,000 people who lost at least 10 percent of their starting weight and kept it off for at least one year (the official definition of weight-loss success), a stunning 83 percent of them lost weight without help. And, half of the members of the National Weight Control Registry — a database maintained by the University of Colorado of about 3,000 successful dieters — did *not* use outside help.

That doesn't mean that you should turn your back on the help available. Although in the minority, some successful losers *did* find the extra support critical to their success.

# Finding a Good Fit from the Start

One size never fits all. So before you sign up for a weight-loss program, ask yourself the following questions. You may not be able to answer all of them with certainty, but do keep these points in mind as you weigh your options:

- Do I need the support of a group to keep me going?
- Do I have the time to commit to attending weekly sessions or meetings for up to a year?
- Can I afford to join a club or program? (See Chapter 16 for more on cost issues.)
- Does the program require special foods and can I afford them? If so, will my eating special foods interfere with my family's lifestyle?
- Am I willing to follow a program's instructions, guidance, and skill-building techniques to find out how to eat in a more healthful way and, if the program requires it, be physically active for the long term?

# Meal-Plan Based Programs

Weight-loss programs based on meal plans can be good options for people who have trouble sticking to a weight-loss plan on their own. A 2003 report in the Journal of the American Medical Association concluded that the structure of commercial programs gave some dieters an advantage that resulted in more weight loss than dieters who attended self-help programs.

Meal-based programs offer a variety of services, from special foods and custom-designed diets and exercise programs to liquids only. Having so many choices can be confusing, however — and sitting in the office of a recruiter for one of these programs can be intimidating. (Recruiters are salespeople, well trained at closing a deal.) By carefully evaluating the programs in this section, you can avoid signing up and then not showing up because you hate the foods that you must eat or because the plan doesn't provide enough supervision.

## Jenny Craig, Inc.

**Philosophy:** The program is based on exercise, lifestyle modification, and a low-calorie diet. Members are advised to eat three meals and three snacks a day and increase physical activity. Prepared packaged foods are available and encouraged especially during the initial phases of weight loss. Rapid weight loss is discouraged. Expected weight loss is 1 to 2 pounds per week.

**Staff:** Registered dietitians design the programs and trained, nonmedical personnel administer them. The nonmedicals must complete a 56-hour training session and participate in monthly continuing education sessions.

**Cost:** Programs and specials vary but generally cost $1 per pound. The food is extra. A one-time enrollment fee is required. The initial weight-loss plan requires that you use their foods, which costs an additional $75 a week.

**Availability:** Centers are located in 46 states and in Puerto Rico, Canada, Australia, and New Zealand. The program can be accessed via the Web.

**Contact:**
11355 North Torrey Road
La Jolla, CA 92038-7910
800-597-JENNY
`www.jennycraig.com`

## Weight Watchers

**Philosophy:** Diets are individualized and are based on a point system instead of calorie counting. Point targets are assigned based on your current weight. You can choose any food you want to eat each day as long as you don't go over your targeted number of points. You can "earn" extra points by exercising. Commercial Weight Watchers food products can be purchased but are optional for program participation. Expected weight loss is 1 to 2 pounds per week. Members can stay enrolled for as long as it takes them to reach their goals. Exercise is encouraged, and group counseling sessions are included. Lifestyle modification is a component of the overall program structure.

**Staff:** Registered dietitians, exercise physiologists, and clinical psychologists developed this program. Leaders (who are Lifetime Members) deliver the program; their initial training requires at least 46 hours of classroom instruction.

**Cost:** For weight loss, you pay a one-time registration fee of $16 to $20 and a weekly fee of $10 to $14. For maintenance, the fee is $10 to $14 weekly for about six weeks until Lifetime Member status is reached. Lifetime Members don't pay a fee.

**Availability:** In North America, 20,000 weekly meetings take place. To find a meeting, use the meeting finder feature on Weight Watchers' Web site. Simply type in your zip code for a list of locations near you. Online meetings are also available.

**Contact:**
175 Crossways Park West
Woodbury, NY 11797
800-651-6000
www.weight-watchers.com

## Health Management Resources (HMR)

**Philosophy:** This is a medically supervised rapid weight-loss program for moderate or high-risk weight-loss patients. It's administered in hospitals and healthcare settings. Participants who use a very low calorie diet (VLCD) of about 500 to 800 calories a day must be under the care of medical personnel. A second option of a 1200-calorie-a-day diet is also offered. Both plans require meal replacement shakes, entrees, and bars. Weekly 90-minute classes are mandatory. Expected weight loss is 1 to 5 pounds per week. Medical screening is required for all participants.

**Staff:** Physicians, registered dietitians, registered nurses, and psychologists developed the program. Programs offering the VLCD have an MD, RN, and health educator on staff.

**Comments:** The side effects of a very low calorie diet may include intolerance to cold, constipation, dizziness, dry skin, and headaches.

**Cost:** Fees vary. Healthy Solutions program fees average $20 per week (shakes and entrees are additional). The VLCD averages $50 a week. Maintenance costs average $80 per month.

**Availability:** The program is available at more than 200 hospitals and medical settings in the United States.

**Contact:**
59 Temple Place, Suite 704
Boston, MA 02111
800-418-1367
www.yourbetterhealth.com

A complication of some of the VLCD programs is gallbladder stones. This is due to the very lowfat nature of the diets and the fact that the individuals who go on these programs tend to be very overweight and are predisposed to developing stones.

## Optifast

**Philosophy:** This medically supervised rapid weight-loss program is administered in hospitals and clinics. The plan requires liquid meal replacements and/or fortified food bars. As weight loss progresses, more regular foods are added. Dieters are assigned to an 800-, 950-, or 1,200-calorie plan. Participation is limited to individuals who must lose at least 50 pounds. The weight-loss portion of the program lasts about three months and transition takes six weeks; participants are transitioned to maintenance after five months. Emphasis is on behavior modification, problem-solving skills, physical activity, and individual counseling.

**Staff:** Group meeting leaders and one-on-one counselors are psychologists or dietitians. Physicians, registered nurses, registered dietitians, and psychologists regularly see each dieter at most locations.

**Cost:** Costs range from $1,500 to $3,000 for the six-month program. The price may include maintenance at some centers.

**Availability:** The program is available in numerous hospitals and clinics in the United States and Canada. Residents in the U.S. can find a clinic on the Optifast Web site by typing in their area codes and zip codes. Residents of Canada can call (800) 986-3855 ext. 4067 for clinic locations. No information on Optifast is available outside the United States or Canada.

**Contact:**
Novartis Nutrition
1441 Park Place Blvd.
Minneapolis, MN 55416
800-662-2540
www.optifast.com

Be aware that long-term weight-loss maintenance on VLCDs is disappointing. Although participants initially achieve impress losses, after five years, the majority of patients regain all their weight.

# Nondiet Programs and Support Groups

Often, the real problems that dieters face aren't only what they eat but *why* they eat the way that they do. The following programs focus on the nonfood factors that may contribute to obesity and stand in the way of weight-loss success. If you could use some peer support while trying to lose weight — but don't require a regimented plan structure or the services of program-provided weight-loss professionals — one of the organizations in this section may be your best choice.

## The Solution

**Philosophy:** The focus of the program is on developing internal skills of self-nurturing and setting limits to achieve balance and freedom from excess. There is a diet plan based on government recommendations and recommendations for exercise. Laurel Mellin, MA, RD, developed the program from her books, *The Solution* and *The Pathway.* The program has been refined to include community and professional support.

**Staff:** Most providers are mental health professionals or registered dietitians; all are "Solution Certified" meaning that they have completed and passed special training classes. The program delivery team consists of registered dietitians and licensed mental health professionals (psychologists, family therapists, social workers, and psychiatrists).

**Comments:** During the maintenance program, clients can return for 12-week sessions at any time. Every three months, a Saturday afternoon maintenance session for all program graduates is held.

**Cost:** Materials must be ordered from the center and costs start at about $100. The initial fees for support groups (four weekly two-hour sessions) are about $150. Cost can run from $250 to $600, depending on needs. The books on which the program is based can be purchased at bookstores.

**Availability:** Course work is done in group meetings and coaching sessions, though the workbooks can be purchased and used privately. One hundred fifty groups meet all over the United States. The program also offers Telegroups and Telecoaching through video-conferencing centers.

**Contact:**
The Institute for Health Solutions
1623A Fifth Avenue
San Rafael, CA 94901
415-457-3331
`www.sweetestfruit.org`

## Overeaters Anonymous (OA)

**Philosophy:** Overeaters Anonymous is based on the 12 steps of Alcoholics Anonymous, a proven model that has helped millions of people with addictive behaviors. The group recommends emotional, spiritual, and physical recovery changes. It makes no exercise or food recommendations.

**Staff:** Volunteer group leaders who meet specific criteria run the meetings. No healthcare providers are on staff.

**Cost:** You have no dues or fees. The group is self-supporting through member contributions.

**Availability:** Groups meet in more than 50 countries in churches, hospitals, and rehab centers.

**Contact:**
World Service Office (WSO)
6075 Zenith Court NE
Rio Rancho, NM 87124
505-891-2664
www.oa.org

## TOPS Club, Inc. (Taking Off Pounds Sensibly)

**Philosophy:** The desire to change comes from within; a supporting environment provides the most effective way to sustain change. The group doesn't impose or set weight-loss goals other than the ones you bring to the group. The group encourages you to remain a part of TOPS as long as you need support.

**Staff:** Each chapter is lead by a volunteer leader. A nine-member board of directors administers the program, and a field staff of regional directors, coordinators, and area captains supports the volunteer chapter leaders.

**Cost:** Annual membership is $20 in the United States and $25 in Canada. This amount includes the monthly magazine. Local chapters charge nominal fees of $.50 to $1 per week.

**Availability:** Two hundred and thirty thousand members meet weekly in 10,300 chapters in the United States, Canada, and around the world. Online membership is available.

**Contact:**
4575 South Fifth Street
Milwaukee, WI 53207
800-932-8677
www.tops.org

## Overcoming Overeating (OO)

**Philosophy:** Compulsive eaters are people preoccupied with food to the extent that it has become self-destructive. They believe that dieting hasn't solved weight problems but caused compulsive overeating. Change comes from self-acceptance and weight acceptance. They don't address eating disorders.

**Staff:** Codirectors Jane R. Hirschmann, MSW, a psychotherapist, and Carol H. Munter, a psychoanalyst, are specialists in eating disorders. The program is based on their 1998 book, *Overcoming Overeating.* Trained social workers or psychologists run programs located outside of New York City.

**Cost:** Workshops run about $45. Private sessions fees are based on a sliding scale; group meeting fees are $25 to $45 and are set by the individual therapist. Audio and videotapes can be ordered for $39.95 and $119.95 respectively, plus shipping and handling.

**Availability:** Centers are located in New York, Chicago, and New England. A referral list by state of therapist and support groups is posted on their Web site. Online e-mail chat groups are ongoing and online chat relays are frequently scheduled.

**Contact:**
National Center for Overcoming Overeating
P.O. Box 1257
Old Chelsea Station
New York, NY 10113-0920
212-875-0442
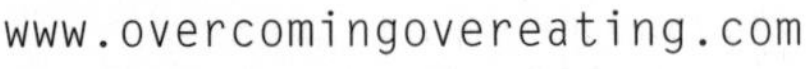
www.overcomingovereating.com

For sites that focus on eating disorders, see Chapter 21.

# Online and E-Mail Programs

The biggest news for diet help is online access to programs. Could they be an aid to your success? Researchers wondered that, too. And as two studies in the Journal of the American Medical Association report, one in 2001 and a new one published in April 2003, the answer is a definite yes, especially if the plans incorporate e-mail with behavioral advice and support.

Keep in mind, plenty of junk science is out there, but the sites that follow are the best.

## Nutrio.com

**Philosophy:** A site that offers expert weight-loss and weight-management assessments, tools, and resources with private and community message boards.

**Staff:** A team of registered dietitians, exercise physiologists, and therapists designed and maintain the site.

**Cost:** Free content is general. Subscription service ($10 activation plus $9.95 a month; discounts available for annual membership) offers one-on-one counseling on nutrition and fitness. Recipes, shopping lists, dining-out guides, and customized meal plans are available. Subscribers can log their nutrition and fitness progress.

**Contact:**
Nutrio.com
2843 Executive Park Drive
Weston, FL 33331
954-385-4700
`www.nutrio.com`

## DietingPlans.com

**Philosophy:** An interactive site that offers expert diet planning, fitness, and one-on-one support from dietitians. Thirty minutes of aerobic activity on three or more days a week is expected. The diet plan is based on the member's personal diet profile, and a virtual trainer aids physical activity.

**Staff:** Dietitians staff the site for one-on-one sessions, and they also answer e-mail.

**Cost:** Subscription is $14.95 per month.

**Contact:**
6060 Center Drive
Los Angeles, CA 90045
800-269-4390
`www.dietingplans.com`

## NutriTeen.com

**Philosophy:** A site geared to 12- to 17-year olds. Each person is given a personal counselor, a dietitian, and a personal trainer who e-mails support and coaching. Parents are required to participate in a separate, integrated program. The plan includes behavior modification, eating healthfully as opposed to a weight-loss diet, and physical activity. The program lasts 12 months.

**Staff:** A board of pediatric doctors, psychologists, dietitians, and fitness experts supervises the program. Registered Dietitians and Certified Personal Fitness Trainers counsel the children.

**Cost:** $99 for a three-month membership.

**Contact:**
NutriTeen
PO Box 1272
Old Chelsea Station
New York, NY 10113
1-866-LOSE-123
`www.nutriteen.com`

## Cyberdiet.net

**Philosophy:** Members receive meal plans and can follow their eating and exercise progress. The site has plenty of information on diet, nutrition, and fitness. Members can access a community of fellow dieters through an online message board and online chats.

**Staff:** The director of nutrition services is a registered dietitian.

**Cost:** The initial charge of $39.95 covers membership (the fee includes a $10 registration fee) for two months. Then, thereafter, the monthly fee is $14.95.

**Contact:**
DietWatch.com, Inc.
336 Atlantic Ave, Suite 301
East Rockaway, NY 11518
`www.cyberdiet.net`

# Determining Which Program Is Right for You

After you consider the different types of weight-loss programs and find one that you think may work for you, make an appointment to visit one of that program's centers for a personal interview. Take along the following list of questions and demand satisfying answers. (You may already know some of the answers based on the information given in this chapter, but having the program reconfirm that information certainly doesn't hurt.) How truthfully and in how straightforward a manner the answers are given can help you decide whether a particular program is right for you.

- What data proves that the program actually works? What has been written about the program's success, besides individual testimonials?
- Do customers keep off the weight after they leave the diet program? (Ask for results over two to five years. The Federal Trade Commission requires weight-loss companies to back up their claims.)
- What are the program's requirements? Are special menus or foods, counseling visits, or exercise a part of the program?
- Does the plan include physical activity recommendations? Will the program include guidance on physical activity for the long term? How?
- What are the approaches and goals of the program?
- What are the health risks?
- If I don't need to purchase special meals, does the plan take into account my personal food preferences? Will I have to give up all my favorite foods? Are the foods available at the supermarket? Will the program help me to discover how to live with its eating plan for the long term? How?
- What are the costs of membership, weekly fees, food, supplements, maintenance, and counseling? What's the payment schedule? Are any costs covered under health insurance? Will the organization give a refund if I drop out or give rebates for successful weight loss and maintenance?
- Will the staff monitor my success at three- to six-month intervals and then modify the program if needed?
- Does the plan have a maintenance program? Is it part of the package or does it cost extra?
- What kind of professional support is provided? What are the credentials and experiences of these professionals? (Detailed information should be available on request.)

# Chapter 20

# Rating the Diet Plans

### In This Chapter

- Checking out the most widely known diets
- Gauging the usefulness of liquid diets and diet bars
- Understanding the effects of fasting

The best news in the diet book industry is the growing popularity of well-researched and scientifically sound weight-loss books written by legitimate nutrition educators. A search of the best-selling weight-loss books from big online booksellers revealed that about 15 percent of the top 20 are scientifically sound. That's great news and a big change from only five years ago. (See Appendix A for these titles and more sources of good dieting advice.)

Yet, pounds of not-so-well-researched diet books continue to be published. Check out any online or traditional bookstore, and you'll see hundreds of these books for sale. A closer look at the contents of many of these books reveals that the diet is a rehash of a previous one. In most cases, the pitch hasn't changed since dieting became an industry. Yet based on the way these diets are written and promoted, you may believe that the author has uncovered a heretofore unheard-of formula that assures weight loss once and for all. Despite these claims, diet success is still a matter of calories in versus calories out.

This chapter explains some of the most common diets — many making encore appearances dressed in new names. It would be easy for us to tell you that none of these diets work and that they have no redeeming health value. But we don't entirely believe that. Some have merit. And when you analyze the thinking behind the plans, you can discover some valuable lessons about eating healthfully.

# Evaluating the Most Popular Diets

The current crop of weight-loss advice making the rounds in bookstores and locker rooms generally falls into one of several categories. Some tout or ban specific foods; others suggest that food can change body chemistry; and still others blame specific hormones for weight problems. This section explains and evaluates the most common diets and gives you the facts behind the fibs.

Just because a diet-book author is a medical doctor and uses the initials MD after his name or has a PhD doesn't mean that all the advice in the book is good nutrition science or nutrition advice. See the sidebar "Is the research legit?" to evaluate whether the research on which a diet is based is legitimate.

## Food-specific diets

The premise of food-specific diets is that some foods have special properties that can cause weight loss, other foods cause weight gain, and combinations of specific foods cause you to lose or gain. But no food is magic and no formulaic combination of foods can change the way you feel and look. So why do some people swear by these diets? Because any food eaten to the exclusion of others — even eating hot fudge sundaes and only hot fudge sundaes — can result in weight loss. Eventually, you get bored and stop eating the allowed food or at least enough of the allowed food to maintain your weight.

Our major criticism of the diets in this group is that none foster healthy eating habits; therefore, sooner or later, you'll have a hankering for something else — anything else, as long as its texture and flavor aren't allowed. You may even have a strong urge (dare we say *craving?*) for celery sticks, but it also may be for steaks.

Nutritionists call the human appetite for a variety of foods *food-specific satiety.* It's nature's way of assuring that you eat a diverse diet and, therefore, get the full spectrum of nutrients. You don't have to eat only hot fudge sundaes to see the dynamic at work. Think of last Thanksgiving's dinner, for example. After eating a full savory, salty meal of turkey, stuffing, gravy, mashed potatoes, rolls, and so on, we bet that you were still tempted to have a slice of sweet pecan or pumpkin pie. That desire for dessert was because your palate was looking for the full complement of flavors. Unless you ate plenty of marshmallow-topped sweet potatoes, your desire for something sweet wasn't satisfied. Sour, salty, and bitter — the other components of flavor in the Western diet — probably were featured in the main course. Sweet comes from dessert.

Including foods that require you to burn more calories to digest them than they contain is another purported theory at work with food-specific diets. It's true that, under laboratory conditions, protein, carbohydrate, and fat require different numbers of calories to digest. (For example, protein burns more of its calories during digestion than carbohydrate and fat do.) In the body, however, other variables, such as how much you exercise and your overall health, determine how many calories you burn during digestion. The truth is that metabolic needs adjust so that only about 10 percent of a day's total calories are used for digestion — regardless of the diet's composition.

The following sections describe some popular food-specific diets that are based on these principles.

### *Eat Right 4 Your Type*

**The author:** Peter J. D'Adamo, ND (naturopathic doctor)

**The premise:** Individuals can use their blood type as a genetic footprint or road map to determine which foods they should be eating. When you eat foods that "agree" with your blood type, you reduce the risk of infections, cancer, heart disease, diabetes, and liver failure. For example:

- People with type A blood have ancestors who were farmers; they should be vegetarians and avoid most meats and dairy products.
- Type Bs can trace their predecessors to nomads and should eat red meat and fish but avoid chicken and shellfish.
- Type Os are genetically linked to hunters and gatherers and should eat plenty of animal protein, but not much carbohydrate, especially wheat.
- Those with type AB blood should eat a diet that's a combination of types A and B.

**The truth:** The theories advanced in this diet book are not documented in scientific literature. Research referred to in the book was performed only by the author and has not been duplicated elsewhere. Many foods are off limits, making the diet extremely inconvenient and boring.

**Lessons to remember:** The genes you inherit from your ancestors may give you some clues to which foods may be especially hazardous or beneficial for you to eat. For example, if your parents and grandparents died from heart disease before the age of 50, you would be wise to eat foods that are low in fat (especially saturated fat) to keep your blood cholesterol in check, maintain a healthy weight, and keep your blood pressure under control.

### *Curves*

**The authors:** Cary Heavin and Carol Colman

**The premise:** The organizing principle is the same as the thinking used at Curves fitness and weight-loss centers around the country. (Basically a fast, 30-minute series of exercises for fitness and weight loss.) The diet is as much of a sales pitch for the franchised clubs as it is a weight-loss program. A quiz based on how much weight you have to lose, your sensitivity to calories or carbohydrates, and your body type determines the best diet plan for you.

**The truth:** Body type and amount of weight you have to lose aren't scientifically based criterion for determining dietary needs. Like it or not, no one is so unique that weight-loss success depends on specific foods. Calories in versus calories out is the bottom line and the only rationale that will help you become a shadow of your former self.

**Lessons to remember:** Exercise must be part of any weight-loss or weight-maintenance plan. And, in order to make a diet work for you, it must be tailored to your individual likes, dislikes, and lifestyle.

### *The Fat Flush Plan*

**The author:** Ann Louise Gittleman

**The premise:** A strict daily prescription of essential fats, protein, and carbohydrates to detoxify the liver and increase metabolism. People gain weight because they have a stagnant lymph system, sneaky food allergies, or hormone imbalance. It's the liver that holds the key to permanent weight loss and certain foods (such as eggs and lemon juice) and avoidance of medications (such as ibuprofen, prescription cholesterol-lowering, antidiabetic, anticonvulsant, and birth control drugs) frees the liver to function more effectively as a fat burner. Many foods are banned in the plan's first two-week protocol.

**The truth:** The initial phase of the diet is a low-calorie one — 1100 to 1200 calories a day — and restricts grains and starchy vegetables. Phase two is a 1500-calorie diet. Most people can lose weight when calories are so low. The business of the liver being a fat furnace and that specific foods can fire it up deserves to be, frankly, flushed! There's no scientific basis for her claims. Gittleman credits her theory to the teachings of Hazel Parcells, an alternative healer, and her personal study of medical textbooks, not tested scientific principles.

**Lessons to remember:** Eating all kinds of foods, even eggs and many colorful vegetables, makes good health sense. Reducing calories is the only way to lose weight and eliminating overly refined white flour and sugar is a good way to start.

## Is the research legit?

Recent diet-book writing commonly quotes experiments, studies, and research. How do you know whether the research to which an author refers is scientifically valid? Understanding the lingo helps. Look for these terms:

- **Associated with:** A connection or an occurrence more frequent than can be explained by mere coincidence, but a cause has not been proven.
- **Blind, single-blind, or double-blind study:** A single-blind experiment includes subjects who don't know whether they're part of the treatment or are receiving a *placebo* (fake treatment). In a double-blind experiment, neither the researchers nor the participants know which subjects are receiving the treatment or placebo while the study is being conducted.
- **Control group:** Usually the group of subjects *not* receiving the treatment in a study to make a comparison to determine whether the treatment is effective.
- **Correlation:** An association that's often defined statistically. It may not prove cause and effect.
- **Meta-analysis:** A technique in which the results of several individual studies are pooled to yield an overall conclusion.
- **Probability:** A chance that the event will occur. Probability can be high or low but doesn't indicate certainty.
- **Prospective study:** Research that follows a group of people over a period of time to observe the effects of diet, behavior, or other factors. Generally, a prospective study is considered a more valid research design than a retrospective study, which relies on the recall of past data or information.
- **Random sampling:** A method of selecting subjects for a study in which all the potential subjects have an equal chance of being selected.
- **Reliable:** A reliable test gives reproducible results when performed on the same group several times.
- **Risk factor:** Anything that shows a relationship to the incidence of disease. It does not necessarily imply cause and effect. It's important to understand what the risk is. If the original risk is 1 in 1 million, then double the risk is only 1 in 500,000. But if the risk is 1 in 100, then double would be 1 in 50, which may be a cause for concern.
- **Statistically significant:** Sometimes this phrase is simply written *significant.* It implies that there is a very small chance that the results would have occurred if there had been no real effect or association.

### *Suzanne Somers' Somersize*

**The author:** Suzanne Somers

**The premise:** Detailed rules define which foods must be combined and which ones shouldn't be eaten together. For example, protein-fat meals and carbohydrate meals shouldn't be combined in the same meal nor consumed within three hours of each other. Fruits must be eaten on an empty stomach. Sugar and starches are severely limited.

**The truth:** The nutrients in many foods are more available to your bodies when combined. Take a sandwich made on whole wheat bread with lean beef topped with tomatoes and lettuce. The fiber in the bread helps the meal digest at a steady rate that keeps energy stable. The vitamin C in the tomatoes helps to absorb the iron from the beef, as well as the iron from the whole grains. If you don't eat carbs with your protein, you miss those kinds of health benefits.

**Lessons to remember:** You must eat. You must not go hungry in order to lose weight. Don't skip meals. Although we wouldn't call them "funky foods," as the author does, eliminating sugar, refined carbohydrates, and alcohol when you're trying to lose weight is basic common sense.

### Body for Life

**Authors:** Bill Phillips and Michael D'Orso

**The premise:** Eat six meals a day with six snacks but only partake of foods from a limited list: Eighteen protein foods and 18 carbohydrate foods, only 2 servings of authorized vegetables and 1 tablespoon of unsaturated fat are allowed per day. Exercise is a vital and daily component.

**The truth:** The diet is overly strict and the foods on the list have no special qualities that aid weight loss.

**Lessons to remember:** Eating small meals on a frequent basis is key to weight control. Having six mini-meals each day is a good strategy to make sure that you feel satisfied. You should never be famished because that leads to overeating at the next meal. Daily exercise will help you change your muscle to fat ratio, and you'll burn calories more efficiently.

## Low-carbohydrate diets

These plans have been around since Dr. Stillman's Quick Weight Loss Diet made its first appearance in 1967 — although we imagine that Dr. Stillman started with William Banting's 1860s low-carbohydrate diet, which is considered the first weight-loss plan ever published.

These diets are based on the idea that carbohydrate is bad, that many people are "allergic to it" or are insulin resistant and therefore gain weight when they eat it. So by eliminating or severely limiting carbohydrate, you can force your body to use the fat it already has in storage for energy instead of adding to those fat stores. The authors of these diets are quick to point out that because people are eating plenty of carbohydrates — which most mainstream nutrition professionals recommend — they're heavier than ever before. What the advocates of these diets *don't* tell you is that people are eating more than the recommended amount of carbohydrates, most of it refined. They're also eating more total calories, too, and *that's* the real reason they're gaining weight.

The American Dietetic Association, and the American Heart Association have cautioned against the use of ultralow-carbohydrate diets, because when carbohydrate intake drops too low, serious metabolic complications can occur. And, recently, the American Medical Association looked at all the research that's been done on low-carbohydrate diets and reported their findings in the April 9, 2003, issue of their journal. Their conclusion: Of the 94 diets involving 3,268 people, weight loss was attributed to reduced caloric level, not the restriction of carbohydrates. They also found that carbohydrate restriction had no effect on the blood cholesterol, glucose, or insulin levels, nor was there an effect on blood pressure.

The following diets are based on the low-carbohydrate premise. Each author has his own spin on the science and the rationale for weight-loss success.

The bottom line, you will lose weight on any of these diets because you're eating less and monitoring your portion sizes.

### The South Beach Diet

**The author:** Arthur Agatston, MD

**The premise:** Weight-loss success depends on eating quality carbohydrates and good fats. In the first two weeks of the diet, you eliminate bread, potatoes, pasta, fruit, and alcohol. Phase two loosens the restrictions to allow selected carbohydrates.

## Putting carbohydrates into perspective

One of the misconceptions about the Food Guide Pyramid (see Chapter 9) that's often repeated in many popular diets is that eating plenty of carbohydrates is recommended. Yes, the idea is to build a base of grain foods but not an unlimited amount of them.

When fat became villainous in the '90s, carbohydrate foods, because they're often fat free, became free foods. That kind of thinking led to overconsumption of carbohydrates. For example, how many people does a one-pound box of spaghetti serve in your house? If it's fewer than four, you're eating too much. There are eight servings in a pound of cooked pasta; having two would be the equivalent of two servings, the same as a sandwich.

The other lost message in the pyramid is that most of the carbohydrate servings are whole grains. However, USDA data shows that we eat less than one serving of whole grains a day.

**The truth:** You'll probably lose plenty of weight on the first phase of this diet, because it's so low in carbohydrates. And, like all carb-restricted programs, most of the initial weight loss will be water weight. Carbohydrate metabolism and storage requires water. Therefore, no carbs, no water. Water loss from restricting carbohydrate equalizes after about 10 to 14 days. Thus, most low-carb diets like this one transition you to a phase-two plan at that point. Even if you continued to stay on phase one, your weight loss would slow.

**Lessons to remember:** Eat fewer simple carbohydrates, such as pasta, rice, and white bread, especially if you prefer them with butter, margarine, or oil.

### The Carbohydrate Addict's LifeSpan Program

**The authors:** Rachael Heller, PhD, and Richard Heller, PhD

**The premise:** The authors believe that you can break your carbohydrate cravings (which is why you're overweight) by limiting the amount of carbohydrates you eat. Two meals each day are made up of high-protein foods with little carbohydrate. You can eat high-carbohydrate foods at the third meal as long as you balance them with more high-protein foods.

**The truth:** There's no magic to eating high- or low-carbohydrate foods other than the fact that they contain different amounts of calories. Most experts agree that giving in to cravings is better than trying to eat around them, because you eventually eat too many calories in trying to avoid the one food that you truly want to eat. Plus, if you follow this diet, you *must* eat a second serving of a protein food if you eat a second serving of a high-carbohydrate food; therefore, eating too many calories is easy. And fat can creep up to dangerously high levels even if you select lean protein foods.

**Lessons to remember:** Because of its emphasis on protein, this diet reminds dieters to eat some protein at every meal to keep hunger at bay. Adding protein to meals gives them more staying power than high-carbohydrate foods alone can.

### Dr. Atkins New Diet Revolution

**The author:** Robert C. Atkins, MD

**The premise:** You can eat as many calories from fat and protein as you want as long as you eat very little carbohydrate. This diet consists of four phases. Phase one is the most dramatic, allowing no more carbohydrate than you'd get in 3 cups of salad — about 4 grams. Phase four allows no more than 40 to 60 grams of carbohydrate a day. But most nutritionists recommend that 55 to 60 percent of your calories come from carbohydrate, which translates into about 234 to 255 grams on a 1,700-calorie weight-loss diet.

**The truth:** Eating high-fat foods, such as burgers, cheese, bacon, butter, and mayonnaise, may sound dreamy, but you can't eat a bun with your double bacon cheeseburger or eat rye bread with your ham sandwich. Beyond the starch cravings that dieters may experience, the body can't burn fat efficiently without the carbohydrates that bread, potatoes, pasta, and other starches provide. As a result, the body produces compounds called *ketones* that accumulate in the blood. Ketones put a strain on the kidneys and can make kidney disease worse. Those who follow this diet often experience constipation, nausea, headache, fatigue, and bad breath. Eating high-fat foods day after day is a sure way to increase your risk of heart disease and cancer, too.

**Lessons to remember:** The goal of losing weight should be to improve your health, not make it worse. Unfortunately, this diet offers little information of value other than that eating fat can help make you feel full.

### Protein Power and the 30-Day Low-Carbohydrate Diet Solution

**The authors:** Michael R. Eades, MD, and Mary Dan Eades, MD

**The premise:** The hormone insulin, if released in great quantities, can cause health problems, such as heart disease, high blood pressure, elevated cholesterol and other blood fats, diabetes, and excess fluid retention, as well as excess weight. By keeping consumption of carbohydrate foods low and therefore the insulin it triggers, your body burns its fat stores instead of feeding them, and your risk of health problems is reduced. The diet and theory are similar to *The Zone* (described later in this section) in that protein requirements are based on lean body mass.

**The truth:** This spin is an example of putting the cart before the horse. The authors confuse the scientific evidence demonstrating that being overweight isn't the result of insulin being out of whack. Rather, being overweight often *causes* problems with insulin. The diet is extremely low in carbohydrate; the 30 grams a day allowed during the initial phase is about 205 to 225 grams less than what's considered healthy even during weight loss. (Nutrition experts recommend that 55 to 60 percent of your calories come from carbohydrates. Therefore, on a 1,700-calorie diet, which is low enough for most people to lose weight, daily carbohydrate intake should be approximately 234 to 255 grams.) Also, this diet minimizes the importance of reducing fat intake.

**Lessons to remember:** Many overweight adults eat too much carbohydrate, because they concentrate too much on reducing fat while ignoring total calorie intake. Many of these folks are heavy consumers of foods that have been engineered to be low in fat, which usually means that they're eating too much carbohydrate in the form of sugar. (When fat is removed from a product, sugar is often added to make up for the loss in taste and texture.) Because many foods that contain plenty of sugar supply calories but few or no nutrients, everyone should keep sugar consumption low, and those who are trying to lose weight should eat it sparingly.

### *Sugar Busters!*

**The author:** H. Leighton Steward, editor

**The premise:** Sugar, not fat, is the cause of extra weight. Foods that cause a spike in insulin supposedly increase the likelihood that their calories will be stored as fat rather than used for energy. Foods to avoid are classified according to their *glycemic index,* a measure of how fast they appear as glucose in the blood. Foods with a high glycemic index, such as white bread and pasta, refined grains, carrots, beets, and bananas, are to be avoided. High-fiber carbohydrates don't promote an insulin surge and therefore may be eaten.

**The truth:** High insulin levels increase the risk of heart disease but no evidence shows that they cause people to store fat. And although it's true that some foods cause a more rapid glycemic response than others when measured independently under laboratory conditions, in the body the composition of the entire meal influences how quickly the foods enter the bloodstream. And for most people who do not have a metabolic disorder such as diabetes, or prediabetes, also known as insulin insensitivity, if bread, pasta, or any other "off-limits" food is eaten alone, the insulin response — even a dramatic rise — is temporary, and the body accommodates it easily.

**Lessons to remember:** Many people eat too much sugar and refined grains and not enough high-fiber foods. Many foods that contain plenty of sugar supply calories but few or no nutrients. Most healthy people should use sugars in moderation, and anyone who wants to lose weight should use sugars sparingly.

### *The Zone*

**The author:** Barry Sears, PhD

**The premise:** To stay within the healthy zone for maximum calorie burn, every meal and snack must be 40 percent carbohydrate, 30 percent protein, and 30 percent fat. That's where the diet's other name, "the 40-30-30 diet," comes from. (Most nutritionists recommend 50 to 55 percent carbohydrate, 15 to 20 percent protein, and no more than 30 percent fat.) The diet, says the author, is based on hormones, not on calories. He claims that most people are insulin resistant, so eating carbohydrates makes them fat. Insulin is a hormone that takes glucose (the product of carbohydrate digestion) from the blood and delivers it to the cells. The author claims that when people eat carbohydrate foods, their bodies produce too much insulin, which causes too many calories to be stored as fat. Therefore, he says, carbohydrates must be kept low, and some are banned altogether.

## Insulin sensitivity explained

Frequently, overweight people have decreased *insulin sensitivity,* which means the cells do not respond to the normal amounts of insulin to move glucose from the blood to the cells for conversion to energy. For them, extra insulin must force the cells to let the glucose in and when it does, all the sugar rushes in and overloads the energy requirements. The extra glucose that's not needed for immediate energy is stored as fat.

Not only are carbohydrates kept to a minimum, but they must also be matched by prescribed amounts of protein (which are calculated on your lean body mass) and fat to keep *eicosanoids* (eye-*koh*-suh-noids) in balance. The author claims that eicosanoids are the chemical moderators that control all hormonal reactions, and the closer you get to your ideal protein-to-carbohydrate ratio, the better you'll balance your good and bad eicosanoids. Supposedly, bad eicosanoids increase insulin production. Good ones moderate hunger.

**The truth:** The pseudoscience on which this diet is based is complicated and unsubstantiated, and has been strongly disputed by the scientific community. Only 20 to 25 percent of adults are insulin resistant, usually because they have some other health problem that causes the condition. Further, insulin resistance often *results from* being overweight. It does not cause it. And although eicosanoids are involved in blood clotting and in the immune system, no evidence shows that this diet (or any other, for that matter) affects their synthesis. Any weight loss that you achieve on this diet is due to the 700- to 1,200-calorie plan, not a hormonal shift. And with so much focus on eating protein, which usually comes bundled with heart-damaging fat, it's easy to get more than 30 percent of your calories from fat — the amount that most health professionals consider healthy.

**Lessons to remember:** Many people, especially women, give up meat to cut calories. Instead, they fill up on carbohydrates. But carbohydrates aren't particularly satisfying by themselves, and they don't satisfy for long. Therefore, eating too many calories from carbohydrates is easy. By adding protein and a bit of fat to every meal, including snacks, you feel satisfied longer. Also, most people eat carbohydrate foods with fat. For example, margarine or butter on bread or rice, pasta with oily sauces.

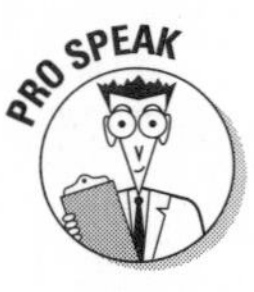


Metabolic syndrome, also known as syndrome X, is a group of conditions that include abdominal obesity (more apple than pear shaped; see Chapter 2), elevated triglyceride levels, low high-density lipoprotein cholesterol, elevated blood pressure, and insulin resistance. Some of the low-carbohydrate diets that specifically limit refined carbohydrates balanced with lean protein and moderate unsaturated fats, combined with moderate physical exercise, may help these patients lose weight.

## High-fiber, low-calorie diets

The thinking behind these diets is that because fiber can't be digested, it doesn't have calories. This is true. And because it takes up so much room in the stomach, it's filling, too. Also true. Therefore, if a diet is really high in fiber, weight loss should be easy.

### Eat More, Weigh Less

**The author:** Dean Ornish, MD

**The premise:** By keeping fat to no more than 10 percent of daily calories and eating basically a high-fiber vegetarian diet, you can reverse heart disease and lose weight.

**The truth:** Studies published in scientific journals have shown that this diet keeps its promises. However, many people find such a lowfat, vegetarian diet too stringent and difficult to stick with for long. Many nutritionists believe that this diet is too low in fat and that meals provide little satiety or long-term satisfaction.

**Lessons to remember:** We can recommend some aspects of this diet. For example, it has some good ideas for healthier food choices. However, it may not be a promising lifelong plan for many people because it's so restrictive. But if you can incorporate some of the lowfat, high-fiber strategies into your normal eating style, you can make positive health changes.

### Good Carbs, Bad Carbs

**The authors:** Johanna Burani, MS, RD, CDE and Linda Rao, MEd

**The premise:** Your body needs carbohydrate for fuel. Although you shouldn't restrict the amount of carbohydrate foods you eat, you should limit the *kinds* of carbohydrate based on the glycemic index. The *glycemic index* is a system of ranking carbohydrate foods according to how fast they're digested and enter the bloodstream as glucose.

**The truth:** Some carbohydrates are digested faster and more completely than others. For example, a white potato is turned into glucose faster than an equal amount of cooked lentils. Glycemic index does change in the company of other kinds of foods, such as fat, or how the food may be cooked. Therefore, glycemic index alone can't determine whether a carbohydrate food fits into your diet or not. (See the truth: Sugar Busters! earlier in this chapter.)

**Lessons to remember:** We eat far too many simple, sugary, and refined carbohydrates and not enough of the fiber-rich ones. Although most people eat only about 11 grams of fiber a day, health authorities recommend consuming 20 to 35 grams of fiber per day. And remember, eating excess calories from fat, carbohydrate, *or* protein makes you gain weight — not just from carbohydrate alone.

# Factoring in Liquid Diets and Diet Bars

Over-the-counter liquid and bar meal replacement shouldn't be used for long-term weight loss. But meal replacement drinks and bars can help some people lose weight, in theory anyway. Such drinks and bars eliminate the need to count calories or worry about portion sizes, so they can simplify a person's life especially during high-risk situations when going overboard on regular foods would be easy. Likewise, because the average dieter typically doesn't consume enough nutrients, a meal replacement is often an improvement over the usual diet. And if meal replacements can help people get out of habitual patterns, such as missing breakfast, drinking a can of a liquid diet or grabbing a bar on the way out the door is an easy adjustment that may prevent overeating later in the day. (For more on selecting a healthy bar, see Chapter 23.)

However, keep in mind that if you have plenty of weight to lose, using meal replacements doesn't ensure success. Data published by the SlimFast company in the *Journal of the American College of Nutrition* 13(6), 1994, a well-respected scientific publication, showed that after more than 2 years on the program, women lost a total of 13 pounds and men lost 14 — not much weight for 116 weeks of dieting! And despite being paid $25 a week to stay on the plan, only 51 percent of the people enrolled stayed on the plan for the entire study. We call that guaranteed failure.

# Fasting

Fasting to cleanse the body and jump-start a weight-loss diet has been recommended for years. But the reality is that fasting deprives the body of nutrients. The result is low energy, weakness, and lightheadedness, not real weight loss. Any loss is water and muscle, not fat, and you'll regain the weight when you start eating again. Fasting does not clear toxins from the body, either — just the opposite: Ketones can build up when carbohydrates aren't available for energy, and that massing of ketones stresses the kidneys and can ultimately be harmful to your health.

# Part VI
# Special Circumstances

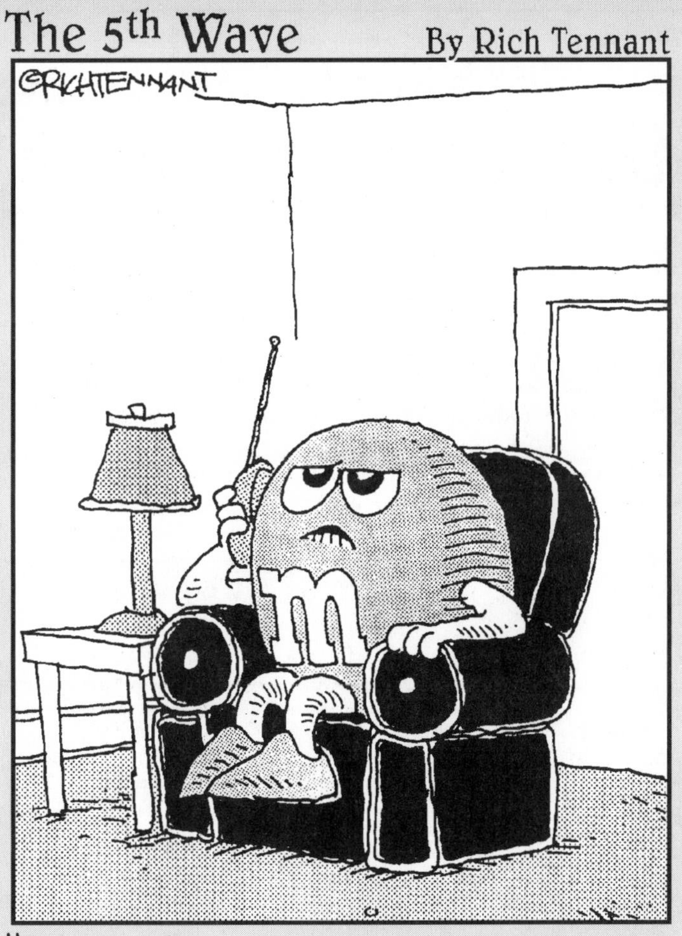


"My body type? I'm an 'M.' But I'd like to get down to an 'N,' maybe an 'H.'"

## In this part . . .

One size never fits all. A successful eating plan is one that's customized, practical, and healthy. The chapters in this part explore the specific health and diet needs for competitive athletes, children, and people with eating disorders. For example, a child's growing body demands special food and exercise considerations that aren't appropriate for a middle-aged man. Likewise, a woman who is 50 pounds overweight and has been inactive for many years needs a different meal and exercise plan than an athlete who bikes 100 or more miles each week. This part also addresses the very special needs of men and women with eating disorders who need counseling, as well as medical, emotional, and physical support.

## Chapter 21

# Eating Disorders: When Dieting Goes Too Far

### In This Chapter

- Determining where eating disorders come from
- Identifying the different types of eating disorders
- Understanding the psychological and medical aspects
- Treating and coping with eating disorders
- Figuring out where to find outside assistance

Eating disorders are a difficult problem to understand if you don't have one. They're difficult to treat and cure, too. And the person with the eating disorder isn't the only one affected; family and friends also feel the pain and anguish. Affecting about 5 million Americans, eating disorders are a serious and growing problem in society today. But just because you go on a diet doesn't mean that you'll get one. The vast majority of dieters don't turn their diet plans and activities into eating disorders. For those who do, however, the mental and physical consequences can be severe.

## Understanding the Origins of Eating Disorders

What causes eating disorders? Contrary to popular belief, eating disorders aren't just about being fat or thin, about food or weight. Instead, eating disorders are typically about self-esteem, depression, power, communication, or self-expression. Many factors can contribute, including society's emphasis on being thin and physically beautiful; the prevalence of dieting in our culture; pressure by oneself or others that people should be perfect; and food and nutrition beliefs.

Often, eating disorders begin when a person is dealing with a major problem or transition in life, such as alcoholism, death, divorce in the family, leaving home to go to school, or getting married. The person feels out of control and helpless and food provides them with unconditional comfort. Experts view eating disorders as a combination of physical, emotional, spiritual, and cultural factors gone awry. Eating disorders are complex and take a long time to treat and cure.

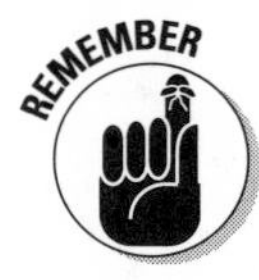


You shouldn't confuse an eating disorder with what's commonly termed disordered eating, however. *Disordered eating* refers to a temporary eating pattern to cope with a temporary stress (exams, visiting in-laws, and so on) or can even be an overly strict weight-loss diet. You may have picked up unhealthy eating habits from friends or in response to unusual situations, such as traveling where you may eat on the run and surviving on "junk food" for days. Conversely, an eating disorder is *not* temporary. It's not a diet. It's an illness.

Although disordered eating can lead to an eating disorder, significant differences exist between the two conditions. Table 21-1, reprinted with permission from the Harvard Eating Disorder Center, highlights these differences.

**Table 21-1 Disordered Eating versus Eating Disorders**

| | *Disordered Eating* | *Eating Disorders* |
|---|---|---|
| Essential distinction | A reaction to life situations. A habit. | An illness. |
| Psychological symptoms | Infrequent thoughts and behaviors about body, foods, and eating that do not lead to health, social, school, and work problems. | Frequent and persistent thoughts and behaviors about body, foods, school, and work problems. |
| Associated medical problems | May lead to transient weight changes or nutritional problems; rarely causes major medical complications. | Can result in major medical complications that may lead to hospitalization or even death. |
| Treatment | Education and/or self-help group can assist with change. Psychotherapy and nutritional counseling can be helpful but are not usually essential. Problems may go away without treatment. | Requires specific professional medical and mental health treatment. Problem does not go away without treatment. |

### Who gets eating disorders

Generally speaking, bright, energetic, attractive, conscientious, hard-working people of all races and economic classes get eating disorders. Ninety to 95 percent are female. They are most often between the ages of 12 and 25, although some cases have been reported in people much younger and much older. People who are vulnerable to eating disorders also may have relationship problems, biological predispositions, and psychological disturbances that change their thinking. Many factors can trigger an eating disorder. The one thing that all those who suffer from eating disorders have in common is a history of dieting.

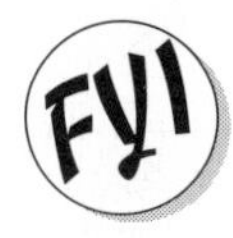


Eating disorders may develop when a person is young, but can recur in middle age. Often the person has suffered silently for many years. By midlife, the disease is more about easing tension, anxiety, and anger than appearance. Worry about passing the disease to their children is what brings many sufferers to seek treatment.

### Psychological problems associated with eating disorders

Tragically, a person with an eating disorder strives for control and self-esteem. But the disease produces the opposite effect. A person with an eating disorder may find that she must struggle with any of the following psychological problems in addition to the physical symptoms:

- Feels hopeless. May give up and sink into fatalism or denial.
- Feels out of control and helpless to do anything about her problems.
- Suffers from anxiety and self-doubt.
- Feels guilt and shame.
- Fears being discovered.
- Has obsessive thoughts and preoccupation with food and eating.
- Struggles with anger and suppressed anger.

## Recognizing the Many Faces of Eating Disorders

Eating disorders come in several forms. Anorexia nervosa, bulimia nervosa, and binge eating disorder are the most common and are described in detail later in this section. For information at a glance, Table 21-2 illustrates the specific similarities and differences among them.

**Table 21-2 Anorexia Nervosa, Bulimia Nervosa, and Binge Eating Disorder: Differences and Similarities**

| | *Anorexia Nervosa* | *Bulimia Nervosa* | *Binge Eating Disorder* |
|---|---|---|---|
| Estimated | Up to 0.5-1.0% | Up to 1.0% | Up to 2.0% prevalence* |
| Male versus female incidence | 5-10% male versus 90-95% female | 5-10% male versus 90-95% female | Unknown |
| Typical age of onset | Early to middle adolescence | Late teens to early 20s | Any age, but usually not recognized until adulthood |
| Weight | Extremely thin and emaciated; less than 85% of normal or ideal body weight | Near-ideal body weight, but often has weight fluctuations | Usually overweight or obese |
| Self-esteem | Low | Low | Low |
| Depression | Common | Common | Common |
| Substance abuse | Rare | Common | Rare |
| Rate of weight loss | Rapid | Repeatedly loses and gains weight or chronically diets without losing weight | Repeatedly loses and gains weight or chronically diets without losing weight |
| Past dieting | Yes | Yes | Yes |

** Determining accurate statistics is difficult because physicians are not required to report eating disorders to a health agency, and because people who have eating disorders tend to deny that they have a problem and are very secretive about their behaviors.*

## Anorexia nervosa

A person may have anorexia nervosa when she diets to the point of weighing only 85 percent of her normal, healthy weight (or a BMI of 17.5 — see the chart in Chapter 3 for more about BMI), fears gaining weight, is preoccupied with food, develops abnormal eating habits, stops menstruating, or, if male, experiences a decrease in sexual drive or interest in sex.

*Anorexia nervosa* is an eating disorder in which a person refuses to maintain her body weight at or above a minimally normal weight for her age and height. The person also has an intense fear of gaining weight or becoming fat, even though she is obviously underweight. Anorexia nervosa affects about 1 out of 100 people between the ages of 10 and 20 years old. Anorexia tends to develop in early to midadolescence when body fat increases from 12 percent before puberty to about 20 to 25 percent after. This increase in body fat is not true weight gain in the adult sense, but a natural biological function of female development. Ninety to 95 percent of anorexics are female and 75 percent of the young women who develop anorexia nervosa do not have a history of being overweight.

In addition to the physical changes that accompany anorexia nervosa, pronounced emotional changes, such as irritability, depression, moodiness, and increasing isolation are also common. In fact, eating disorder experts have developed a profile of personality and family traits characteristic of a person with anorexia nervosa. Anorexics tend to be compliant, approval seeking, conflict avoiding, perfectionist, socially anxious, and obsessive/compulsive, with average or above-average intelligence. Their family environment may include a mother who is overprotective, critical, intrusive, and domineering, and a father who is passive, withdrawn, and emotionally absent from the family. Although not every person who develops anorexia exhibits all or even some of these traits — nor may her family — they help paint a picture of the issues that many anorexia nervosa sufferers must struggle to overcome.

Do you (or someone you know) have any of the following symptoms? The more "yes" answers, the greater the likelihood that you (or she) may have anorexia nervosa.

- Skips meals, takes only tiny portions, and will not eat in front of other people.
- Eats in ritualistic ways, such as cutting up food into extremely small bites or chewing every bite excessively, and creates strange food combinations.
- Grocery shops and cooks for the entire household but will not eat.
- Always makes excuses not to eat: "not hungry," "just ate with a friend," "feeling ill," and avoids mealtime or situations involving food.
- Becomes "disgusted" with former favorite foods, such as red meat and desserts.
- Will eat only a few "safe" foods; boasts about how healthy the meals she does consume are; drastically reduces or completely eliminates an entire group of foods, such as carbohydrates or fats.
- Says that she's too fat, even when this is not true, and has a distorted body image.

- Becomes argumentative with people who try to help.
- Has trouble concentrating.
- Denies anger, making statements such as, "Everything is okay; I'm just tired and stressed."
- Withdraws into self, becoming socially isolated.
- Often exercises excessively and follows a rigid routine.
- Wears baggy clothing to hide thinness.

## Bulimia nervosa

*Bulimia nervosa* is characterized by recurrent episodes of binge eating followed by purging behaviors, such as self-induced vomiting, misuse of laxatives or diuretics, fasting, or obsessive exercise, in an attempt to prevent weight gain from occurring as a result of the bingeing. Bulimia occurs in adolescents and young adult women but is relatively uncommon in men, and typically develops in the late teens or early twenties. Fifty percent of bulimics have or had anorexia nervosa.

Some authorities believe that as many as 10 percent of women are affected over their lifetimes. Clinically speaking, a person with bulimia nervosa binges at least twice a week, eats large amounts of food in a relatively short period of time, and then purges to rid her body of the unwanted calories. More than half of bulimics are severely depressed and often suffer from alcohol and drug abuse in addition to their eating problems. Unlike the anorexic, who is excessively thin, the bulimic's weight is usually average or slightly above average and often fluctuates.

Do you (or someone you know) have any of the following symptoms? The more "yes" answers, the greater the likelihood that you (or she) may have bulimia nervosa.

- Gorges, usually in secret, and may also buy special binge food; is uncomfortable eating around others
- Makes excuses to go to the bathroom after meals
- Buys large amounts of food that suddenly disappear
- Displays unusual swelling around the jaw and cheeks; knuckles may be scraped or calluses formed on back of hand from inducing vomiting
- Has discolored or stained teeth due to vomiting
- Eats large amounts of food on the spur of the moment and feels out of control, unable to stop eating
- Withdraws from friends

- Doesn't seem to gain an excessive amount of weight given the amount of food regularly consumed
- Often exercises excessively
- Runs water to cover the sound of vomiting, may use mouthwash and breath mints excessively, and may have a foul-smelling bathroom
- Can't explain the disappearance of food in the home or residence hall setting
- May engage in drug or alcohol use and/or in casual or even promiscuous sex
- Experiences mood swings; may experience depression, loneliness, shame, and feelings of emptiness (although may pretend to be cheerful)

### Binge eating disorder

Binge eating disorder can happen at any age, but it's often not recognized until adulthood. It's similar to bulimia nervosa, but without purging activities. Victims of binge eating disorder eat large amounts of food at least twice a week, often in a relatively short time. They eat to escape from emotions, yet food makes them feel out of control. They often avoid social situations where food may be served but are preoccupied — even obsessed — with food, dieting, and their body weight. Most binge eaters are overweight or obese and may have obesity-related disorders such as high blood pressure, high blood cholesterol levels, or type 2 diabetes.

Do you (or someone you know) have any of the following symptoms? The more "yes" answers, the greater the likelihood that you (or that someone you know) have binge eating disorder.

- Frequently eats an abnormally large amount of food in a discrete period of time
- Eats rapidly
- Eats to the point of being uncomfortably full
- Often eats alone and in private to hide eating; in front of others, eats only small amounts
- Shows irritation and disgust with self after overeating
- Does not purge by vomiting, abusing laxatives, or vigorously exercising
- Is usually sedentary

### Athletes with eating disorders

Eating disorders are surprisingly common among both professional and amateur athletes. Men and women who participate in sports and other activities that emphasize appearance and a lean body, such as ballet and other forms of dance, figure skating, gymnastics, running, swimming, horse racing and riding, and rowing are susceptible, too. Wrestlers are especially vulnerable. In fact, some of the first studies on binge eating disorder were done on them. Before a match, it's common for wrestlers to binge to carbo-load and then purge so that they can qualify for a lower weight class.

Female athletes run a twofold risk of developing an eating disorder. They face all the usual conflict about their bodies, appetites, and needs for approval. But athletes also face the demands of sports that prize low body fat and unrealistic body shapes, sizes, and weights. For males, the pressures are different, which may account for their lower risk. Dieting is the primary risk factor for developing an eating disorder, and generally speaking, fewer men diet than women. Plus, many more of the male-dominated sports require strength and mass than traditionally female-dominated sports, so thinness isn't as much of an issue.

Bingeing only at night isn't uncommon and may not be an eating disorder. People with Night Eating Syndrome (NES) are often more than 100 pounds overweight, and eat more than half of their daily calories between dinner and breakfast. Unlike Binge Eating Disorder (BED), which is characterized by brief episodes, NES continues for many hours. Nocturnal Sleep-related Eating Disorder (NS-RED) is another kind of binge eating, but the person is often not fully conscious when eating. NS-RED is believed to be a sleep disorder, not an eating disorder.

## Seeing What Triggers Eating Disorders

Eating disorders may be triggered for many different reasons. Dieting is one possible reason, some people argue, because the disorders share dieting as a common thread. They think that if dieting didn't exist, there would be far fewer eating disorders and argue that people wouldn't get caught in the following cycle:

- Severe calorie restrictions make them ravenously hungry.
- They overeat in response to the unbearable hunger (*bulimia nervosa* and *binge eating disorder*).
- They panic about gaining weight, which brings them back to dieting and all the physical and psychological consequences that accompany food restriction. (See Chapter 5 for more on the hunger mechanism.)

Of course, not all dieters develop eating disorders. And many of the reasons that people develop eating disorders may have little to do with food or dieting.

## Psychological factors

The label *perfectionist* describes many people with eating disorders. They demand success and excellence from themselves. Their achievements are many, but they may feel inadequate, defective, and worthless. Some people with eating disorders try to take control of themselves and their lives by managing their food and their weight, which gives them a sense of accomplishment. In addition, they see everything as good or bad, black or white, fat or thin. And if thin is good, thinner is better. Some are searching for an identity. Dieting gives them the sense of self: "I am a successful dieter, therefore I matter. I diet, therefore I am."

## Biological factors

Genetics (at least in part) determine personality, and some personality types are more vulnerable to eating disorders than others. People who have low self-esteem and/or are socially anxious, value perfectionism, avoid conflict, and constantly seek approval from others are more likely to develop an eating disorder than are others who don't possess these traits. Bulimia tends to run in families that have a higher incidence of mood disorders and substance abuse, especially alcohol, which also have genetic components.

### Men get eating disorders, too

Only 5 to 10 percent of people with anorexia nervosa are male, and 10 to 15 percent of bulimics are male. Males tend to develop anorexia nervosa at older ages than females do. No statistics about the number of male binge eaters have been collected yet, but some researchers believe that males and females binge in equal numbers.

The factors that precipitate eating disorders in a male are similar to causes for females:

- History of being obese or overweight or dieting
- Involvement in sports that require thinness, such as running, track and field, horseback riding, wrestling (reduced weight means competing in a lower weight category), and body building (body fat and fluid reserves are depleted to increase definition)
- Involvement in professions that value thinness, such as modeling and acting
- Living in a culture or among people who value attractiveness and may judge men as critically as women

## Drug use in eating disorders

Hundreds of double-blind studies have shown that treatment with antidepressants can help reduce bulimic behavior and binge eating by about half. Doctors first started using antidepressants to treat eating disorders when they realized that many people with bulimia are depressed. And as with depression, many kinds of medications can be effective.

Only a doctor can prescribe the correct dose and type of medication by evaluating a patient's history, current medications (if any), and how quickly and thoroughly symptoms are relieved. Close monitoring until the drug of choice is determined is crucial. The medication often takes several weeks to take effect.

## Familial factors

The families of people with eating disorders often are overprotective and strict and have trouble resolving conflict. These families may value achievement and success and discount doubt and anxieties. Imperfections are criticized. These families may place a premium on physical appearance, making overt or teasing comments about someone's shape and size. Though not genetically linked, 50 percent of bulimic sufferers have a history of early sexual abuse.

## Social factors

Experts such as L. K. George Hsu, MD, professor of psychiatry at Boston's Tufts University, believe that culture influences the onset of an eating disorder. The public continues to believe that body weight and shape is determined by willful, conscious self-control.

People today are flooded by messages that being thin has its advantages. Like it or not, in society, thinness is equated with attractiveness, and with that comes power, success, and popularity. Additionally, people have an abundance of food and an ever-increasing variety of cuisines and foods to choose from. It's an easy — and cheap — way to indulge, and advertisers often encourage it. People graze, never actually sitting down to a meal. Instead of eating socially with friends and families, hectic schedules drive folks to eat alone. There are few "rules" for defining what makes an appropriate meal. Cereal for dinner? Sure. Cold pizza to start the day? Why not? And in the face of so many choices and opportunities for lack of "discipline," society considers loss of control over eating to be morally wrong. Fat people are labeled as failures — lonely, weak, and stupid. And so the conflict of appetite versus control begins.

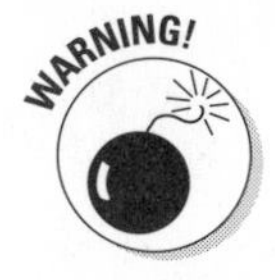


Web sites that promote and glamorize anorexia nervosa (known as pro-ana) or bulimia nervosa (code word: pro-mia) are proliferating and are popular among adolescents. Professionals are worried. And parents and friends take note: Instead of offering treatment options, pro-ana and pro-mia sites exist to pass along techniques and tips to encourage sufferers to "perfect" and perpetuate their diseases.

# Surveying the Medical Consequences of Eating Disorders

Make no mistake: Eating disorders — particularly anorexia nervosa — can be deadly. The following lists explain the many medical consequences of eating disorders.

Anorexia nervosa may cause the following problems:

- The heart muscle changes, and its beat becomes irregular, potentially leading to cardiac arrest and death.
- Dehydration, kidney stones, and kidney failure may result in death.
- Liver damage (made worse if substance abuse is also a factor) may result in death.
- Menstruation often stops, even before extensive weight loss. This is called *amenorrhea* and can lead to infertility and bone loss or osteoporosis.
- Muscles waste away, resulting in weakness and loss of function.
- Slowed digestion caused by a lack of energy and diminished body function results in bowel irritation and constipation.
- Permanent loss of bone calcium leads to fractures and lifelong problems of osteoporosis.
- The person becomes intolerant to cold (especially in the hands and feet), and has sunken eyes, hair loss, bloating, and dry skin.
- The immune system weakens.
- Skin becomes dry and blotchy and has an unhealthy gray or yellow cast.
- Anemia and malnutrition may result.
- Fainting spells, sleep disruption, bad dreams, and mental fuzziness may result.

Five to 20 percent of anorexics will die.

In addition to the complications in the preceding list, the following common medical complications associated with bulimia nervosa result from repeated cycles of bingeing and purging:

- Loss of muscle mass from excessive vomiting may occur.
- Vomiting and abuse of laxatives and diuretics flush sodium chloride and potassium from the body, resulting in an electrolyte imbalance. *Arrhythmia* (irregular heartbeat) can result, which can ultimately lead to heart failure and death.
- Stomach acids in vomit can erode tooth enamel, resulting in damage such as cavities and discoloration. The acids can go into the salivary glands in the month, causing swollen glands in the neck, stones in the salivary ducts, and "chipmunk cheeks."
- Self-induced vomiting can result in irritation and tears in the lining of the throat, esophagus, and stomach.
- Laxative abuse can create a dependence and result in an inability to have normal bowel movements.
- Abuse of medications to help induce vomiting, such as ipecac, can result in toxicity, heart failure, and death.
- Peptic ulcers may occur.

The medical consequences of binge eating disorder are most often associated with obesity and include the following:

- High blood pressure, elevated cholesterol levels, and elevated triglyceride levels, which may cause hardening of the arteries and heart disease
- Increased risk of bowel, breast, and reproductive cancers
- Increased risk of diabetes
- Increased risk of arthritic damage to the joints

# Treating Eating Disorders

Treatment works for at least 60 percent of people with eating disorders. They can return to and maintain healthy weights and eat normally. They can develop healthy relationships with people, raise families, and build careers.

But despite often-intense treatment, about 20 percent don't recover fully. These people remain focused on food and their weight. They can't feel comfortable with friends or romantic relationships. They work, but usually don't have meaningful careers.

The remaining 20 percent don't improve, even with treatment. Their lives continue to revolve around food and weight. Unfortunately, without proper treatment, up to 20 percent of people with serious eating disorders will die. But with therapy, the number of fatalities drops drastically to 2 to 3 percent.

The treatment for eating disorders is individual and specific to the person suffering. Because many factors contribute to the development of an eating disorder, a team approach makes for the best treatment. The professionals on the healthcare team include doctors, registered dietitians, psychologists or psychiatrists, and social workers. Counseling includes many stages, some in individual sessions and some in groups. But in general, the goals of treatment by the healthcare team include:

- Return to and maintenance of normal or near-normal weight
- Ability to eat a varied diet of normal foods (not just low-calorie, nonfat, and non-sugar items) and the elimination or major reduction of irrational food fears
- Restoration of relationships with family members and friends
- Application of problem-solving and coping skills

## Anorexia nervosa

More than 25 percent of patients with anorexia nervosa require inpatient hospitalization until they reach 85 percent of their ideal body weight. Outpatient programs are another good option for those who have not lost so much weight. Psychotherapy, family counseling, and medical nutrition therapy to help regain lost weight are part of the team approach needed to take on this disease. Drug therapy hasn't been effective in treating anorexia nervosa, although drugs may be prescribed to treat depression and other psychological problems common to patients with this disease.

## Bulimia nervosa

The treatment of bulimia nervosa is usually conducted on an outpatient basis. Psychotherapy is effective, especially in a group setting. Family counseling and medical nutrition therapy are also an important part of the treatment plan. Many psychiatrists prescribe antidepressants to treat bulimia nervosa, because they may help reduce the frequency of purging episodes. One type of drug for treating depression is proving useful as at treatment for bulimia, as well. The drugs are known as SSRIs or *selective serotonin reuptake inhibitors,* such as Prozac or Zoloft.

### Binge eating disorder

Treatment for binge eating disorder is similar to that used for treatment of bulimia nervosa, often including psychotherapy (especially cognitive behavioral therapy), family therapy, and medical nutrition therapy. Antidepressants may be an effective treatment as well.

## What to Do If Someone You Know Has an Eating Disorder

If someone you know has an eating disorder, you can help. The problem is that the person who has the eating disorder may deny having a problem. That denial may leave you, the supporter, feeling powerless, confused, frightened, or even angry.

It helps to understand that people with anorexia refuse to believe that their eating patterns are abnormal. Binge eaters and those with bulimia are more likely to recognize that they have a problem, but they may still be skittish about seeking treatment. People with eating disorders may deny that they are too thin or that they purge or vomit, despite the mounds of evidence that you may be tempted to present to them. *Don't* push them — and *don't* show them documentation of your case.

Instead, first realize that eating disorders require professional treatment. Do some background research on treatment, referral centers, and support groups in your area (check with your local school system, university, medical center, or mental health center for recommendations and help). Ask your family doctor for an eating disorder referral. If you're a student, see the school nurse or school-counseling center.

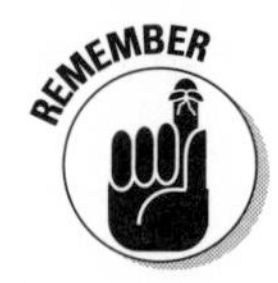


If you decide to talk to the person about the eating disorder, it's critical to do so in a nonthreatening, caring, and nonjudgmental way. Some important dos and don'ts:

- *Do* listen and be supportive.
- *Do* care and nurture.
- *Do* provide information.
- *Do* encourage professional help.
- *Don't* be judgmental.

- *Don't* dwell on eating, weight, or appearance.
- *Don't* insist that the person eat, not eat, or change attitudes about eating.
- *Don't* nag, criticize, or shame the person.
- *Don't* try to police or control the person.
- Most important, *don't* ignore the problem. Instead, help the person get the help that she needs.

Remember, too, that recovering from an eating disorder takes a long time. There's no such thing as an overnight success. Just because symptoms are no longer visible doesn't mean that the disorder is cured. Changing behaviors and attitudes about food can take months or years. So hang in there — and be the support that your friend or loved one so desperately needs.

# Knowing Where to Find Help

If you or someone you know is suffering from an eating disorder, look to these sources.

**American Dietetic Association**
216 W. Jackson Blvd.
Chicago, IL 60606
www.eatright.org
Call 800-366-1655 for a referral to a registered dietitian in your area who specializes in eating disorders. For general questions, call 800-366-1655.

**Anorexia Nervosa and Related Eating Disorders (ANRED)**
P. O. Box 5102
Eugene, OR 97405
541-344-1144
An eating disorder information clearinghouse. You can download all the information via the Internet at www.anred.com.

**The National Women's Health Information Center (NWHIC)**
8550 Arlington Blvd.
Suite 300
Fairfax, VA 22031
www.4woman.gov
A health information clearinghouse and referral service. Call 800-994-9662 (800-994-WOMAN); 888-220-5446 (TDD) Monday through Friday from 9 a.m. to 6 p.m. eastern time.

**The National Association of Anorexia Nervosa and Associated Disorders (ANAD)**
Box 7
Highland Park, IL 60035
847-831-3438
www.laureate.com
Offers free eating disorder information and prevention services, hotline counseling, support groups, and referrals to healthcare professionals.

## Chapter 22

# What to Do If Your Child Is Overweight

### In This Chapter

- Understanding why many children are overweight
- Figuring out whether your child is overweight
- Providing parental support
- Answering common questions

If you walk into a middle school classroom in North America, at least 3 of the children in a class of 20 will be overweight. Like the adult population the world over, children are getting fatter. In fact, the number of overweight children has doubled over the last 20 years. Because overweight children have a good chance of becoming overweight adolescents, and overweight adolescents have a good chance of becoming overweight adults, they're at an increased risk for a number of health problems, including diabetes, heart disease, high blood pressure, and stroke. In addition to health worries, fat children face painful social pressures from their peers.

If you're concerned about your child's weight, read this chapter and discuss your child's situation with your pediatrician. But think twice about starting your youngster on a weight-loss plan. Childhood weight issues are complex and varied. Don't impose adult diet or body standards on your growing child; serious emotional, psychological, and physical damage can result. Consult with your pediatrician first.

## Identifying Why Children Are Overweight

Children become overweight due to genetic tendencies, lack of physical activity, unhealthy eating habits, or a combination of these factors. In some rare cases, an endocrine disorder is to blame. Your pediatrician can perform an exam and blood test to rule out this possibility or to design a treatment program if needed.

## It's just baby fat, isn't it?

Your child's excess pounds are just baby fat, right? The answer may depend on *your* weight. A study of 854 children in the state of Washington found that obese children under 3 years old whose parents weren't obese probably wouldn't be obese as adults. An obese child's chances of becoming an obese adult more than doubles if his parents are obese. And the longer a child remains overweight, the greater the likelihood that he'll grow up to be an obese adult. Chapter 4 provides more detailed information about the critical time periods for childhood weight gain and how they relate to adult obesity.

# Nurture or nature?

Sometimes, the apple doesn't fall far from the tree. If a parent or sibling is overweight, chances are that the child will be, too. The odds of a child becoming overweight increase dramatically if both parents are overweight. But why?

Researchers have been asking that question for some time. In a series of studies on twins, researchers found that the likelihood of becoming fat is estimated to be between 65 and 75 percent if you have a family history of obesity. (For comparison, the genetic risk for breast cancer is about 45 percent.) Researchers found that when identical twins were placed in separate adoptive homes, the twins' bodies looked more like each other's and those of their biological parents than the bodies of their adoptive parents — the homes in which they were raised. More recent work on twins shows that twins often share similar metabolic rates, eating styles, and food preferences, too, even when they're raised separately. Some experts have criticized the twin studies for assuming that all environmental conditions are the same, which may or may not be true.

Genes alone don't sentence a child to a life of obesity. Many experts think that the way a child is raised is even more important. If nature is the genetic pool that humans swim in, then nurture is the location of that pool and the way it's maintained. Ethnic background, geographical location, and socioeconomic status may influence weight. In fact, contrary to the twin studies, many genetic experts argue that the inherited component of weight is much closer to 30 percent on average, compared to the 65 to 75 percent chance purported by the researchers who studied the twins. They argue that so many factors may be involved in determining weight that pinpointing the precise determinant is hard. They also point out that the role of genes varies from person to person — it may be 5 percent for one person, 95 percent for another.

### All juices are not created equal

Fruit flavor in a juice doesn't necessarily mean fruit nutrition. Today's supermarkets display tons of juice-based beverages, and the nutritional value each provides varies. Some products you may think are loaded with juice don't contain much juice at all. A few tips on choosing juices:

- **Be aware that all juice and juice products contain water and sugar.** A drink labeled 100 percent fruit juice contains naturally occurring sugars (fructose), whereas juice drinks, cocktails, and other beverages also have added sugars, such as high-fructose corn syrup. (See Chapter 7 for more information on the connection between high-fructose corn syrup and obesity.)
- **Read the label.** Government regulations require that all juice-based beverages state the amount of juice they contain. If you opt for a product that's not 100 percent juice, you may be getting an item that contains mainly added sugar and water, with a bit of fruit flavoring thrown in for good measure. But know that 100 percent juice is not necessarily nutritionally superior. Because some juice beverages have added nutrients, they may provide more vitamin C, for example, than a product that's 100 percent real juice. However, a noteworthy difference between fruit juices and fruit drinks is that fruit juices often contain other important nutrients that fruit drinks aren't fortified with, such as folate in orange juice.

## A marked lack of activity

It's crystal, in-your-face clear that a lack of physical activity leads to excess weight in both children and adults. Interesting is the correlation between the amount of time that a child watches television and his weight. The more TV that a child watches, the heavier he is. Experts think that this phenomenon is twofold. First and foremost, while children watch TV, they're inactive, and therefore, burning few calories. Second, commercials often encourage consumption of high-calorie foods — and eating too many of them, of course, can result in weight gain. This also can be true for kids who spend plenty of time at the computer.

## The dangers of current eating trends

In childhood, and in adulthood, the more fat that people consume, the more calories they consume, too. And in turn, the more weight they tend to gain. That's because, bite for bite, a gram of fat delivers more than twice the number of calories than a gram of protein or carbohydrate does. Research performed at Brigham Young University [reported in the *Journal of the American Dietetic Association* 97(9), 1997] measured the amount of fat consumed by 262 children aged 9 and 10. Then the researchers compiled data on the children's weights, the parents' weights, and the level of the children's activity. The greater the amount of fat the youngsters ate, the more they weighed, even after genetics and activity level were factored in. The higher the amount of carbohydrates and fiber the children ate, the lower their weights. Fiber-rich carbohydrates are associated with lower body weights and a reduced risk of cancer and heart disease in adults as well.

Unfortunately, more children are eating their meals away from home (not including brown-bag lunches) and those meals are often higher in fat and the portions are larger than most children need. Often, these meals are eaten at fast-food restaurants, where fiber-rich carbohydrates, such as fruits, vegetables, and whole grains, are hard to come by. Other common food-away-from-home sources include stores, day-care centers, and school cafeterias.

Another trend is the shift from drinking milk to consuming more noncitrus juices, juice drinks, and other calorie-dense beverages like soda. Not only has milk been squeezed out of children's menus, but the consumption of these other beverages that provide calories — and little else — has increased rapidly. The statistics are staggering; by the time a child reaches 5 years-old, her milk consumption will start to slide, so that by 18 years old, soft drinks and juice drinks will reduce milk intake to a skimpy ¾ cup a day. The researchers who conducted and analyzed the data are worried because the most frequently consumed beverages are low in all nutrients except sugar.

Some juice is fine, but drinking it all day long is not — no matter if it's a juice drink or 100 percent juice. Not only can constantly washing the teeth with juice lead to dental cavities, but also consuming more than 12 ounces of it a day is associated with reduced height and increased obesity in 2- and 5-year-old children. (See *Pediatrics* 99, 1997.) Although counting a 4-ounce to 8-ounce glass of 100-percent fruit juice as one or two fruit servings per day is fine; in reality, juice accounts for 50 percent of all the fruit consumed by children. And juice isn't the best way to get all your fruit servings, because it doesn't provide fiber, which most children — and adults — don't get enough of in their diet. Table 22-1 shows how several popular juices compare nutritionally.

**Table 22-1 Nutritional Comparison of Some Fruit Juices**

| | *Orange Juice* | *Grapefruit Juice (Unfortified)* | *Apple Juice* | *Grape Juice (Unfortified)* |
|---|---|---|---|---|
| Vitamin C | Excellent source | Excellent source | Not significant | Not significant |
| Potassium | Good source | Good source | Good source | Good source |
| Folic acid | Excellent source | Good source | Not significant | Not significant |

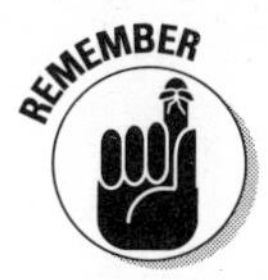


Remember to count both juice and milk as servings from their appropriate food groups — they contain calories, but also some important vitamins and minerals. If you're looking to quench your child's thirst, go with water — it's refreshing, and calorie free, to boot.

# Determining Whether Your Child Is Overweight

Simply looking at your child should give you a pretty good idea of whether your child is on the plump side. And your pediatrician will confirm or contradict your suspicions by using one of several tools, such as a growth chart, graph, or formula.

You may have used the charts in Chapter 3 to figure out if your Body Mass Index (BMI) indicated that your weight is a health risk. BMI is the standard used to measure a child's weight-related health risk, too. However, you must use charts specifically designed for children. Children's BMI charts, unlike those for adults, are based on age and gender. Ask the staff at the pediatrician's office to show you your child's charts. Or you can use the formulas and charts that follow to do the calculations yourself.

To calculate your child's BMI, use the same formula that's in Chapter 3 as follows:

1. **Convert your child's weight from pounds to kilograms.**

   Weight (in pounds) ÷ 2.2 = weight (in kilograms).

   For example, 75 pounds ÷ 2.2 = 34 kilograms.

2. **Convert your child's height from inches to meters.**

   Height (in inches) ÷ 39.37 = height (in meters). For example, 48 inches ÷ 39.37= 1.22 meters.

3. **Calculate your child's Body Mass Index using the gender and appropriate chart.**

   Figure 22-1 can be used for girls and Figure 22-2 is for boys.

BMI is usually calculated in kilograms and meters, but if you feel more comfortable using pounds and feet, this formula will work for you:

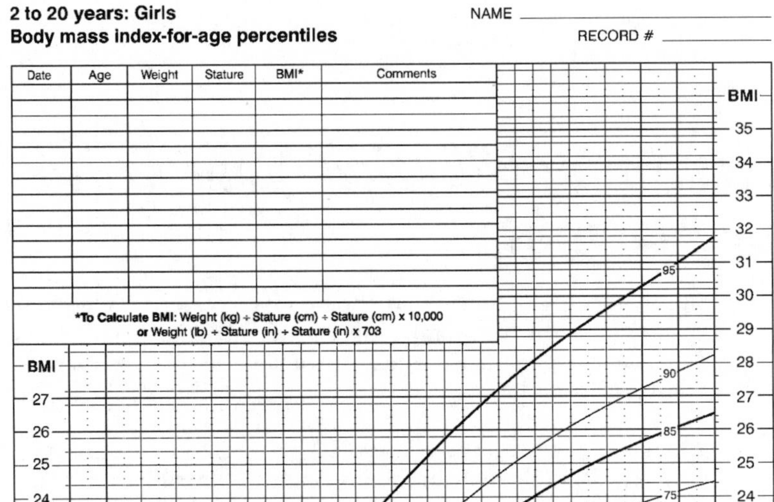


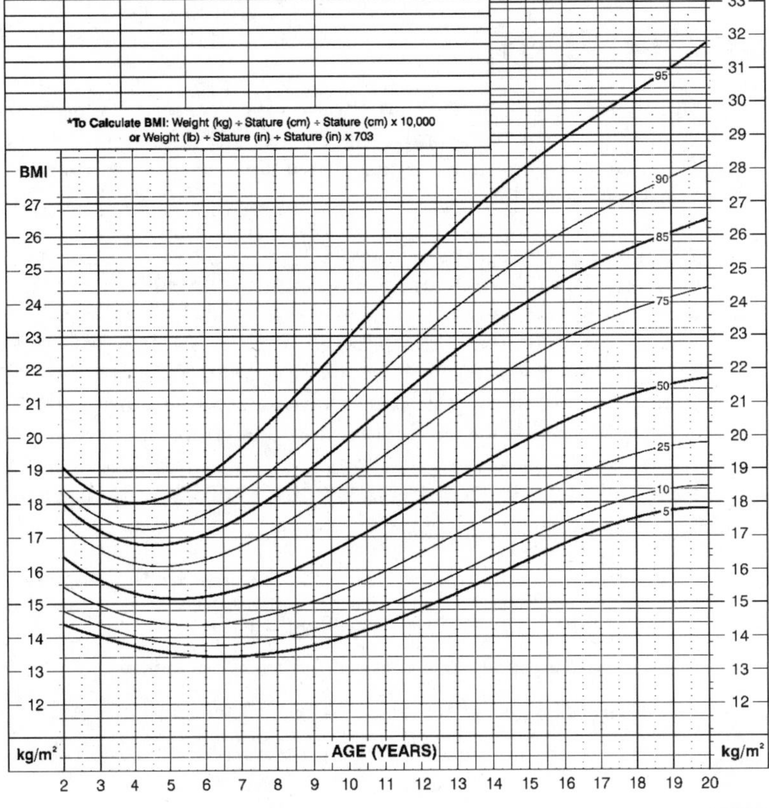


Published May 30, 2000 (modified 10/16/00).
SOURCE: Developed by the National Center for Health Statistics in collaboration with the National Center for Chronic Disease Prevention and Health Promotion (2000).
http://www.cdc.gov/growthcharts

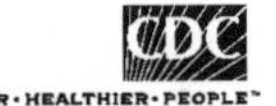


**Figure 22-1:** Compare your daughter's BMI to the numbers on this table to determine what percentile her BMI falls into.

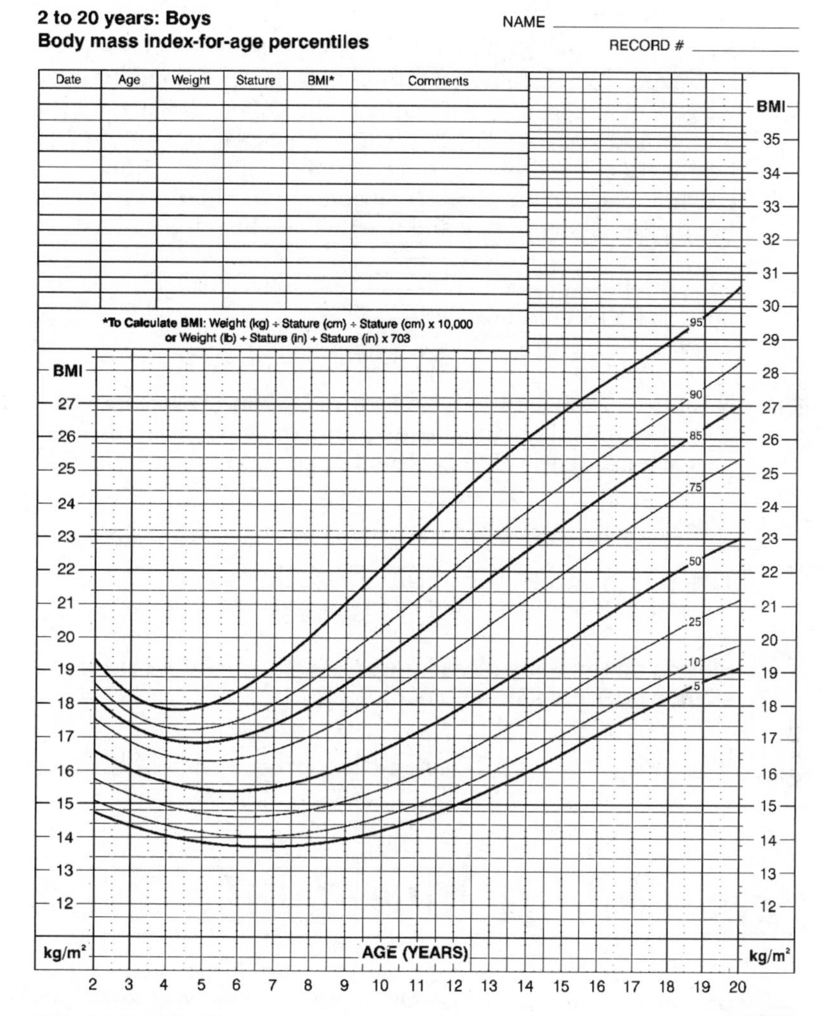


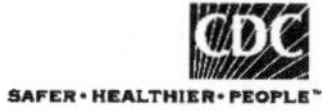


**Figure 22-2:** Compare your son's BMI to the numbers on this table to determine what percentile his BMI falls into.

$$\frac{\text{weight in pounds} \times 704.5}{\text{height in inches} \times \text{height in inches}} = \text{BMI}$$

As a general rule, a child whose BMI is over the 85th percentile for age and sex, needs to be evaluated for hypertension and high blood fats, because his weight is dangerously unhealthy. If the child's BMI is over the 95th percentile for age and sex, a thorough medical assessment is needed. Many of the health concerns that are equated with midlife are showing up in overweight children. So, it's important to become your child's advocate to ensure that her doctor is identifying and treating any health problems early on.

For example, suppose 11-year-old Jacob weighs 105 pounds and is 61 inches tall. His BMI would be calculated like this: 105 pounds ÷ 61 inches ÷ 61 inches x 704.5 = 19.8 BMI.

Next, find Jacob's age, 11, on Figure 22-2, body mass index-for-age percentiles for boys, and follow the line up until you reach 20.5, his BMI. Because his BMI falls just above the 85th percentile line, Jacob is overweight.

Now check out one more example:

Julie is 15 years old. She weighs 135 pounds and is 5 foot 2 inches, or 62 inches tall. Her BMI would be calculated like this: 135 ÷ 62 ÷ 62 x 704.5 = 24.6 BMI.

Plotted on the Body Mass index-for-age percentile chart for girls, Julie also is slightly over the 85th percentile.

Both Jacob and Julie would be healthier if they tried to hold their weight where it is, and let their heights catch up.

# If Your Child Is Overweight

It's certainly hard for a child who is overweight — getting teased or called names or being the last person picked for the kickball team. It's difficult for the parent, too. No parent wants to see his or her child left out of social events or hurt. If your child is overweight, you can help. But remember, the goal of weight control in children is just that: control, *not weight loss.* Instead of trying to help a child reduce her weight, let height catch up to weight by maintaining a slow rate of weight gain. The only exception is if the child's health is in danger because of the extra weight — and that's a decision to make with a physician.

In its 1998 position paper, the American Pediatric Association's Expert Committee recommended that children with a BMI over the 95th percentile for age and sex lose weight. But, this weight loss should be s-l-o-w-l-y achieved — no more than 1 pound loss per month. We strongly recommend that children be put on weight-loss diets only under a physician's orders and that the child and her family work closely with a registered dietitian.

Don't restrict food if your child is overweight. Restricting food sets up a binge mentality and metabolism similar to what a person experiences during starvation. Even after the restriction is lifted, the bingeing doesn't stop. Besides, no one has the right to withhold food from another person, even a child.

From a parenting perspective, restricting food is a natural response to dealing with a weight issue. Many parents perceive this as helping or being supportive of their overweight child. In some respects it's counterintuitive to not restrict food or not to bring errors of judgment to the child's attention. But the goal here is to coach your child to recognize intrinsic cues — her own hunger and sense of fullness. The only way to do that is to let the child decide for herself how much to eat.

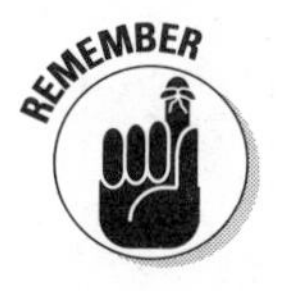


Food isn't the only thing that affects your child's weight — many psychological aspects factor into being overweight as a kid, too. If you want to help your child control weight, you can do many things to ensure that her self-esteem remains high.

## Nurture a positive body image

Children pick up behaviors by watching grown-ups. If you show your children nutritious eating habits, they're more likely to follow your example. If you're constantly dieting and criticizing your body, they'll begin to disrespect theirs, too.

A study conducted by *Glamour* magazine on 4,000 young women (reported in the November 1994 issue) examined the effects that their mothers' dieting had on their eating habits. The subtle messages that daughters of dieters received from their parents greatly affected them. The more often a mother dieted, the greater the likelihood that her daughter dieted, too, regardless of the child's age. The study also revealed that a father's teasing about his daughter's body often had a stinging effect on body image and dieting behavior.

Let your children know that they are loved and perfect just the way they are. If they don't feel criticized by you for their size or shape, they'll become able to accept and feel good about themselves. Let them share their thoughts about their size with you. Help them to discover that people come in all shapes and sizes and that their outsides have nothing to do with their insides. Chapter 21 offers more information about how self-esteem and a positive body image affect how people deal with food and the prevention of eating disorders.

Focus on the tangible things that the child excels at — notice and acknowledge when her room is cleaned, she helps a friend, or finishes her homework without being told. This allows the child to view herself in a positive way.

## Encourage physical activity

Sure, getting physical helps balance calories. But it also helps develop coordination and self-confidence. And habits that start now are more likely to follow your child into adulthood. Get the whole family involved in physical activity. The following list offers some ideas on how to do that:

- Take walks together after dinner.
- Plan nature walks, hikes, and canoe trips for the whole family.
- Encourage your child to join school or community athletic programs — but only if she enjoys the activity. If it's not fun, the child won't do it, and it won't engender lifelong habits. Volunteer to coach or, at the very least, go to games and practice sessions.
- Take up sports that the whole family can do, such as inline skating, cross-country or downhill skiing, and backpacking.
- Get a pedometer for each family member. It's a tangible way to promote and encourage physical activity.
- Get a rope and start jumping. Stage a family tournament.
- Encourage children to ride bikes and swim at an early age, and show them how. Dust off your bike, too; put on your suit and get into the pool with your kids.
- Turn off the TV. Better yet, unplug it. And limit computer and video game time.
- Ask your child what he liked best about doing a favorite activity. You may be surprised to find out that you're the draw. Exercise can provide a focused opportunity for conversation between the two of you.

Be sensitive about your child's size when selecting activities. Some activities will be difficult. Her size may make movement difficult, uncoordinated, and embarrassing. And don't use physical activity as a form of punishment. One of the reasons many adults say they don't like to exercise is because as children they were made to work out as a form of discipline. Keep exercise fun. Studies show that the exercise habits made in youth are the habits you're most likely to keep as you become adults. It is important to find sustainable activities that your kids enjoy.

## Ways to enhance your child's body image

You know many wonderful and unique things about your child. Have you shared them with him lately? Consider the following list. Your opinions can color your child's body perception in subtle ways.

- Examine *your* expectations of your child's body.
- Examine *your* own beliefs and prejudices about body weight.
- Link respect for diverse body shapes and sizes with diversity of race, ethnicity, and so on.
- Realize that it's okay to criticize a child's behavior, but it's not okay to criticize the child.
- Take the opportunity to praise a child's behavior, and make the compliment specific.
- Don't model poor behavior by criticizing your own body shape, make excuses for not exercising because of your weight, or talk about your need to diet.
- Encourage eating only in response to hunger.

## Honor your child's body

As a parent, your job is simple — in theory, anyway. You must provide the what, when, and where food is eaten. Your child's job is to decide whether she will eat and how much. Whether your child is normal, underweight, or overweight doesn't matter. An overweight child should not be treated differently from other children. This is the mantra of Ellyn Satter, RD, ACSW, who's done some landmark work helping parents help their children develop normal, healthy eating habits. The following information is adapted from her work:

A parent's responsibility is to:

- **Provide healthy food choices.** The Food Guide Pyramid (see Chapter 9) is a good place to start. When you plan a snack or meal, make sure that it includes protein, carbohydrate, and a little bit of fat. A carbohydrate-only meal or snack — such as noodles or an apple — satisfies quickly, but it doesn't have the staying power that protein and fat do. A hamburger patty or a handful of peanuts, which are mostly protein and fat, may have staying power but don't provide immediate satiety. Yogurt and peanuts, cheese and fruit, or peanut butter and waffles are well-rounded snacks.

Serve foods that are reliable sources of fiber, such as vegetables and whole grains, often. These foods have fewer calories than fiber-free foods that are high in fat and sugar, such as pastries and ice cream. Nutrition experts use this formula to determine kids' fiber needs: Take the child's age (up to 20 years old) and add 5. That's the number of grams of fiber needed daily. So a 6-year-old needs at least 11 grams of fiber per day and an 11-year-old needs 16 grams.

Providing children with food regularly but not constantly is also important. Children need to eat about every three hours; younger tykes may need to eat even more frequently. For adolescents who can eat more at one time, four hours between meals is fine. Don't allow children to eat all day with no beginning or end to the meal. Children, like adults, eat out of boredom. An open kitchen policy and a ready supply of tempting edibles encourage all-day eating. Instead, schedule and serve snacks and meals at predictable times. Make snacks substantial enough to be filling but not so large that they ruin an appetite for an upcoming meal.

- **Manage the environment as much as you can.** What foods you serve and when you serve them are important. *Where* is the third leg of a parent's responsibility. Following are some tips for establishing a good mealtime environment:
  - Limit eating to one or two rooms in the house — preferably the kitchen and dining room.
  - Insist that children sit while eating.
  - Eat your meals together as a family as much as possible. Keep the TV off and books and toys out of sight to encourage conversation.
  - Sit and eat with your child. You create a healthy social environment and serve as a role model, too.
- **Be a good example.** Eat the same foods that you expect your child to eat. If you want her to drink lowfat milk, you should have some, too — not a soda. Eat slowly and allow your child to set her own pace. That shows respect for her individual eating rhythm.

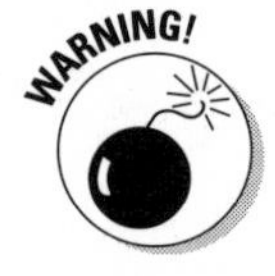


- **Never use food as a reward or punishment.** This approach will backfire. Studies on children and their parents show that if food (such as dessert) is given as a reward for eating another food (such as a vegetable) or if food is withheld as a punishment for not eating vegetables, then the children's desire to eat the vegetables decreases.
- **Remember that it's a child's responsibility to decide whether to eat — not yours.** A child may not be hungry at one meal but may make up for it and eat heartily at the next. Trust her body to decide. Studies that measure children's intake show a tremendous variability over the course of a day. However, when researchers calculated the calories consumed over several days, the results showed little difference in total calories from one day to another.
- **Let a child decide when to stop eating.** People are born with an innate sense of knowing when to eat and when to stop. Unfortunately, outside influences have taught most adults to ignore these signals. The best

approach that you can use to help children control their weight — now and in adulthood — is to encourage them to trust, honor, and listen to their own internal hunger and fullness signals. Offering advice (such as "I think you've had enough") or regulating the amount of food that a child is allowed to eat fosters distrust and fear of hunger and may leave a child powerless and unable to take responsibility for her own body.

# Frequently Asked Questions

If you have questions about your child's diet, you're not alone. Most parents, at one time or another, are concerned that they may not be doing the right thing when it comes to feeding their kids. You may have asked yourself these same questions.

## What should I do when my child's classmates taunt him about his size?

It's undoubtedly hard for a child — and his parents — when he feels left out. His peers may tease him, too. Other children can be cruel when a person is "different" and not realize how terrible they can make an overweight child feel. Take the time to talk regularly to your child about his feelings. Assure him that the inside of a person — not the outside — counts and that you love him no matter what his weight. Overweight children need support, acceptance, and encouragement from loved ones. They also need tools. Although it's necessary to be sympathetic, caring, and supportive, your child needs problem-solving skills to build self-reliance. Ask questions like: Do you think that there was another way to handle those comments? How do you think you can handle that situation if it happens again? Is there a way that I can help you?

## What do I do when my child refuses to eat vegetables?

Just like adults, children should aim for five servings of fruits or vegetables a day. They're good sources of fiber, they're packed with vitamins and minerals, they're low in fat, and they're important for good health and development. Even if your child isn't crazy about vegetables, you can get her to eat them — and happily — by using these tips:

- **Offer to cut raw veggies as snacks.** Many kids prefer uncooked vegetables to cooked ones and especially like to dip them. Try bean dip, hummus, salsa, or plain, lowfat yogurt flavored with seasonings as an accompaniment.
- **Know that bright colors and crisp textures are kid winners.** Steam or microwave veggies in a small amount of water to avoid overcooking them. You want them to be firm to the bite.
- **Sneak them in!** Add peas to mac and cheese; add shredded carrots or other vegetables to spaghetti sauce, lasagna, chili, tuna salad, or even peanut butter.
- **Bake them in.** Try lowfat zucchini and carrot muffins — your kids won't know what hit them!
- **Stir in finely chopped vegetables.** Add them to meatloaf, ground turkey, ground beef, rice, or mashed potatoes.
- **Start a garden.** Most kids eat vegetables that they grow themselves — and are proud to share the bounty with the rest of the family. You can even grow lettuce in a warm, sunny window in the middle of winter.

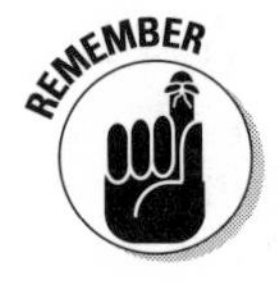


Research indicates that children need plenty of exposures to a new or novel food before it's accepted. Therefore, you may want to set up some family rules where everyone (mother and father included) should taste every item on their plate. You can use the child's age to determine the number of bites. Setting an expectation increases the likelihood of acceptance — without tasting the food, a child will never be able to like the food.

## How do I keep my child from trading her healthful lunch for a candy bar?

Parents have been asking this question for years. A candy bar is a big temptation to most kids, and after kids are out of your sight, they're out of your control, for the most part. However, you *can* help them eat healthfully even when you're not around to monitor their eating by packing items that they enjoy eating. Children often enjoy eating a little bit of many things — it adds surprise and fun to their meals. Plan easy-to-eat foods, such as baby carrots, cherry tomatoes, cucumber slices, and pepper strips along with a lowfat dip. If you have the time, use a cookie cutter to turn an ordinary sandwich into an extraordinary shape. Score the rind of an orange or tangerine so that it's easier to peel or offer fruit salad. Lowfat pudding or a few lowfat cookies are fine, too.

Most important, if you get children to help plan and prepare their own lunches, they're more likely to keep them than trade them — after all, they made them!

### Out of sight, out of mind

The sight and smell of food can be a powerful appetite turn-on — a huge temptation for overweight children who may be especially sensitive to food cues. You don't have to ban all high-calorie foods from the house, but do limit the temptation by putting away the cookie jar, or not filling it. Have bowls of fruit ready instead. The point is not to take the fun out of food, just to offer healthier, less calorie-dense options more often than nutrient-poor ones.

## What are some low-calorie and healthful snacks that children can eat in the car?

Unless you must be in the car during a regularly scheduled meal or snack time, don't feel that you need to provide food. Filling idle time in the car with eating gives food too much entertainment value. You don't want to condition your children to equate riding in the car with eating, which trains them to ignore their appetites and eat for the wrong reasons. Food should be served so that children eat and only eat. When they focus their attention exclusively on the meal, without distractions, they're far more likely to recognize their innate but subtle appetite clues of hunger and satiety.

However, when schedules don't allow for dining-room meals, your youngsters will welcome snacks. Staying hydrated is most important, especially if the heat or air conditioner is running nonstop. Water is the best choice. Whole-wheat crackers, not-too-sweet cookies (such as ginger, vanilla, or graham crackers), and fruit are the healthiest snacks to carry.

## What's wrong with skipping breakfast?

Many parents allow their children to skip breakfast. In fact, research presented in 2002 by the NPD group (formerly known as the National Products Diary) showed that households that skip breakfast most often are the ones with children. What a shame! Parents may reason that the children aren't hungry in the morning, and by skipping breakfast they avoid a bunch of calories. However, eating breakfast is important because it shifts the body out of starvation mode and into action. When a body thinks that it's starving, it hoards energy by slowing down the burning of calories. Concentration becomes difficult. A child often becomes cranky and isn't able to run, play, or jump with much enthusiasm. A school-aged child won't do well in morning lessons.

The healthiest breakfasts are a combination of whole grains, some form of lowfat or fat-free milk, yogurt or cheese (for calcium and protein), and a little fat. Like any meal, avoid eating sweet breakfast foods without balancing them with fiber, protein, or fat because the sugar load can backfire in an energy crash. Be practical: Breakfast can be as simple as a granola bar or half a tuna sandwich and milk or as homespun as a warming bowl of hot cereal sweetened with raisins. That your child eats something every morning — even if it's a slice of cold left over pizza — is what's important.

## How much fast food is too much?

One or two meals of burgers, fries, and shakes aren't going to ruin a week's worth of eating healthfully. But keep in mind that fast foods lack variety and generally contain too much fat and salt and little fiber. The environment isn't conducive to relaxed eating. And the prepackaged serving sizes don't encourage eating and stopping based on internal clues.

One way to add variety is to offer many vegetable-rich, crunchy, fresh foods at breakfast, lunch, and snack time. Another way is to expand the kinds of restaurants you visit. Try Mexican food one night, pizza another, and a seafood dinner occasionally, and add in Asian cuisine. Not only do these various cuisines allow your children to open their taste buds to new foods and experiences and add adventure to their meals, but they also add variety — which means that they'll get a wide array of vitamins and minerals in addition to enjoying their food.

# Chapter 23

# Weight Loss for Athletes

### *In This Chapter*

- Identifying your unique physique
- Determining your nutrition needs
- Translating your eating plan into meals
- Drinking enough water

If you're a competition-level athlete — or someone who loves one — don't pass by this chapter. Athletes have special dietary needs, particularly when they want to lose weight. Therefore, some of the information in other chapters won't give you the kind of help that you're looking for.

For example, most of the information in Chapter 3 is too basic when applied to you. Likewise, the general principles in Chapter 10 apply, but the specifics may not take your optimal protein and carbohydrate needs into account. And Chapter 12 is written for the person who doesn't engage in physical activity or at least not enough of it, which is hardly a problem for an athlete.

We don't address detailed physical activity for athletes in this chapter, because it's beyond the scope of this book. Your coach or trainer will have training advice for you. But you can turn to this chapter whenever you have questions about how to eat to optimize your performance while keeping your weight under control.

So who's an athlete? For the purposes of this discussion, we refer to anyone who is extremely active and dedicated to excelling in a particular physical activity. We include ballet dancers, ballroom dancers, horseback riders, gymnasts, acrobats, and clowns. Shopping for equipment regularly at a sports superstore doesn't automatically make you an athlete for this discussion. For example, we don't consider billiard players, stock-car drivers, and bowlers to be athletes.

# Putting Body Weight into Perspective

*Lean and mean* doesn't apply to all athletes. If you lined up a marathon runner, a jockey, a speed skater, a weightlifter, a pole-vaulter, a linebacker, a gymnast, and a sumo wrestler right next to each other, the variation of heights and weights would be vast. The amount of fat on their bodies varies tremendously, too. Obviously, athletes come in as many shapes and sizes as the general population.

The standard reference for healthy weight is the Body Mass Index (BMI). BMI is a ratio of height and weight. (See Chapter 3 for information on how to calculate BMI.) A BMI between 19 and 24.9 is considered normal, 25 to 29.9 is overweight, and a BMI of more than 30 is obese. A BMI under 18.9 is too low and may be just as unhealthy as a BMI over 25.

Generally, as BMI increases so does the percentage of a person's weight that is fat. Increased body fat is associated with increased health risk. For athletes, however, BMI doesn't provide enough information about your health status or optimal body composition for your sport. For example, a large and muscular athlete, such as a defensive lineman, who is extremely lean but not fat, can have a BMI in the overweight range.

## Assessing body composition

The percent of an athlete's body that's fat mass (FM for short) versus the percentage that's fat-free mass (FFM) is a more useful tool than BMI, because body composition directly relates to your athletic performance. Your age, gender, race, diet, and training regimen impacts how much body fat you have.

Before you make any changes in your training schedule or eating habits, get an accurate body composition analysis. Several ways to do this include:

- Underwater weighing
- Skin-fold thickness
- Bioelectrical impedance

See Chapter 3 for details about how these procedures are done.

## Matching body composition to performance

Women have higher percentages of body fat than men, because female reproductive hormones require more fat. Women with healthy weights are generally between 15 and 25 percent body fat and men fall into the 10 to 20 percent range. But for the athlete, optimal body fat may be 10 to 20 percent for women and 5 to 12 percent for men.

Table 23-1 sums up the difference between percent body fat in the general population and what's considered ideal for optimal athletic performance.

**Table 23-1 Percent Body Fat in Athletes and Nonathletes**

| | *Women* | *Men* |
|---|---|---|
| Athlete | 10 to 20 percent | 5 to 12 percent |
| Normal (optimal) | 15 to 25 percent | 10 to 20 percent |
| Overweight | 25.1 to 29.9 percent | 20.1 to 24.4 percent |
| Obese | Over 30 percent | Over 25 percent |

Skaters, gymnasts, and dancers, who are judged for their aesthetic appearance as much as their physical skill, strive to achieve minimum body fat. Runners, too, find that they run better when their body fat is low — because it means that they have less mass to move. Swimmers, on the other hand, find body fat helps them with buoyancy.

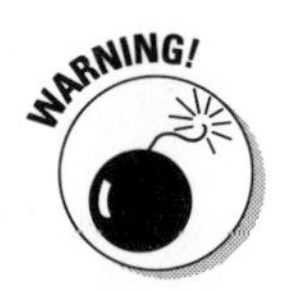


You *can* have too little body fat. If a woman's body fat falls below 12 percent of her total body weight, hormone production can be compromised, and menstruation can be interrupted, and therefore the risk of *osteoporosis* (thinning bones, which is directly related to hormonal status) is high. Body fat below 10 percent in women and 4 percent in men may be an indication of an eating disorder. (See Chapter 21 for more information about eating disorders.)

Specific body compositions aren't recommended for individual sports but generalizations have been made through observation of elite athletes. These generalizations are summarized in Table 23-2.

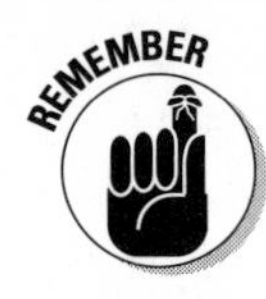


These are observations, not recommendations. Additionally, they're observations *in adults* and should not be used as standards for adolescents.

**Table 23-2 Observed Body Composition Characteristics of Athletes***

| *Sport* | *% Body Fat* | |
|---|---|---|
| | ***Men*** | ***Women*** |
| Ballet | | 12–22 |
| Baseball/Softball | 13 | 14–24 |
| Basketball | 7–14 | 15–24 |
| Bicycling | 8–13 | 8–15 |
| Field Events | | |
| Decathlon | 3–13 | |
| Pentathlon | | 8–14 |
| Throwing | | 19–35 |
| Discus | 12–21 | |
| Shot | 12–21 | |
| Jumping | 6–10 | 10–15 |
| Field Hockey | | 14–25 |
| Football | | |
| Defensive backs | 5–14 | |
| Running backs and wide receivers | 5–13 | |
| Linebackers | 9–19 | |
| Offensive line | 12–19 | |
| Defensive line | 13–24 | |
| Quarterbacks | 8–21 | |
| Gymnastics | 4–9 | 16–17 |
| Lacrosse | 8–17 | 14–24 |

| *Sport* | *% Body Fat* | |
|---|---|---|
| | *Men* | *Women* |
| Racket sports | | |
| Tennis | 6–16 | 20–24 |
| Squash | 7–15 | |
| Skating | | |
| Ice hockey | 5–14 | |
| Speed skating | 5–10 | 11–20 |
| Skiing (Nordic) | 5–9 | 18–21 |
| Soccer | 5–14 | 15–27 |
| Swimming | 6–12 | 12–20 |
| Track | | |
| Distance runners | 2–8 | 11–18 |
| Sprinters and hurdlers | 3–13 | 7–14 |
| Triathlon | 7–17 | 15–18 |
| Volleyball | 7–13 | 14–21 |
| Weight lifting and bodybuilding | | |
| Olympic lift | 8–12 | |
| Power lift | 8–10 | 20–23 |
| Bodybuilding | 8–10 | 12–15 |
| Wrestling | | |
| Adult | 5–13 | |
| Sumo | 26–28 | |

**Adapted from Sports Nutrition, A guide for the Professional Working with Active People, 2000. Data has been rounded to the nearest whole number.*

# Estimating Nutrient Needs

As we say earlier in this book, to lose weight you must take in fewer calories than you expend. Nonathletes who want to lose weight can simply determine how many calories they're eating at their present weight and then reduce that number by eating less and exercising more. See Chapter 8 for the exact details. Simple enough, right?

However, for athletes, reaching weight-loss goals while maintaining optimal body composition to maintain performance without negatively impacting your health takes more than just counting calories. For you, the amounts of carbohydrate and protein must be calculated specifically while staying within the proper calorie range.

## Establishing weight-loss goals

For athletes, reducing percent body fat should be the focus of weight-loss efforts rather than reducing total body weight, otherwise optimum performance will be compromised. In some cases, total weight may not even change, when percent body fat goes down and muscle goes up. (Muscle weighs more than fat.) Therefore, assessing body composition is crucial as you determine your weight-loss goals.

We can use Emily to illustrate. Emily is a 24-year old runner who's training for a marathon. She feels she could improve her performance if she lost some weight. Until a few years ago, she weighed about 120. Emily is 5 feet and 4 inches tall and now weighs 135 pounds. Her present estimated body fat is 23 percent. Her body fat goal is 15 percent. All body fat goals in this section are based on mean body percentages from Table 23-2 earlier in this chapter.

Here's how she would calculate her optimal weight:

1. **135 (current weight) x 23 percent (current % body fat) = 31 pounds of fat**
2. **135 (current weight) – 31 (weight that's fat) = 104 pounds of lean**
3. **FFM (fat-free mass) goal = 85 percent (difference between body fat goal and total body)**
4. **104 (current pounds of FFM) ÷ 85 percent = 122 (Emily's goal weight)**

Emily's weight-loss goal is to reach 122 pounds and reduce her percent body fat from 23 percent to 15 percent.

Another example is Geoff. He's a cyclist but hasn't been able to make much progress in his speed or endurance despite a rigorous training schedule. He now weighs 185 pounds. His present estimated body fat percentage is 15 percent but his goal body fat is 10 percent.

He calculated his optimal weight thus:

1. **185 (current weight) x 15 percent (current % body fat) = 28 pounds of fat**
2. **185 (current weight) – 28 (weight that's fat) = 157 pounds of lean**
3. **FFM (fat-free mass) goal = 90 percent (difference between body fat goal and total body)**
4. **157 (current pounds of FFM) ÷ 90 percent = 174 (Geoff's goal weight)**

Geoff's weight-loss goal is 174 pounds and to reduce his percent body fat from 15 percent to 10 percent.

Now plug in your own numbers:

1. **_______ (current weight) x ___% (current % body fat) = ____ pounds of fat**
2. **____ (current weight) – ____ (weight that is fat) = ____ pounds of lean**
3. **FFM goal =___% (difference between body fat goal and total body)**
4. **____ (current pounds of FFM) ÷ ____% = _____ (Your goal weight)**

## Estimating calorie needs

After you know what your weight-loss goal is (and remember it may not be a different number than it is now), you can calculate your total daily calories and the ideal amounts of carbohydrate, protein, and fat.

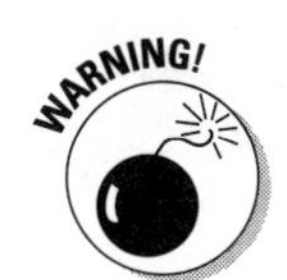


Cutting calories drastically impairs your performance. Therefore, you should always maintain weight (but shift your percentage of fat to lean) while you're training and use the "off season" for weight loss. If you must lose while training (because you're a year-round athlete), weight loss should be very, very gradual: ½ to 1 pound a week. Losing weight more quickly causes loss of *muscle glycogen* (the form of energy that is stored in the muscles) and muscle tissue loss as well. Rapid weight-loss diets that are low in carbohydrates are particularly dangerous for athletes. Most of these diets cause water loss, which can lead to impaired cardiac function, inability to maintain body temperature, and muscle cramping.

To figure out how many calories you need to lose weight, first calculate how many calories you're eating now. To do this, review the information in Chapter 8 about keeping a food journal for several days to tally your daily calories.

Another way to calculate your caloric needs is based on formulas. To use the formula method, first find your Basic Metabolic Rate (BMR), which is the number of calories you need to maintain heartbeat and breathing. Flip back to Table 8-1 in Chapter 8 to get your BMR. Then multiply it by the activity factor that applies to you in Table 23-3.

**Table 23-3 Activity Factors**

| *Exercise Level* | *Description* | *Factor* |
|---|---|---|
| Very Light | Extremely sedentary, largely bed rest | 1.2–1.3 |
| Light | No planned activity, mostly office work | 1.5–1.6 |
| Moderate | Walking, stair climbing during the day | 1.6–1.7 |
| Heavy | Planned vigorous activities | 1.9–2.1 |

As you can see from Table 23-3, most athletes fall in the *heavy* range for physical activity. Therefore, their BMR would be multiplied by 1.9–2.1.

If you recall our examples from the previous section using Emily and Geoff, here's how to calculate their calorie intake:

For Emily:

> 1,398 (Emily's BMR calculated from Table 8-1) x 2.0 (activity factor) = 2,796 current calorie intake.

For Geoff:

> 1,854 (Geoff's BMR calculated from Table 8-1) x 2.0 (activity factor) = 3,708 current calorie intake.

Plug in your own numbers here:

> _____ your BMR x ____ your activity factor = current calorie intake.

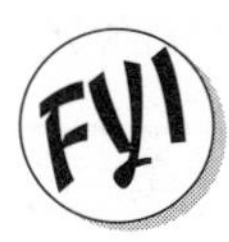

We shortened the method to calculate calories in this chapter by eliminating one of the suggested steps outlined in Chapter 8. The numbers given in Table 23-3 reflect the 10 percent needed for digestion. Because it's already incorporated in the table, we skipped that step. When you know how many calories it takes to maintain your weight, you can subtract the number of calories for weight loss. One pound contains 3,500 calories, so if you want to lose 1 pound of weight a week, you'd deduct 3,500 calories from your week's calorie total. Another way to look at it is to divide the calories by 7 to get the number of calories that you need to cut per day.

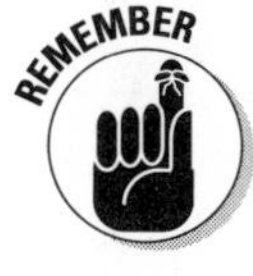


The recommended weight loss for athletes in training is ½ to 1 pound per week.

So, here's the breakdown:

**Calorie deficit per week:** 3,500 (calories in a pound) x ½ to 1 = 1,750–3,500

**Calorie deficit per day:** 1,750–3,500 ÷ 7 (days in a week) = 250–500

## Estimating carbohydrate needs

Working muscles need energy. Carbohydrate is the form of energy that muscles prefer. Carbohydrates are stored in the body in limited amounts as glycogen in muscles and the liver. When an exercising body uses all its glycogen, the athlete *hits the wall* and can no longer maintain exercise intensity. The technical term is *glycogen depletion.* Athletes describe it as feeling sluggish or stale. Often they think it's because they've overtrained. But the real culprit is usually insufficient carbohydrate intake.

In Chapter 10, we discuss calculating carbohydrate requirements (and protein and fat for that matter) based on a percentage of your total calories. Most athletes should get at least 60 percent of their calories from carbohydrates — the same as the general public. Some elite athletes, who have more specific energy needs, should base their requirements on their body weight.

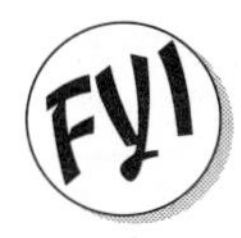

Carbohydrate needs are greater during training than for competition. The old practice of "carbo-loading" before an event doesn't enhance performance as effectively as maintaining glycogen stores while training.

Table 23-4 helps you estimate your carbohydrate requirement based on your weight. Generally, athletes require 3.1 to 4.5 grams of carbohydrate per day per pound of body weight. To put that into perspective, nonathletes need only 1.8 to 2.3 grams per pound per day. Determine how heavily you're training, then multiply the recommended grams of carbohydrate by your body weight to determine your daily carbohydrate requirement.

| Table 23-4 | Carbohydrate Needs for Athletes |
|---|---|
| *Training Level* | *Grams of Carbohydrate per Pound per Day* |
| 1 hour of training per day | 2.7 to 3.1 grams |
| 2 hours of training per day | 3.6 grams |
| 3 hours of training per day | 5 grams |
| 4 hours of training or more per day | 5.5 to 5.9 grams |

## Estimating protein needs

Like carbohydrates, your protein needs are calculated based on your weight and your level of physical activity. Endurance exercise increases protein and carbohydrate requirements. Building muscle takes added protein, too. And because one of the goals of weight loss for athletes is increasing muscle mass, a special protein is recommended for athletes who diet.

Table 23-5 lays it all out for you. Notice there is no separate recommendation for *maintaining* muscle. Nor is there a recommendation for protein higher than 1 gram per pound of body weight because there is no proven benefit that higher levels enhance muscle building — despite recommendations and testimonials dispensed in the locker room.

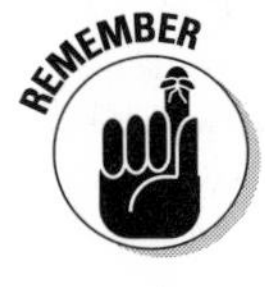


Muscle building takes adequate protein plus adequate calories.

| Table 23-5 | Protein Needs for Athletes |
|---|---|
| *Activity Level* | *Grams of Protein per Pound per Day* |
| Recreational adult (noncompeting) | 0.5 to 0.75 |
| Competitive athlete | 0.6 to 0.9 |
| Muscle building | 0.7 to 0.9 |
| Weight loss | 0.7 to 1.0 |

## Estimating fat and calorie needs for weight loss

To estimate grams of fat and total calories you can eat that will allow you to build muscle and lose body fat, we'll do a few calculations using the calories you're eating now and the number of grams of carbohydrate and protein you need.

Go back to Emily's and Geoff's weight-loss and training goals as examples. (If you need a refresher on the numbers used in these examples, check out the section, "Establishing weight-loss goals" earlier in the chapter). We'll start with Emily.

Her current weight is 135 pounds, and we calculated that she'll run faster if she lowers her total body weight and has less body fat. Because she's training for a marathon, she's working out on most days of the week, and we don't want to interrupt her progress by letting her lose too much weight too fast. In fact, she should lose only ½ to 1 pound a week.

To calculate Emily's fat and calorie needs, start with her carbohydrate requirement. According to Table 23-4, Emily needs 440 grams of carbohydrate each day because she runs or weight trains at least 1 hour a day.

> 135 (pounds) x 3.1(the high end of training 1 hour per day) = 419 grams carbohydrate (it's actually 418.5 which we rounded up to 419)

Using Table 23-5, we calculate that her protein requirement is 130 grams per day.

> 135 (pounds) x 1.0 (recommended protein for dieting) = 135 grams of protein

Now that we know how many grams of carbohydrate and protein Emily needs, we can figure out how many calories they represent. So, we need to multiply their grams by 4 because there are 4 calories in 1 gram of carbohydrate and 1 gram of protein.

> 419 (grams carbohydrate) + 135 (grams protein) x 4 (calories per gram) = 2,216 carbohydrate and protein calories

So how many calories from fat can Emily eat and still lose weight? We know from the calculations in the "Estimating calorie needs" section earlier in the chapter that Emily's current intake is 2,796 calories. So, subtract her carbohydrate and protein calories from her current total calories, and then take another 250 from the result, which is the number of calories Emily will have to cut to lose a ½ pound a week safely.

Then, divide the remaining calories by 9 (one gram of fat has 9 calories) to get her total fat grams. Finally, go back to Emily's current calorie level and subtract the amount of her weight-loss calories to get her new total calories.

Here are the steps to follow:

1. **2,796 (current calories) – 2,216 (carbohydrate and protein calories) – 250 (for ½ pound weekly weight loss) = 330 calories**
2. **330 (calories remaining) ÷ 9 (calories in a gram of fat) = 37 grams fat**
3. **2,796 (current calories) – 250 (for ½ pound weekly weight loss) = 2,546 calories**

So Emily's diet looks like this:

> 2,546 calories, 419 grams carbohydrate, 135 grams protein, 37 grams fat

You can figure Geoff's diet the same way. Because he's not in training for a specific event, he can afford to lose weight a little faster than Emily can. For Geoff, 1 pound per week is safe. So he can reduce his total calories by 500 per day. And because he's not training as vigorously as Emily, he doesn't need her carbohydrate quota either. Following the same progression we used for Emily's calculations, Geoff's would go like this:

1. **185 (current weight) x 2.7 (low end of 1 hour training; see Table 23-4 for info) = 500 grams carbohydrate (we rounded up from 499.5)**
2. **185 (current weight) x 1.0 (protein for weight loss) = 185 grams protein**
3. **500 (grams carbohydrate) + 185 (grams protein) x 4 (calories per gram) = 2,740 carbohydrate and protein calories**
4. **3,708 (current calories) – 2,740 (calories from carbohydrate and protein) – 500 (for 1 pound week weight loss) = 468 calories**
5. **468 (remaining calories) ÷ 9 (calories per fat gram) = 52 grams**
6. **3,708 current calories – 500 = 3,208 (calories for 1 pound a week weight loss)**

Therefore, Geoff can lose weight and gain muscle if he eats a daily diet of:

> 3,208 total calories, 500 grams carbohydrate, 185 grams protein, and 52 grams fat

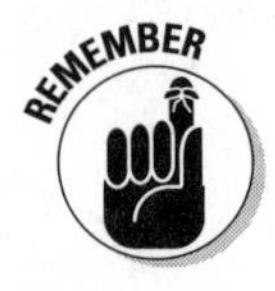


Both Emily and Geoff should monitor their progress by getting their percent body fat calculated once a month. You should do the same to make sure you're getting the optimal amounts of nutrients while you lose weight. Call a nearby hospital for a referral to a site where you can have your body fat measured. A trained technician at your fitness center can calculate your body fat, too.

You can use this space to determine your diet prescription:

1. **____ (current weight) x ____ (carbohydrate needs) = ____ grams carbohydrate**
2. **____ (current weight) x 1.0 (protein for weight loss) = ____ grams protein**

3. ____ (grams carbohydrate) + _____ (grams protein) x 4 (calories per gram) = _____ carbohydrate and protein calories.
4. ____ (current calories) – _____ (calories from carbohydrate and protein) – 500 (for 1 pound week weight loss) = ____ calories
5. ____ (remaining calories) ÷ 9 (calories per fat gram) = ____ grams
6. ____ current calories – 500 = _____ (calories for 1 pound a week weight loss)

# Using the Athlete's Pyramid to Plan Your Meals

In Chapter 9, we configured the USDA's official Food Guide Pyramid to better serve people who want to lose weight by creating the Weight-Loss Pyramid (refer to Figure 9-5). To match the needs of athletes, we've reconfigured it again. Figure 23-1 can be used as a general guide for competitive athletes, because it represents a diet that gets 60 percent of its calories from carbohydrates.

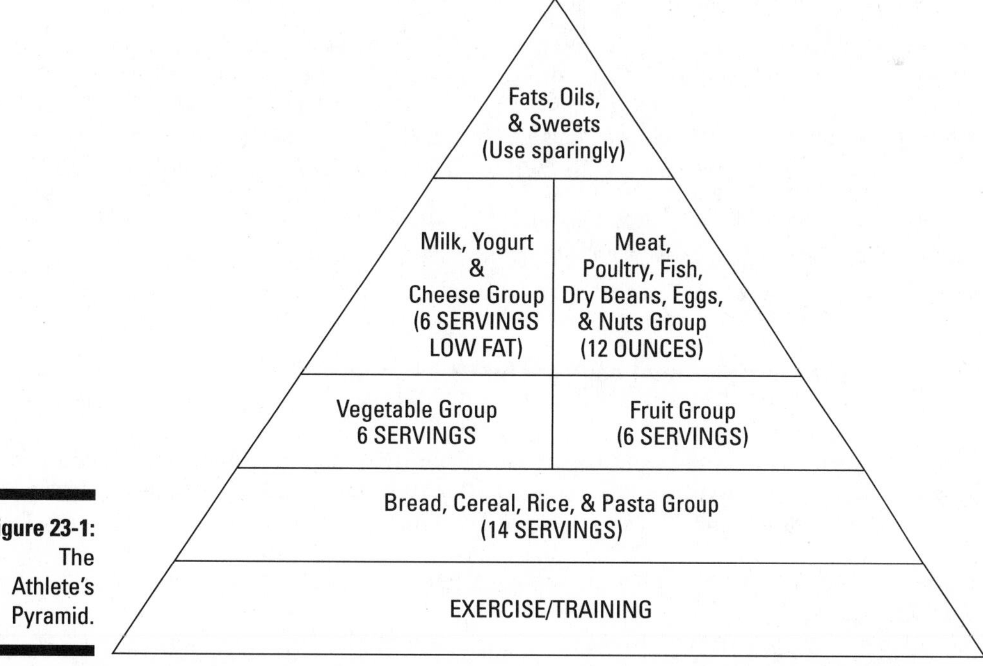


**Figure 23-1:** The Athlete's Pyramid.

## Buying a better bar

Bars used to dominate the energy supplements category. Now gels are squeezing in, and stores are flooded with energy drinks, too. But no federal standard exists for fitness products as it does for say, ice cream. Federal standards dictate that the stuff in any container that calls itself *ice cream* must have a similar amount of fat, sugar, and flavorings. In contrast, labels on bars, gels, and drinks marketed as *performance enhancers* use terms such as *energy, sustained energy,* or *40-30-30* (which represents that 40 percent of the calories come from carbohydrate, 30 percent of calories come from protein, and 30 percent from fat). These labels mean nothing legally. Perhaps that's because few research studies have been done to test the effectiveness of these products to improve athletic achievement. However, sports foods clearly do have a place in an athlete's diet, if only to provide a portable snack.

One study reported in the *Journal of the American Dietetic Association* (January 2000) evaluated candy bars, high-energy bars, moderate-energy bars, and white bread. The researcher was testing how quickly the foods were converted into glucose and how much glucose was delivered. All the foods delivered their peak glucose at roughly the same time — 45 minutes after eating. But the high-energy bar caused the highest glucose levels; the white bread and candy bar delivered an equal amount of glucose but less than the high-energy bar; the moderate carbohydrate bar produced the lowest overall glucose response.

When it comes to fueling an athlete, the higher and sooner the glucose peak, the more energy that's available. But what goes up must come down. Endurance athletes who want sustained energy rather than a burst prefer foods that deliver a more moderate dose of glucose over a longer period of time. When shopping for a sport food, use these general guidelines:

- Foods labeled *energy* and *high-energy* contain the highest amounts of carbohydrate, usually in the form of high-fructose corn syrup. These foods make ideal refueling foods after a long workout.
- Sustained energy foods have fiber and protein added to them to slow and moderate glucose response. Look for nutrition labels that indicate that the product has 3 to 5 grams of fiber, at least 14 grams of protein, and not more than 45 grams of carbohydrate. Foods labeled 40-30-30 qualify as sustained energy products.

For the most nutrient bang per bite, be sure that the bread group servings are mostly whole grains, and the milk and dairy that you drink are low in fat.

Then take a look at the specifics in Chapter 9, especially the information describing portion sizes, so you can match the Athlete's Pyramid as precisely as possible. Table 23-6 can be your guide.

**Table 23-6 Food Group Servings for Various Calorie Levels**

| | *About 2,500* | *About 3,000* | *About 3,500* |
|---|---|---|---|
| Bread group servings | 12 | 14 | 16 |
| Vegetable group servings | 5 | 6 | 10 |
| Fruit group servings | 4 | 6 | 8 |
| Milk group servings | 3 | 3 | 4 |
| Meat group* <br>* The meat group is calculated in ounces because what qualifies as a protein serving varies so widely between the foods in that group. | 10 ounces | 12 ounces | 14 ounces |
| Fats, oils, and sweets | USE | VERY | SPARINGLY |

# Staying Hydrated

Part of any athlete's diet program should include plenty of fluids. We're talking water — and plenty of it — before, during, and after exercise.

The following is a good guideline:

- **Before exercise:** 2 cups of water 1 to 2 hours before working out, plus another 2 cups 10 to 15 minutes before
- **During exercise:** ½ cup every 15 minutes
- **After exercise:** 2 cups

Sport drinks that contain carbohydrates (usually in an easily digestible form) plus *electrolytes* (sodium and potassium to help regulate body temperature) are advised if you exercise more than one hour at a time.

Sport drinks help replace spent calories and minerals lost in sweat. They're preferred over fruit juices and sodas, which have highly concentrated carbohydrates that can cause diarrhea during vigorous exercise and don't contain the electrolytes that sport drinks do.

# Part VII

# The Part of Tens

The 5th Wave
By Rich Tennant
©RICHTENNANT
Say it with Chocolate
St. Valentine's Day
February 14

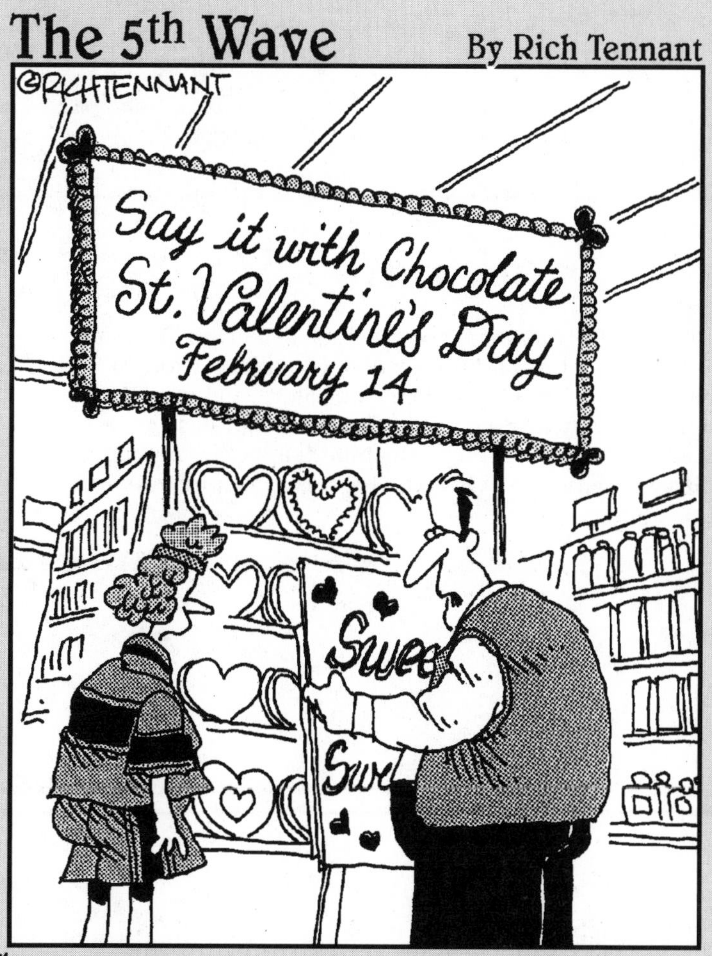

"Of course you're better off eating grains and vegetables, but for St. Valentine's Day, we've never been very successful with, 'Say it with Legumes'."

## In this part . . .

Every *For Dummies* book includes a Part of Tens, full of quick tips and tidbits of useful information. In this part, you can find tips for cutting calories, living healthfully, and staying committed to your weight-loss goals. You'll also find out the truth about ten dieting myths, plus a variety of diet-friendly recipes to inspire you in the kitchen.

# Chapter 24

# Ten Myths about Dieting

### *In This Chapter*

- Recognizing that when you eat isn't a factor
- Debunking notions about vegetarian diets and fasting
- Revealing the truth about eating fat free

Everyone's heard them: the little tricks and "wisdoms" that people say can make or break a diet. In this chapter, you can find some of the most common beliefs and the truth behind the hype.

## Eating Late Packs on the Pounds

The *kinds* of foods you're eating put on the weight, not the clock. Your body doesn't process calories differently after dark. However, the foods that people tend to go for in front of the TV after dinner — chips, ice cream, chocolate treats, and the like — are usually high in fat and calories. How often have you snacked on celery sticks while watching a pay-per-view? Also, many people eat continuously from dinner to bedtime. It's the kind of chaotic eating pattern that assures weight gain and prevents weight loss.

## Consuming Fewer Calories to Achieve a Breakthrough

You may share the common misconception that eating fewer calories can help you break through a weight-loss plateau. However, if you eat fewer than 800 to 1,000 calories a day, your body will turn down its thermostat to conserve every calorie it can get. It doesn't know whether you're starving on a desert island or starving to wear a teeny-weeny bikini on a desert island. The only way to keep your metabolism purring is to exercise. When weight loss slows, walk a little longer, work out more frequently or more intensely, and don't forget to eat.

# Never Have Seconds

Instead of using a plate of food or a predetermined serving size as a yardstick for how much you should eat, try taking hunger and fullness cues from your body. Eating according to your appetite is much healthier. And when you eat slowly, recognizing when you've had enough is much easier.

Keep in mind that there's a difference between appetite and hunger. *Appetite* has more to do with flavor preferences; *hunger* is a biological manifestation of the body's real need for food. If it's been a while since you and your appetite have seen eye to eye on how much to eat, try this: Serve yourself only half of what you think you want to eat. If you're still hungry after eating at a leisurely pace, go for it — in moderation, of course.

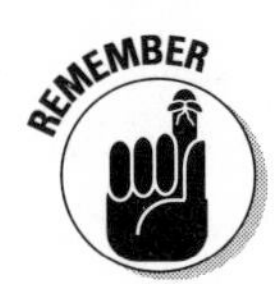


Also recognize that you're hungrier on some days than on others. So when you're really, truly hungry, it's fine to eat more. Remember that one meal doesn't define eating healthfully. What you eat over the course of a day or several days, does.

# Denying Your Cravings

Maybe you've heard people suggest that your cravings are all in your head. Sometimes, the faster you give in and have a small portion of the food that you're craving, the better off you are. You can pack on many calories by trying to eat around the one thing that you truly want. Have a small serving of the food you crave and get over it.

# Don't Eat Between Meals

Most people need to eat every three to four hours to avoid getting too hungry, which often leads to overeating. Dividing your calories into three meals and two or three snacks, instead of only three meals, can keep you well fueled for the day. Try planning two or three snack-size portions (for example, a piece of fruit or two fig cookies plus lowfat or fat-free milk or yogurt) into your day's food choices. Doing so may help lessen your hunger pangs so that you're less likely to overeat at the next meal.

## Eating Breakfast Makes You Hungry All Day

Many typical breakfast foods — Danish, toast with jelly, and bagels, for example — are mainly carbohydrates in their simplest form. These foods, while initially satisfying, are out of your system in about 30 minutes, and you need (and want) to eat again. That's why many people say that breakfast kicks off nonstop eating throughout the day.

Breakfast foods that have some protein and a little fat, in addition to complex carbohydrates and sugars, stay with you longer and give you the energy you need to make it through the morning. Whole-grain cereal with lowfat or fat-free milk, an egg on toast, and even a fruity breakfast shake made with lowfat or fat-free milk are good choices.

## To Lose Weight, Become a Vegetarian

Being vegetarian doesn't ensure that you'll lose weight. Like any other method of eating, a vegetarian diet can be high in fat and cholesterol, low in fiber, or both. Many vegetarian foods, including cheese and nuts, are high in fat and calories. So cutting out meat and replacing it with other equally fatty (or even more fatty) vegetarian foods isn't only a bad diet move, but it may also increase your chances for nutritional deficiencies — especially if you don't plan your diet well.

## Fasting Drops the Pounds

Some dieters will tell you that fasting for a few days drops the pounds quickly and shrinks your stomach. You may drop pounds if you fast, but some of that weight is muscle and most of it is water. You need to eat protein foods, such as lean meat, eggs, lowfat or fat-free milk, or legumes (beans and peas), or you'll be thin and flabby, not thin and shapely.

Some health-conscious dieters share the misconception that fasting cleans out your system. But actually, the opposite is true. When the body doesn't get food, body chemicals called *ketones* build up over time. That process puts a burden on the kidneys, which can be harmful to your health. Not to mention that it gives you really bad breath, too.

## You Can Eat Everything That's Fat Free

Don't believe that you can eat anything that you want as long as it's fat free. Fat-free foods aren't calorie-free foods; check the Nutrition Facts panel on the food label. Many have just as many calories as the original versions, and a few have even more, because plenty of sugar (among other ingredients) is needed to replace the way fat tastes and feels in your mouth. In the end, the total number of calories in a food is what's important.

A little fat is good, because it can help you eat less by giving a meal staying power, which keeps you from feeling hungry too quickly. Instead of a sandwich made with fat-free mayonnaise and fat-free cold cuts, make one with a teaspoon of real mayonnaise and lowfat meat; it will stay with you longer than a fat-free meal.

## Some Foods Burn More Calories Than They Contain

You may have heard this myth in regard to apples, grapefruit, and other fruits. Unfortunately that's like returning from a trip before you left. It's physically impossible. Your body burns calories as it digests and metabolizes foods, but it's only about 10 percent of the calories you need each day.

# Chapter 25

# Ten Ways to Cut Calories

***In This Chapter***

- Reading food labels
- Eating measured portions slowly from plates
- Employing healthy cooking techniques

A food's fat content is important, but when it comes to weight loss, total calories are *more* important. So many of the lowfat products on the market aren't calorie reduced. For example, 2 tablespoons of reduced-fat peanut butter have the same number of calories as the regular kind. And replacing a tablespoon of butter on a bagel with 2 tablespoons of jelly eliminates the fat but doesn't change the number of calories. In this chapter, you can find some calorie-cutting tricks to live by.

## Paying Attention to the Nutrition Facts

Seemingly healthy foods can be surprising sources of calories and fat, so make sure to check out the details on the Nutrition Facts panel on the food label. A container of ramen noodles, for example, packs 15 grams of fat and 400 calories; a bran muffin can top 10 grams of fat and 250 calories. Portion sizes can be deceptively small, too. A serving of sugar-sweetened iced tea contains 60 calories, but each bottle often contains two servings. And a serving of ice cream or other frozen dessert is a skimpy ½ cup.

## Limiting Alcohol

Alcohol, although fat-free, delivers 7 calories per gram or about 70 calories per ounce (2 tablespoons). The higher the proof, the more calories alcohol has: 80-proof alcohol averages 65 calories per ounce, and 100-proof alcohol comes in at 85 calories per ounce. The average light beer or 5-ounce glass of wine contains about 100 calories. A typical regular beer has about 150 calories. And don't forget, usually the nibbles served with alcohol are high in calories.

In addition to the calorie wallop, alcohol whittles away your resolve to stay in control of your eating. And any cardiac benefits you may derive from drinking, such as that seen in men who drink a daily glass of red wine, are not nearly as important as those you derive from weight loss and exercise.

## Switching to Smaller Plates

Serve yourself on a salad-size plate, about 8 inches in diameter, rather than on a dinner plate, which is typically 10 to 12 inches in diameter. Your portion sizes will be closer to those suggested in the Food Guide Pyramid (see Chapter 9) and more in tune with the number of calories you should be eating.

## Asking for the Kid Size

It may seem like a bargain, but is an extra 240 calories for 39 cents really a good way to spend your calorie budget? That's the difference between a small order of fries and a large one. Kid-size popcorn at most movie theaters contains 150 calories, but a large size can top 1,000 *without* the butter-flavored topping. A child-size soda (8 ounces) has about 95 calories; a large soda measuring 36 ounces or more contains at least 400.

## Eating Proper Portion Sizes

Nibbling from packages of crackers and shaving "tastes" from the brownie pan or forkfuls of cake from the platter can add up to plenty of calories and more than you think you've eaten. Portion out everything you eat onto a plate or into a small bowl and put the package or pan away.

Use measuring cups and spoons to portion out a serving onto your dinnerware. Study and memorize how it looks. What does ½ cup of ice cream look like in your dessert dishes? One cup of whole-wheat cereal in your breakfast bowl? One cup of pasta on your dinner plate? Five ounces of wine in your stemware? You can mark your dinnerware and glassware with a dot or dash of nail polish to remind yourself. If you have oversized dinnerware, use the salad or dessert plates. You may even consider buying a luncheon set, which has smaller plates.

## Dining in the Dining Room

When you bring plates to the table already filled, you won't be tempted to pick from serving bowls and platters in front of you. You're also forced to go out of your way for seconds and thus have the chance to reconsider. An added benefit: Because you don't have to dirty serving bowls and platters, you have fewer dishes to wash.

## Eating Slowly

Your brain takes a full 20 minutes to register the fact that your stomach is full. Try putting your fork down and taking a sip of water between bites. Chew your food well and don't load up your fork or spoon until you swallow what's in your mouth. Doing so enables you to more easily recognize when you're full.

## Filling Up on Plant Food

Fruits, vegetables, and whole grains without butter, dressings, or sauces take up stomach space, leaving less room for denser, high-calorie foods. They also take more time to chew and eat. Consider the fact that a teeny little pat of butter has as many calories as 3 cups of broccoli or that a 1-inch cube (1 ounce) of cheddar cheese has the same number of calories as 1 cup — that's 8 ounces — of bran flakes.

## Switching to Lowfat Dairy Products

Dairy is one place where going with the reduced-fat, lowfat, or fat-free variety makes sense, because the calories are significantly reduced in the lowfat version. For example, an 8-ounce glass of whole milk contains 150 calories, but the same amount of fat-free (skim) milk has only 85. One ounce of regular cheddar cheese has 114 calories, but reduced-fat and lowfat varieties contain 80 and 49 calories, respectively.

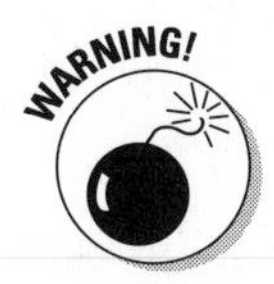


Note one exception, however: Dairy products, such as ice cream and flavored yogurt that are marketed as reduced-fat, lowfat, or fat-free often contain added sugar to make up for the loss of flavor and texture that fat provides. Don't be fooled into thinking that they provide fewer calories, too. Always check the calorie content on the Nutrition Facts panel of the food label.

## Remembering That Dull Is Better

Not dull as in *boring,* but dull as in *not shiny.* At the salad bar, shiny means a thick coating of oily (high-calorie) salad dressing. Vegetables that shimmer usually have butter added to them. Muffins that leave a grease slick on your napkin have more calories than ones that don't. Bread or rolls that are slick with butter . . . you get the idea.

## Cooking Meats with Methods That Start with the Letter B

Broil, barbecue, bake (on a rack), or braise meats, and you save many calories over frying, sautéing, and stewing, because the fat (and therefore its calories) has a chance to drip away from the meat.

Cooking chicken and other poultry with the skin on and removing it after it's been cooked is fine, because the meat absorbs little of the fat but stays moist.

# Chapter 26

# Ten Strategies to Keep the Weight Off

### In This Chapter

- Understanding what a healthy weight is
- Keeping the weight off successfully
- Finding friends to cheer you on

We hope that you've made some good progress with your weight-loss program and that you're eager not to lose ground. A weight-maintenance program should be a priority after the initial six months of a weight-loss diet. Weight maintenance isn't a matter of "going off your diet" — it's a matter of keeping your eating and activity habits up to a healthy standard.

In some ways, the strategies you need for maintenance are no different from those that you used to lose weight in the first place. But in other ways, the strategies *are* different. Maintenance means keeping at it forever. Stop, and you'll slide right back up to where you started — or worse yet, even higher.

## Staying at a Healthy Weight

Notice I said a healthy weight — not a supermodel's or a movie star's weight. It's not even staying at the weight you were at in high school. A healthy weight is the weight that you can reasonably attain and maintain without going crazy. For example, most people would say that a 5-foot, 4-inch woman who has brought her weight down to 125 pounds has reached a healthy weight. But would you consider her weight healthy if you knew that she had to restrict her calorie intake so much that she couldn't relax around food for fear of losing control? That she had to exercise vigorously for at least two hours a day and sometimes more for fear of ballooning up to her old weight? That this lifestyle robbed her of time with her family and friends? And that maintaining her weight was the sole focus of her life? That's not healthy. That's neurotic.

## Have you reached a reasonable weight for you?

If you have your heart set on a particular point on the scale that's lower than you are now, ask yourself how reasonable it is for you to reach and maintain that weight. You can answer that question by looking at your current weight-loss success and your diet history. Ask yourself the following questions:

- What's the lowest adult weight you were able to maintain for at least one year?
- Think of a time that you were at a lower weight than you are now. How difficult was it to reach that weight and stay there? How much exercise did you have to do? How few calories did you have to eat?
- Considering your starting weight and clothing size, what's the largest clothing size in which you feel comfortable and think that you look pretty good?

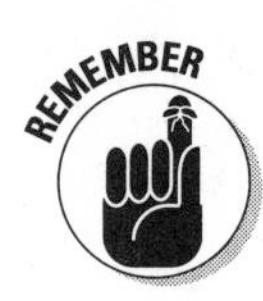


To maintain a healthy weight, you must maintain a healthy lifestyle — balancing your diet with exercise, stress reduction, and relationships in a healthy manner. As you work through your weight-loss plan and look forward to staying at your new, lower weight, consider the points in this chapter. They're the real measures of a healthy weight.

## Being realistic

Assigning a number as your ideal weight, based on information from a height-and-weight chart, isn't really a healthy way to judge your progress. Although the charts do serve a useful purpose as guides to a healthy weight range, specifying a number as *ideal* connotes that any number higher than that isn't good enough. Establishing an ideal weight sets you up in pass/fail mode instead of giving you credit for progress made. Thinking of your weight in terms of what's *reasonable* for you is healthier.

For more information about adjusting your attitude and getting realistic about your weight, see Chapter 3.

## Being adventurous

Changing your attitude about yourself and your body may be the most beneficial step you can take. If your weight keeps you from enjoying activities, let the issue go. Have you ever said, "I'll go on vacation when I'm 125 pounds again" or "I'll try water-skiing when I'm thinner" or "I'll go for a hike in the woods when I'm in better shape"? Don't wait until you reach your goal weight. If you do, you're missing out on plenty of living. Don't miss out on life, because you're hiding behind your weight. You can try many activities no matter what your weight — in-line skating, ballroom dancing, ice skating, skiing, hiking, or biking, just to name a few.

Be adventurous with your eating as well as with your activities. Try a new fruit that you've never tasted. If you always eat bananas and apples but are so bored with them that you don't eat your recommended number of fruit servings, break out of your rut. Try a papaya or a kiwi. Reach for different grains, too. White long-grain rice is nice, but don't miss out on the short, medium, aromatic, and brown rice varieties. And then you have *quinoa* (pronounced *keen*-wa), barley, and cracked wheat. Experiment with recipes. Check out Chapter 28 for plenty of tasty, adventuresome ideas.

## Being flexible

You need to be flexible about what you consider to be weight-loss success. You also need to be flexible about what you consider to be a successful dieting or exercise day. Sure, you need to set goals, but you also need to accept that some days you aren't going to make them. Adding a week's worth of healthy meals and exercise to another week and another and another — even if you don't meet your goal on a few days in between — is how you build success.

If you can't work in your normal walking route one day, try to stay active in other ways. For example, park your car in the parking space that's farthest from the door. Be sure to take the stairs rather than the elevator. Any kind of exercise counts. If you're stuck at a family party or business meal and every dish in sight is a caloric disaster, don't throw in the towel and overeat. Enjoy small amounts of the foods that are offered and then be especially diligent at the next meal or the next day.

## Being sensible

"I'm never going to eat another pepperoni pizza again!" Doesn't that sound silly? Ban words like *never* and *always* from your eating and exercise plans. These ultimatums put you just bites away from failure. Better to have one small serving and enjoy every bit or share a serving with a friend or pack half of it in a doggie bag for another meal on another day.

Exercising a little every day is better than trying to make up for a missed day or week by overexerting yourself. Chances are, you won't enjoy the exercise as much if you're overdoing it, and you'll probably be so sore afterwards that you'll miss the next few days of activity as well. No pain, no gain isn't our motto. Take it slow and steady and *enjoy* yourself — that's what's most important.

### Being active

Don't you just love folks who say things like "We won the baseball game," when they mean that the team they were rooting for on TV won? Or the people who say that they're going to walk the dog and then go outside and watch the dog walk around the yard while they stand in the driveway? These people are spectators, not participants.

We use many other expressions that make us sound active: "Mow the lawn" (or do we sit on the mower?); "wash the clothes" (or do we put them into the washing machine?); "shovel the snow" (or do we push the snow blower?); "run to the store" (or do we drive the car?) — you get the idea. These passive activities sound like actions, but they're really not.

If you're guilty of using more active language than actually being active, change your behavior. Look for ways — big and small — to fit activity into your day: Climb the stairs, hide the remote, don't use your kids as slaves to fetch things, walk during your lunch break instead of sitting, play ball instead of watching, walk to the school bus stop instead of driving to meet the kids. Park farther from the store instead of circling to find the closest spot, and toss the remote. Clip a pedometer to your belt and aim for 10,000 steps a day. See Chapter 12 for more on pedometers.

## Getting Some Tips from Losers

Many people lose weight, but most people don't keep it off. The number of people who regain lost weight after 5 years is as high as 95 percent. A depressing number, for sure, but don't let that statistic stop you from trying. That 95 percent figure only reflects the people who have been in weight-control studies and official programs, not the vast number of people who lose weight on their own and keep it off.

The National Weight Control Registry, a database maintained at the University of Colorado, has followed a group of people who had success losing weight by using a variety of methods. The requirement for inclusion in the registry is a 30-pounds-or-greater weight loss that's maintained for at least 1 year. But the actual numbers are far better. Of the 3,000 participants, the average weight loss is 60 pounds, which the participants have maintained for more than 6 years!

These people obviously can share ideas about taking weight off, but they have even more ideas about maintaining the loss. Interestingly, some of their advice flies in the face of conventional weight-loss wisdom — like weighing yourself on the scale every day. But the take-home message here is that these people have found certain strategies that work for them. What have you found that works best for you? Keeping an exercise log or food diary? Exercising in the morning versus the evening? Planning meals for the week ahead of time? People who keep their weight off have their own personal tricks. The key to successful weight maintenance is to put them into practice.

## Trying, trying, and trying again

The average woman goes on 15 diets in her lifetime and loses about 100 pounds. But she regains about 125! Experts call it *yo-yo dieting* or *weight cycling.* At one time, health authorities believed that each time a person's weight yo-yos, weight loss becomes more difficult in the future. The individual loses more muscle, needs fewer calories to maintain the weight, and becomes more frustrated. The bottom line seemed to be that you're better off not trying to lose weight and that going on repeated diets is dangerous.

One major study published in *The Journal of the American Medical Association* 275(5), 1994, looked at 43 studies and found no convincing evidence that weight cycling in humans has adverse health effects on body composition, energy balance, risk factors for cardiovascular disease, or the success of future efforts at weight loss. Proof positive is the fact that 90 percent of the people in the National Weight Control Registry had tried to lose weight previously — in fact, each person had lost and regained an average of 270 pounds! Yet they were able to lose weight and keep it off, once and for all — even after years of yo-yo dieting.

## Weighing in

When you're trying to maintain weight loss, monitoring your weight closely is the best approach. Successful maintainers are able to catch a 5- or 10-pound weight creep and take immediate action. Many people in the National Weight Control Registry say that they weigh themselves every day. During the weight-loss phase, weighing daily can be disappointing, so experts recommend that you get on the scale no more than once a week. But when you're in maintenance, you may find it helpful to more closely monitor the scale so that you can make adjustments to your eating plan before a 1- or 2-pound gain becomes the 5 pounds you just can't seem to lose.

During your maintenance phase, continue to weigh in, so to speak, on what you eat, too. Some successful maintainers continue to monitor what they eat by keeping food records. And they stick with a lowfat, low-calorie eating plan.

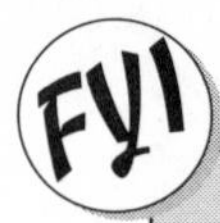

## Is yo-yo dieting a no-no?

Yo-yo dieting is going on and off and on and off a diet so that weight goes up and down the scale, bouncing from one weight to another. After finding that rats who lost and regained weight had more body fat than those whose weights remained stable, researchers concluded that the more humans diet to lose weight, the less healthy they become. But a subsequent review of that study and many other studies proved otherwise. The entire body of research concludes that yo-yo dieting does *not*

- Make future weight loss more difficult
- Increase body fat
- Change the location where body fat is stored
- Lower energy expenditure
- Increase preference for fatty foods
- Change blood pressure
- Change blood cholesterol or triglycerides
- Change insulin or glucose metabolism

However, the psychological effects of weight cycling can be distressing. Some research has found that weight cyclers who tend to binge, binge more when they cycle.

## Solving problems

People who can keep their weight stable are good problem solvers. They find ways to fit exercise into their schedules. They uncover techniques to eat lowfat foods. They work balance and moderation into their eating plans and exercise routines.

## Move

Physical activity is a key predictor of weight-loss maintenance success. (See Chapter 12 for more information about the importance of exercise.) Besides helping you to lose weight, regular physical activity is a super stress reducer. (Less stress means less eating in response to stress.) You'll have more energy, not less. (Many people eat when they're dragging and feeling tired.) If you walk with a friend(s), you'll have good quality time, too.

Don't try to make up for a slow day with an overly active one. But if you do go overboard with an activity that's too strenuous, still try to do something the next day, even if it means a slow walk. The important thing is to do some kind of exercise every day. That's how you make it a habit.

## Be a team player

People are social animals. After all, what's the purpose of life if not to be in relationships with other people? Finding someone to lean on is important. But in order to get support, you must give it as well. Maybe your support person is not a fellow dieter, but he needs to rely on you sometimes, too. You can't take without giving, or your support will walk. Follow these tips to be a good team player:

- **Show up.** Whether you make plans to meet your support person at a regular time or you have a more relaxed and informal arrangement, be there. Don't have other activities planned that take away from the agenda. You're there for each other, so be there in mind, body, and spirit.
- **Really listen.** Listening takes effort. A phone call can work sometimes. But if possible, meet the other person and talk face to face. See the person as well as hear his words. Visual clues can yield plenty of information. Look for expressions or body language that supports or contradicts what you're hearing.
- **Don't judge.** Maybe what you're hearing sounds silly or just plain dumb. But hang in there. When your partner tells you that there's no time to exercise, the judgmental response is, "You're looking for excuses." The nonjudgmental reaction is, "What would make it easier for you to find the time?" Nonjudgmental statements are supportive and lead to discussion. Judgmental ones are conversation stoppers.
- **Be supportive.** Offer moral support by showing that you understand. Share similar experiences and give constructive suggestions if you can think of ways to help.

## *Getting support*

You can't lose weight without support nor can you maintain your loss without help. Most successful weight losers are motivated by their own personal needs, but they do have support from friends, spouses, family, or a group of like-minded dieters. They can turn to these people for help with managing the stress in their lives, solving problems, and scheduling time for exercise by handing off household or child-care responsibilities. People who lend support also can serve as cheerleaders and provide attaboy (or attagirl) encouragement. Don't go it alone!

# Chapter 27

# Ten Rules for Eating Healthfully

*In This Chapter*

- Counting out your servings
- Recognizing the value of breakfast and water
- Uncovering the truth about salt and caffeine

Eating low-cal is definitely a healthy habit. But there's more to good living than just counting calories. The nutrients in the foods you eat can make or break your efforts to live healthfully, so choose your calories by the company they keep. In this chapter, you can find ten easy guidelines to remember.

## Eating Vegetables and Fruit Daily

At a minimum, you want to eat three servings of vegetables and three servings of fruit every day. Most people don't eat enough vegetables — especially the leafy-green and deep-orange ones. On average, Americans eat the equivalent of only about one-quarter of a serving a day. About half eat no fruit at all on some days. Vitamin pills can't replace the vitamins, minerals, and other nutrients in produce. But not to worry, because servings are actually quite small: Half a cup of most cooked vegetables, one cup of salad, or a piece of fruit qualifies as one serving.

Don't drink all your fruits in the form of juice. You'll miss out on fiber if you do, and you'll easily consume too many calories. A mere four ounces of juice equals one serving of fruit, and most people drink much more than that at a time.

## Getting Enough Whole Grains Daily

Most people eat less than one serving of whole grains a day. That's too bad, because you get more vitamin E, vitamin B6, magnesium, zinc, copper, manganese, and potassium in whole grains. These nutrients help protect against heart disease, diverticulosis, cancer, and diabetes. Whole grains are the best source of fiber, too. For example, the fiber difference between a single slice of whole-wheat bread and one of white is 2 grams.

Twenty to 35 grams of fiber are recommended for daily consumption. So you want to make sure that you eat at least three servings of whole grains each day.

# Serving Up Beans, Lentils, or Peas

Eat at least four servings of beans, lentils, or peas each week. Like most vegetables, beans, lentils, and peas are good sources of fiber and *phytochemicals* (plant nutrients) that help cut the risk of cancer, heart disease, and diabetes. But unlike other vegetables, they have enough protein to substitute for a serving of meat, poultry, or fish.

# Eating Regularly

Eating three meals daily, along with two or three snacks, is best. You generally need to eat every three to four hours. Research has shown that people who snack are often less likely to overeat than those who restrict their eating. The body is also better able to absorb and use the nutrients in a meal than it can when presented with the feast-or-famine scenario of the typical three-meals-a-day, no-snacks pattern. So go ahead and snack, just make sure your snacks are as balanced as your meals, meaning that they have some carbohydrate, such as three or four whole wheat crackers; some protein, like a spoonful of peanut butter; and some fat. (There's plenty of that in the peanut butter, too.) Almonds and a fruit, lowfat yogurt with whole grain cereal, or even a hard-cooked egg with salsa and half a cup of corn chips all make good balanced snacks as well.

# Eating Breakfast

Missing this meal is a big mistake. After an overnight fast, your body needs fuel to move. Otherwise, metabolism slows, which reduces how many calories you burn. Many studies have shown that children who skip breakfast have difficulty concentrating during the day. It's true for adults, too. And here's another good reason not to miss breakfast: The National Weight Control Registry of more than 3,000 successful weight losers eat breakfast on most days of the week. These are people who lost an average of 60 pounds and kept it off for an average of 6 years. I don't know about you, but I think that's a pretty convincing endorsement for a bowl of flakes and lowfat milk!

## Limiting Soft Drinks

Sure, you may prefer swigging soft drinks to water, juice, or milk. But cola-type soft drinks (as well as many citrus-flavored sodas) pack a dose of caffeine with lots of sugar and calories without contributing nutrients, except perhaps water. Sugar-free versions don't add empty calories, at least, but when soft drinks replace fat-free milk in your diet, you're missing out on one of the best sources of calcium you can get. That's a shame, because most adults don't get enough of that bone-building mineral.

## Drinking Water

Studies show that when you think you're hungry, often you're actually thirsty, because dehydration is a major contributing factor to fatigue, which leads some people to seek food for energy. The rule is 1 liter (about 4 cups) per 1,000 calories. That translates to about eight 8-ounce glasses a day for people who eat about 2,000 calories.

It's hard to drink too much water. But if it's difficult for you to drink water, know that fruits (which are mostly water) can count toward your day's total. So does your coffee and tea. And, yes, even soda, but please reread, "Limiting Soft Drinks," the earlier section in this chapter, about the problems with drinking too much of it. The color of your urine can be an indication of how much water you're drinking. If it's very dark and you're not taking a medication that colors your urine, you're not drinking enough liquids. Your urine is a *very pale* yellow when you're properly hydrated.

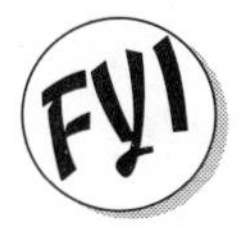


The average adult loses about 2½ quarts of water a day: 4 to 6 cups in the urine, 2 to 4 cups as perspiration, 1½ cups through breathing, and about ⅔ cup in the feces. Roughly 3 to 4½ cups of your daily water comes from solid food.

## Limiting Caffeine

Limit caffeine to two servings or less a day. That's two cups of coffee or tea or other caffeine-containing beverage. Coffee is the main source of caffeine in the American diet, although chocolate, tea, cola and some citrus-flavored soft drinks (such as Mountain Dew), and some over-the-counter pain relievers contribute to a day's total. Caffeine speeds up your heart rate and can make you feel jittery and anxious. It also can contribute to dehydration due to its diuretic effect, which causes your body to lose water.

# Limiting Your Salt

Processed and prepared foods — not the saltshaker — are the greatest source of salt and sodium in people's diets. High-sodium diets in women are associated with increased risk of osteoporosis, a potentially harmful situation for dieters whose calcium levels tend to be below recommended levels. Eating an abundance of salt doesn't make you gain body fat or keep you from losing it, but it does cause water retention, which shows up on the scale, albeit temporarily.

To keep your body running smoothly, you need only about 500 milligrams of sodium a day. That's about the amount in ¼ teaspoon of salt. Eating a diet with so little sodium probably wouldn't taste good, but try keeping your sodium intake to the advised level of 2,400 milligrams or less per day.

Your tongue's preference for salt can be overcome. It takes only about two weeks to prefer the taste of unsalted foods.

# Limiting the Amount of Saturated Fat

Saturated fat isn't simply a calorie counter's concern. It contains the same number of calories as other kinds of fat, but it raises your blood cholesterol level and increases your risk of heart disease. Animal products and tropical oils (palm kernel, palm, and coconut, for example) contain mainly saturated fat. As a general guideline, saturated fat is solid at room temperature. Examples include butter, stick margarine, and the fat in meat and cheese.

Chapter 28

# Ten Recipes for a Healthier Lifestyle

### In This Chapter

- Limiting calories with careful preparation
- Varying recipes for every taste and season
- Making snacks with staying power
- Giving in to some tempting delights

**Recipes in This Chapter**

- Hummus
- Mango Salsa
- Cream of Broccoli Soup
- Tuna and White Bean Salad
- Glazed Fish Fillets
- Chicken in Mustard Sauce
- Oven-Fried Chicken
- Chili Burgers
- Garlicky Mashed Potatoes
- Lemon Cake
- Fruit Tart

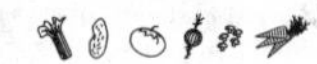

Supermarkets are full of ready-to-cook foods that are low in calories and low in fat. They're great in a pinch, but store-bought always costs more than homemade. Sure, packaged foods can save you time, but the recipes don't take much more of a commitment than most package directions require. And how can you improve on the taste that homemade cooking delivers?

This chapter includes a selection of appetizers, entrees, and, of course, desserts. Think of them as the basics of low-calorie cooking and then improvise and make them your own way. You can try the suggestions that we include to create new taste combinations, too. Also, look to Chapter 14 for more ideas for cooking lean and light.

## Planning Your Meals, Calorie-Wise

Table 28-1 offers some guidelines to consider as you plan your meals for the day. A person on a diet of 1,500 calories a day (a fair weight-loss level for most women) or 1,700 calories a day (a high weight-loss level for most men) should keep these daily nutrient recommendations in mind. But remember, too, that what you eat over the course of several days, not just on one day, counts.

**Table 28-1 Compare and Save**

| *Nutrient* | *1,200 Calories* | *1,500 Calories* | *1,800 Calories* |
|---|---|---|---|
| Protein | 30 grams | 37 grams | 45 grams |
| Carbohydrate | 180 grams | 225 grams | 270 grams |
| Fat | < 40 grams | < 50 grams | < 60 grams |
| Saturated fat | 13 grams | 16 grams | 20 grams |
| Cholesterol | < 300 milligrams | < 300 milligrams | < 300 milligrams |
| Fiber | At least 20 grams | At least 20 grams | At least 20 grams |
| Sodium | < 2,400 milligrams | < 2,400 milligrams | < 2,400 milligrams |

It helps to know how much of your daily nutrient requirements a particular recipe supplies, so you can plan the rest of the day's meals accordingly. Therefore, we supply a nutrient analysis for each recipe in this chapter, listing the amount of each of these nutrients that the recipe provides. The analysis doesn't include optional ingredients, such as salt to taste or parsley for garnish, however.

# Dipping into Appetizers, Snacks, and Sauces

## Hummus

Use this recipe for a dip with a selection of raw vegetables or as a sandwich spread — it's great in a pita topped with plenty of shredded lettuce and chopped tomato. Or turn it into a wrap and roll it in a tortilla with a sprinkle of hot sauce, a dusting of sesame seeds, and sprouts. Because it's made with beans, hummus is a solid yet meatless source of protein. Try this recipe using soybeans or white beans for the chickpeas and play with the seasoning. You can use lime juice instead of lemon, and cilantro in place of parsley.

***Preparation time:*** *15 minutes*

***Cooking time:*** *None*

***Yield:*** *2 cups*

*2 garlic cloves, peeled*

*1½ cups cooked chickpeas, or 1 can (15½ ounces) chickpeas, rinsed and drained*

*¼ cup tahini (sesame paste), or smooth peanut butter*

*3 tablespoons freshly squeezed lemon juice*

*1 teaspoon extra-virgin olive oil*

*¼ teaspoon ground cumin*

*¼ teaspoon salt, or to taste*

*⅓ cup chopped fresh flat-leaf parsley*

1. Mince the garlic by dropping it through the feed tube of a food processor or blender while the motor is running.
2. Stop the motor and add the chickpeas, tahini, lemon juice, olive oil, cumin, and salt. Process until smooth, stopping the motor occasionally to scrape down the sides of the bowl. Add the parsley and set the blender or processor on pulse just until combined.

*Per Serving: 50 calories, 2 grams of protein, 5 grams of carbohydrate, 3 grams of fat, 0.5 grams saturated fat, 0 milligrams cholesterol, 1 gram fiber, 35 milligrams sodium.*

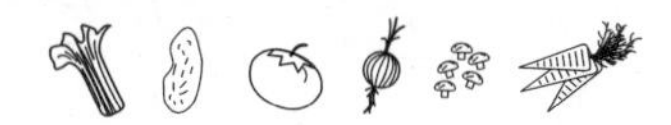

## Mango Salsa

If you think of a plain, broiled chicken breast as the little black dress of the kitchen, then salsa is the pearls, taking the dish from boring to stunning with just a garnish. This recipe features mango or papaya, but you can substitute tomatoes, tomatillos, or even pears or peaches. Experiment!

***Preparation time:*** *15 minutes*

***Cooking time:*** *None*

***Yield:*** *About 2 cups*

*1 mango (or papaya), peeled and cubed (about 1¾ cups)*

*1 to 2 jalapeño peppers, seeded and minced*

*1 scallion, minced, or 2 tablespoons minced white onion*

*2 tablespoons chopped fresh mint, or coriander*

*2 tablespoons freshly squeezed lime juice*

*1 garlic clove, peeled and minced*

*Salt to taste*

*Pepper to taste*

Combine all the ingredients and mix well.

*Per Serving: Per ¼ cup: 20 calories, 0.5 grams protein, 5 grams carbohydrate, 0 grams fat, 0 grams saturated fat, 0 milligrams cholesterol, 1 gram fiber, 2 milligrams sodium.*

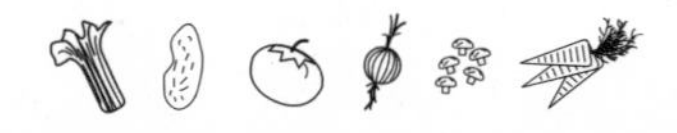

## Cream of Broccoli Soup

This recipe is basic but hardly boring. In the summer, use zucchini or summer squash in place of the broccoli when gardens and stores are overrun with them. Carrots work well, too; be sure to cook them thoroughly. You'll want to adjust the seasoning if you vary the vegetable: Tarragon is nice with zucchini or squash, and dill marries well with carrots.

***Preparation time:*** *15 minutes*

***Cooking time:*** *10 minutes*

***Yield:*** *6 servings*

*4 cups chicken broth*

*1 bunch fresh broccoli, coarsely chopped, or 2 10-ounce packages frozen chopped broccoli*

*1 tablespoon butter*

*1 pear, peeled and chopped*

*1 medium onion, peeled and chopped*

*1 teaspoon chili powder*

*1 cup nonfat yogurt*

*Orange zest for garnish*

1. Heat the chicken broth to boiling in a large saucepan over high heat. Add the broccoli and return to boiling. Cook until tender, about 10 minutes for fresh broccoli or 5 minutes for frozen.
2. Melt the butter in a large skillet over medium heat. Sauté the pear, onion, and chili powder in the butter until the pear is tender, about 5 minutes. Stir the sautéed ingredients into the chicken broth and broccoli.
3. Remove from the heat, cool slightly and then puree in a blender or food processor until smooth. Garnish each serving with a dollop of yogurt and a little orange zest.

*Per serving: 115 calories, 8 grams protein, 13 grams carbohydrate, 4 grams fat, 2 grams saturated fat, 7 milligrams cholesterol, 4 grams fiber, 595 milligrams sodium.*

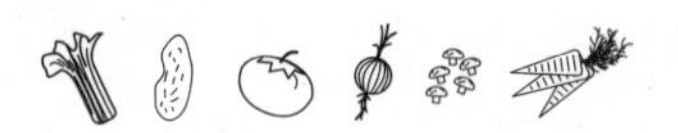

# Main Dishes and a Few Sides

## Tuna and White Bean Salad

To turn this tuna salad into a hearty meal, serve it on a bed of salad greens and garnish it with tomato wedges.

Surprisingly, a can of water-packed white-meat tuna has about 30 more calories and 4 grams more fat than the same amount of water-packed light tuna. Even after being drained, oil-packed light tuna has about 145 more calories than water-packed, and oil-packed white tuna has about 110 more calories than the water-packed varieties.

***Preparation time:*** *15 minutes*

***Cooking time:*** *None*

***Yield:*** *6 servings*

*1 can (16 ounces) white beans, rinsed and drained*

*2 cans (6½ to 7 ounces, each) water-packed light tuna, drained*

*2 tablespoons extra-virgin olive oil*

*2 tablespoons freshly squeezed lemon juice*

*2 tablespoons grainy mustard*

*1 tablespoon red wine vinegar*

*1 tablespoon balsamic vinegar*

*1 garlic clove, peeled and minced*

*1½ teaspoons sugar*

*Salt to taste*

*Pepper to taste*

*¼ cup finely chopped fresh basil leaves*

1. Combine the beans and tuna in a large bowl and set aside.
2. In a small bowl with a whisk or in a small jar with a tight-fitting lid, combine the oil, lemon juice, mustard, vinegars, garlic, sugar, salt, and pepper and beat or shake until well blended. Pour the mixture over the tuna and beans.
3. Just before serving, fold in the basil.

*Per serving: 200 calories, 19 grams protein, 20 grams carbohydrate, 5 grams fat, 0.5 grams saturated fat, 15 milligrams cholesterol, 4 grams fiber, 231 milligrams sodium.*

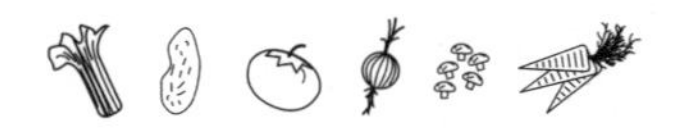

## Glazed Fish Fillets

You can marinate pork tenderloins or chicken breasts with the glaze in this recipe, too. Even slices of eggplant, dressed with the glaze before grilling, are a tasty option.

Don't serve the leftover marinade; it contains uncooked fish or meat juices that can make you sick if you eat them. If you want to use the leftover marinade, boil it for about 5 minutes first.

***Preparation time:*** *5 minutes*

***Marinating time:*** *20 minutes*

***Cooking time:*** *10 minutes*

***Yield:*** *6 servings*

*3 tablespoons sugar*

*⅓ cup soy sauce*

*1 teaspoon roasted sesame oil*

*½ teaspoon coarsely ground black pepper*

*¼ teaspoon crushed red pepper flakes*

*1½ pounds salmon fillets*

*3 tablespoons finely chopped mint, basil, and/or cilantro*

1. Measure the sugar, soy sauce, sesame oil, and peppers into a resealable bag. Swish to blend. Add the fish and return to the refrigerator for 20 minutes.
2. Heat the oven to 450 degrees F. Lightly coat a baking pan with vegetable oil cooking spray. Place the fillets skin-side down on the pan. Roast the fish for 5 to 7 minutes, or 10 minutes per inch of thickness. The fish is done when it's barely opaque and flakes when tested with a fork.
3. Remove from the oven and immediately sprinkle the minced herb(s) over the top.

*Per serving: 215 calories, 26 grams protein, 2 grams carbohydrate, 11 grams fat, 2 grams saturated fat, 82 milligrams cholesterol, 0 grams fiber, 406 milligrams sodium.*

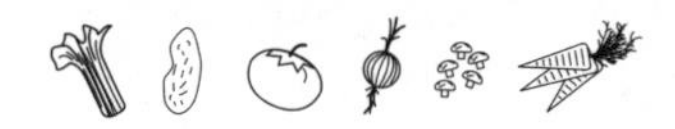

## Chicken in Mustard Sauce

Looking for something new to do with chicken breasts? Try this rich-tasting, creamy recipe. The secret ingredient that makes the sauce so velvety without cream is the mustard. And the combination of its pungent bite and the sweetness of the apples is sublime. This recipe is also delicious made with pork chops instead of chicken breasts.

***Preparation time:*** *15 minutes*

***Cooking time:*** *15 minutes*

***Yield:*** *4 servings*

*4 chicken breast halves, boned and skinned*

*1 tablespoon olive oil*

*1 cup apple juice*

*1 medium onion, peeled and thickly sliced*

*1 garlic clove, peeled and minced*

*1½ teaspoons fresh thyme leaves, or ½ teaspoon dried*

*2 tablespoons Dijon mustard*

*1 apple, cored and thinly sliced*

1. Place the chicken breast halves between two sheets of waxed paper. With the broad side of a heavy knife, pound the chicken breasts to flatten them to about ½ inch thick.
2. Heat the oil in a large skillet over high heat until hot. Add the chicken and sauté for about 3 minutes on each side or until golden.
3. Add the apple juice, onion, garlic, and thyme. Cover and cook for 10 minutes or until the chicken is fork-tender.
4. Remove the chicken and keep it warm. Heat the liquid remaining in the skillet to boiling. Blend in the mustard. Add the apple slices and cook until heated through. Pour the sauce over the chicken.

*Per serving: 245 calories, 27 grams protein, 16 grams carbohydrate, 7 grams fat, 1.5 grams saturated fat, 73 milligrams cholesterol, 1 gram fiber, 256 milligrams sodium.*

## Oven-Fried Chicken

You can use corn flakes or breadcrumbs to coat chicken, but we found the nuttiness of whole-wheat crackers a nice change.

***Preparation time:*** *20 minutes*

***Cooking time:*** *35 minutes*

***Yield:*** *6 servings*

*5 ounces low-fat, unsweetened, whole wheat crackers, such as Melba toast*

*1 tablespoon paprika*

*½ teaspoon dried thyme leaves*

*½ teaspoon crushed rosemary leaves*

*½ teaspoon salt*

*2 large egg whites*

*½ cup nonfat ranch dressing*

*6 chicken breast halves, skin (but not bones) removed*

1. Heat the oven to 425 degrees F. Set a wire rack on a baking sheet and lightly coat it with vegetable oil cooking spray.
2. In a blender or food processor, combine the crackers, paprika, thyme, rosemary, and salt and process to make coarse crumbs. Transfer the crumbs to a shallow bowl.
3. Whisk the egg whites in a bowl until frothy and then blend in the ranch dressing.
4. Dip the chicken breast halves in the eggs and dressing and then in the crumbs. Set them bone-side-up on a rack. Lightly coat the chicken with vegetable oil cooking spray. Turn and lightly spray the other side.
5. Bake for 30 to 35 minutes or until the crumbs are browned and crisp and the chicken juices run clear when tested with a fork.

*Per serving: 190 calories, 17 grams protein, 23 grams carbohydrate, 2 grams fat, 0.5 grams saturated fat, 36 milligrams cholesterol, 2 grams fiber, 606 milligrams sodium.*

## Chili Burgers

You can trim the fat off a steak, but removing the fat from ground beef isn't always easy. Making burgers leaner and lower in calories requires a bit of kitchen wizardry. In this recipe, we add beans to reduce the calories and season the burgers with Southwestern flavor. Serve them with some toe-tingling salsa instead of plain old ketchup.

This recipe also includes chili peppers, which can burn you. The oils that reside in the white membrane where the seeds are attached are powerful. Be sure to wash your hands well with soapy water before touching sensitive body parts! Or wear rubber gloves while you handle chilies.

Finally, to prevent food poisoning, always cook ground beef until it's no longer pink inside. An instant-read thermometer inserted in the center of the meat should read 160 degrees F.

***Preparation time:*** *25 minutes*

***Cooking time:*** *10 minutes*

***Yield:*** *6 servings*

*1 teaspoon olive oil*

*1 small onion, peeled and finely chopped*

*1 jalapeño pepper, seeded and minced*

*1 garlic clove, peeled and minced*

*1½ teaspoons ground cumin*

*¾ cup black beans, rinsed, drained, and slightly mashed*

*1 slice firm white bread, torn into crumbs*

*1 egg white*

*2 tablespoons tomato paste*

*¾ pound extra-lean ground beef*

*½ teaspoon salt*

*½ teaspoon pepper*

*6 sandwich rolls*

*6 lettuce leaves*

*2 tomatoes, sliced*

1. Heat the grill or broiler.
2. In a small skillet, heat the oil. Cook the onion, jalapeño, garlic, and cumin in the oil until fragrant, about 3 minutes. Remove from the heat.
3. Combine the beans, bread, egg white, and tomato paste in a medium bowl. Mash into a paste with a fork or potato masher. Add the ground beef, salt, pepper, and sautéed ingredients. Mix thoroughly.
4. Shape into four ¾-inch-thick burgers. Grill or broil until the burgers reach 160 degrees F in the center (test the temperature with a meat thermometer), about 5 minutes per side. Serve on rolls with lettuce and tomato.

*Per serving: 350 calories, 19 grams protein, 28 grams carbohydrate, 9 grams fat, 3.8 grams saturated fat, 14 milligrams cholesterol, 5 grams fiber, 636 milligrams sodium.*

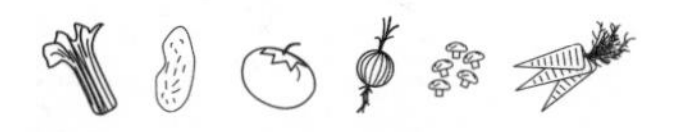

### Garlicky Mashed Potatoes

One of the secrets to making mashed potatoes low calorie is to use naturally buttery-tasting yellow potatoes. Another trick is to use lightly browned butter, which boosts its flavor.

***Preparation time:*** *15 minutes*

***Cooking time:*** *15 minutes*

***Yield:*** *6 servings*

*2 pounds Yukon Gold or baking potatoes, peeled and cut into chunks*

*4 garlic cloves, peeled and halved*

*2 teaspoons butter*

*1 cup buttermilk*

*Salt to taste*

*Pepper to taste*

1. Place the potatoes and garlic in a large saucepan with enough lightly salted water to cover. Heat to boiling over high heat. Reduce the heat to low; cover and simmer until fork-tender, about 10 to 15 minutes.
2. Meanwhile, in a small skillet or saucepan over low heat, heat the butter, swirling the skillet until the butter begins to brown, about 1 minute. Stir in the buttermilk and heat through but do not boil or the milk will curdle.
3. Drain the potatoes well and mash them with a potato masher or electric mixer. When smooth, blend in the buttermilk and browned butter and add salt and pepper to taste.

*Per serving: 170 calories, 4 grams protein, 35 grams carbohydrate, 2 grams fat, 1 gram saturated fat, 5 milligrams cholesterol, 2 grams fiber, 63 milligrams sodium.*

## Giving In to Your Sweet Tooth

### Lemon Cake

Remember this recipe for picnics, potluck dinners, or whenever you need a dessert that travels well. This cake also makes a tasty after-school or midafternoon snack with a dollop of vanilla yogurt and a spoonful of berries.

***Preparation time:*** *15 minutes*

***Cooking time:*** *About 35 minutes*

***Yield:*** *12 servings*

*2 tablespoons butter*

*⅔ cup buttermilk*

*1½ cups all-purpose flour, plus more to dust the pan*

*2 teaspoons baking powder*

*½ teaspoon baking soda*

*½ teaspoon salt*

*3 lemons*

*2 large eggs*

*1 cup granulated sugar*

*1 tablespoon canola oil*

*1 teaspoon vanilla extract*

*1¼ cups confectioners' sugar*

1. Heat the oven to 350°F. Lightly coat a 6-cup Bundt pan with vegetable oil cooking spray; dust with some flour and shake out the excess.
2. In a small skillet or saucepan over low heat, heat the butter, swirling the skillet until it begins to brown, about 1 minute. Pour the browned butter into a bowl, add the buttermilk, and set aside.
3. Sift the 1½ cups flour, baking powder, baking soda, and salt into a bowl; set aside. Grate 2 teaspoons lemon zest (just the yellow part) from the lemons and then squeeze enough juice to make ½ cup; set the zest and juice aside.
4. In another bowl, beat the eggs, sugar, and oil until they become thick and pale, about 3 to 5 minutes. Blend in the vanilla, lemon zest, and 1 tablespoon of the lemon juice; set aside the remaining juice.
5. With a rubber spatula, fold about ¼ of the dry ingredients and then ⅓ of the liquid ingredients into the beaten eggs, folding just until blended. Repeat adding ingredients alternately. Spoon the batter into the prepared pan and bake for 30 to 35 minutes or until a toothpick inserted into the cake comes out clean. Let cool on a wire rack for 5 minutes before removing from the pan.
6. Meanwhile, whisk together 1 cup of the confectioners' sugar and the reserved lemon juice to make a syrup. While the cake is still warm, poke holes all over it with a wooden skewer. Spoon the lemon syrup over the cake. Just before serving, dust with the reserved confectioners' sugar.

*Per serving: 205 calories, 3 grams protein, 40 grams carbohydrate, 4 grams fat, 1.5 grams saturated fat, 0 milligrams cholesterol, 0 grams fiber, 247 milligrams sodium.*

## Fruit Tart

Rather than a two-crust pie, this recipe has one and a half crusts. Use your own recipe for a single crust pie or start with a ready-made pie crust as we do here. Vary the fruit depending on the season. For example, instead of apples and raisins, try pears with dried cranberries or peaches and pistachios.

***Preparation time:*** *20 minutes*

***Cooking time:*** *45 minutes*

***Yield:*** *8 servings*

*1 refrigerated rolled ready-made pie crust (not a preshaped frozen shell)*

*1 lemon*

*1½ pounds tart cooking apples, such as Rome, Empire, or Granny Smith, peeled and thinly sliced (about 4 medium to large)*

*½ cup raisins*

*⅓ cup sugar*

*1 tablespoon butter*

*2 tablespoons all-purpose flour*

*1 large egg white*

1. Heat the oven to 400 degrees F. Lightly coat a large baking sheet with vegetable oil cooking spray.
2. Unfold the pie crust on a lightly floured work surface. Using a lightly floured rolling pin, roll it out into a 15-inch circle. Transfer it to the baking sheet.
3. Grate ½ teaspoon lemon zest (just the yellow part) from the lemon and then squeeze 1 tablespoon of juice. Toss the peel and juice with the apples and raisins.
4. Set aside 1 teaspoon of the sugar. In a small bowl, combine the butter, flour, and remaining sugar with the tines of a fork until it resembles oatmeal and then add it to the apples.
5. Place the apples in the center of the pie crust. Beat the egg white with 1 tablespoon water and brush it over the pasty and exposed apples; sprinkle the tart with the reserved teaspoon of sugar.
6. Bake for 30 minutes or until the crust is golden. Place a sheet of aluminum foil loosely on the top of the pie and bake for about 15 minutes longer or until the apples are very tender when tested with a fork. Let the pie cool for about 15 minutes in the pan and then run a metal spatula under it and remove it to a serving plate.

*Per serving: 200 calories, 3 grams protein, 27 grams carbohydrate, 9 grams fat, 2.5 grams saturated fat, 5 milligrams cholesterol, 1 gram fiber, 146 milligrams sodium.*

# Appendix

# Weight Management Resources

In this appendix, you can find books, Web sites, and organizations that can help you search for more information about weight management.

## Books

With so many books about diet and nutrition out there, telling what's legit from what's not is sometimes hard to do. Check out a few of our all-time favorites:

- *American Dietetic Association's Complete Food & Nutrition Guide,* 2nd Edition, by Roberta Larson Duyff, MS, RD, FADA, CFCS. John Wiley & Sons, 2002.
- *ADA Guide to Healthy Eating for Kids: How Your Children Can Eat Smart from 5 to 12,* by Jodie Shield, MEd, RD, and Mary Catherine Mullen, MS, RD. John Wiley & Sons, 2002.
- *Cooking Thin with Chef Kathleen: 200 Easy Recipes for Weight Loss,* by Kathleen Daelmans. Houghton & Mifflin, 2002.
- *How to Get Your Kid to Eat . . . But Not Too Much,* by Ellyn Satter, RD. Bull Publishing Co., 1987.
- *Intuitive Eating: A Revolutionary Program that Works,* by Evelyn Tribole, MS, RD, and Elyse Resch, MS, RD. Griffin Trade Paperbacks, 2003.
- *Nutrition For Dummies,* 3rd Edition, by Carol Ann Rinzler. Wiley Publishing, Inc., 2004.
- *The Solution: For Safe, Healthy, and Permanent Weight Loss,* by Laurel Mellin, MA, RD. Regan Books, 1998.
- *Strong Women Stay Healthy,* by Miriam Nelson, PhD. Bantam Doubleday Dell Publishing, 2000.
- *The Volumetrics Weight-Control Plan,* by Barbara J. Rolls, PhD. HarperTorch, 2002.
- *The Way to Eat,* by David Katz, MD, MPH, FACPM, and Maura Harrigan González, MS, RD. Sourcebooks Trade, 2002.

# Newsletters and Magazines

Newsletters and some magazines are a great way to keep up on the latest nutrition information. They frequently include articles about eating healthfully, weight loss, and recipes, among other topics of interest.

## Consumer Reports on Health

P. O. Box 52148
Boulder, CO 80322
800-333-9784
www.consumerreports.org

## Environmental Nutrition

P. O. Box 420235
Palm Coast, FL 32142
800-829-5384
www.environmentalnutrition.com

## Tufts University Health & Nutrition Letter

P. O. Box 420235
Palm Coast, FL 32142-0235
800-274-7581
healthletter.tufts.edu

## University of California at Berkeley Wellness Letter

University of California, Berkeley Wellness Letter
Subscription Department
P.O. Box 420148
Palm Coast, FL 32142
386-447-6328
www.berkeleywellness.com

## Eating Well Magazine

823A Ferry Rd,
Charlotte, VT 05445
800-337-0402
www.eatingwell.com

## Cooking Light

2100 Lakeshore Drive
Birmingham, AL 35209
205-445-6000
www.cookinglight.com

# Web Sites

You can find a ton of information out in cyberspace about nutrition and health, but view it with a wary eye. As with books, telling whether the information a Web site provides is from a knowledgeable, sound source or simply from someone who *thinks* they know about nutrition can be difficult. The sites listed in this section provide balanced, accurate information about diet, nutrition, and health. For ways to evaluate products and services recommended on Web sites not listed, see Chapter 19.

## Bam

www.bam.gov

This is a site from the Centers of Disease Control that's kid friendly and mother approved. In comic-book style, the info is fun rather than punitive or pedantic. The focus on this site is action through kid-friendly sports, not diet. Using five comic-book kids as their guides, children who log on can find out about improving their performance in their chosen sports from other real-life children who have excelled in the activity. Though not specifically geared to weight loss, this site delivers a healthy solid message to children who need to lose weight: Move it to lose it.

## Calorie Control Council

www.caloriecontrol.org

This site can help you reduce your fat and calorie intake, figure out what weight is healthy for you, and attain and maintain that weight. It also provides information about low-calorie, reduced-fat foods and beverages and the ingredients that they contain.

## Children's Nutrition Research Center (CNRC)

www.bcm.tmc.edu/cnrc

The CNRC is one of six U.S. Department of Agriculture's human nutrition research centers for the nutrient needs of healthy children and pregnant and nursing women.

## Food and Drug Administration

www.fda.gov

This government site tells you more than you'd ever want to know about food and drugs, including information about dietary supplements, additives, food labeling, and kids' and women's health.

## Food and Nutrition Information Center

www.nal.usda.gov/fnic/

The nutrition gateway at the National Agricultural Library of the U.S. Department of Agriculture will lead you to all kinds of food and nutrition help. Click on the Consumer Corner for info on everything from science to healthy recipes, to nutrition related projects to do with children. You can even find a link for teachers.

## Shape Up America

www.shapeup.org

Go to this site to find information about safe weight management and physical fitness, including a free Body Mass Index calculator. You can also visit the Cyberkitchen and enter your height, weight, age, and activity level to determine an appropriate daily calorie intake for yourself.

## Tufts University Nutrition Navigator

www.navigator.tufts.edu

This online rating and review guide to Internet nutrition information is designed to help you find accurate, useful nutrition information that you can trust. A great resource for helping determine whether sites are legitimate — and it provides links only to those sites it approves.

## Weight Control Information Network

www.niddk.nih.gov/health/nutrit/win.htm

The national information service of the National Institute of Diabetes and Digestive and Kidney Diseases (NIDDK) of the National Institutes of Health (NIH) provides science-based information on obesity, weight control, and nutrition in an easy-to-read fact sheet format.

## WebMD

www.webmd.com

This is a multitiered site with all kinds of medical and health information. Navigate your way to the diet and health pages, and you'll find the weight-loss center. You can find pounds of information and inches of copy to help you on your weight loss program.

# Organizations

The following organizations provide information about a variety of health topics, ranging from exercise to nutrition to the special needs of children.

## Professional associations

### American Obesity Association

This organization is focused on changing public policy and perceptions about obesity. Policy makers, media professionals, and just plain folks use the site to find obesity-related information.

American Obesity Association
1250 24th Street, NW
Suite 300
Washington, DC 20037
202-776-7711
www.obesity.org

### American Academy of Pediatrics

The American Academy of Pediatrics (AAP) is dedicated to the health, safety, and well-being of all infants, children, adolescents, and young adults. It has 57,000 members who are pediatricians, pediatric medical subspecialists, and pediatric surgical specialists.

141 Northwest Point Boulevard
P. O. Box 747
Elk Grove Village, IL 60009
800-433-9016
www.aap.org

### American Dietetic Association (ADA)

With nearly 70,000 members, the American Dietetic Association is the nation's largest organization of food and nutrition professionals. Their mission is to promote optimal nutrition, health, and well-being.

National Center for Nutrition and Dietetics
120 South Riverside Plaza, Suite 2000
Chicago, IL 60606
800-366-1655
www.eatright.org

## Eating disorders

When it comes to eating disorders, being informed is always a good idea. This section lists some organizations that can help.

### Anorexia Nervosa and Related Eating Disorders (ANRED)

This nonprofit organization provides information about anorexia nervosa, bulimia nervosa, binge eating disorder, and weight disorders.

P.O. Box 5102
Eugene, OR 97405
541-344-1144
www.anred.com

### National Association of Anorexia Nervosa and Associated Disorders (ANAD)

ANAD offers free eating disorder information and prevention services, hotline counseling, support groups, and referrals to healthcare professionals.

Box 7
Highland Park, IL 60035
847-831-3438
www.aureate.com

### Harvard Eating Disorders Clinic

This research center, an affiliate of Harvard Medical School, studies eating disorders, their treatment, and prevention. You can find plenty of helpful information on what eating disorders are, where to find treatment, and how to help a person suffering from one.

Harvard Eating Disorders Center
WACC 725
15 Parkman Street
Boston, MA 02114
617-236-7766
www.hedc.org

### Overeaters Anonymous (OA)

OA is an international self-help group for anorexics, bulimics, and compulsive overeaters. The office answers calls, distributes meeting lists, gives general information about the program, and sells literature.

P. O. Box 44020
Rio Rancho, NM 87174-4020
505-891-2664
www.overeatersanonymous.org

## Exercise

**American College of Sports Medicine (ACSM)**
P. O. Box 1440
Indianapolis, IN 46206-1440
317-637-9200
www.acsm.org/sportsmed

**American Council on Exercise (ACE)**
5820 Overlain Dr., Suite 102
San Diego, CA 92121-3787
800-825-3636
www.acefitness.org/index.html

**President's Council on Physical Fitness and Sports**
701 Pennsylvania Avenue, NW
Suite 250
Washington, DC 20004
202-272-3421

**American Heart Association Fitness Center**
7272 Greenville Avenue
Dallas, TX 75231-4596
800-242-8721
www.justmove.org

## Nutrition

**American Dietetic Association (ADA)**
National Center for Nutrition and Dietetics
120 South Riverside Plaza, Suite 2000
Chicago, IL 60606
800-366-1655
www.eatright.org

**American Diabetes Association (ADA)**
1701 North Beauregard Street
Alexandria, VA 22311
800-342-2383
www.diabetes.org

### Surgical centers for obesity

**American Society of Bariatric Physicians (ASBP)**
5600 South Quebec Street
Suite 109-A
Englewood, CO 80111
303-779-2526
www.asbp.org

**American Society for Bariatric Surgeons (ASBS)**
6717 NW 11th Place
Suite C
Gainesville, FL 32605
352-331-4900
www.asbs.org

## Recipes

Eating with your health in mind *can* be delicious! Just check out these Web sites that offer recipes — perfect whether you're looking for a quick work-night meal or planning a more extravagant dinner party.

### FATFREE: The LowFat Vegetarian Archive

www.fatfree.com

Even if you're not a vegetarian, you can appreciate the interesting veggie-based recipes for soups, casseroles, desserts, appetizers, and more — more than 2,500 in all. Many — but not all — recipes are fat free.

### AOL Kitchen Assistant

www.aol.com, Keyword: Food

On this Web site, you can search recipes by lowfat, low-calorie, low-salt or other weight-loss criteria. The collection of 60,000 recipes come from Time, Inc. magazines such as *Health, Real Simple, Cooking Light, Southern Living, Sunset,* and *Oxmore House.*

# Index

## • A •

## • B •

## • C •

## • E •

## • F •

## • G •

## • H •

## • I •



## • J •



## • K •



## • L •



## • M •

## • N •



## • O •

## • P •

## • T •



## • U •



## • V •

## • W •

## • Y •



## • Z •